Clinical
Guide
to
Pediatric
Anesthesia

Clinical Guide to Pediatric Anesthesia

Karen Zaglaniczny, PhD, CRNA

Director of Graduate Nurse Anesthesia Program and of
Perioperative Services, Education and Research
William Beaumont Hospital
Royal Oak, Michigan
Adjunct Associate Professor
Oakland University
Rochester, Michigan

John Aker, MS, CRNA

Chief Nurse Anesthetist
Department of Anesthesia
University of Iowa Hospitals and Clinics
Iowa City, Iowa

W.B. SAUNDERS COMPANY
A Division of Harcourt Brace & Company
Philadelphia   London   Toronto   Montreal   Sydney   Tokyo

W.B. SAUNDERS COMPANY

A Division of Harcourt Brace & Company

The Curtis Center
Independence Square West
Philadelphia, Pennsylvania 19106

Library of Congress Cataloging-in-Publication Data

Zaglaniczny, Karen L.
    Clinical guide to pediatric anesthesia / Karen Zaglaniczny, John
Aker.
        p.   cm.
    Includes bibliographical references.
    ISBN 0-7216-8117-4
    1. Pediatric anesthesia Handbooks, manuals, etc.   I. Aker, John.
II. Title.
    [DNLM: 1. Anesthesia—Child Outlines.   2. Anesthesia—Infant
Outlines.   WO 218.2 Z18c 1999]
RD139.Z34   1999
617.9'6798—dc21
DNLM/DLC
                                                                99-26384

CLINICAL GUIDE TO PEDIATRIC ANESTHESIA   ISBN 0-7216-8117-4

Copyright © 1999 by W.B. Saunders Company

Printed in the United States of America

Last digit is the print number: 9   8   7   6   5   4   3   2   1

To the anesthetists
who are privileged to practice
pediatric anesthesia
and to the children
who benefit from their expert care

Contributors

John Aker, MS, CRNA
Chief Nurse Anesthetist, Department of Anesthesia, University of Iowa Hospitals and Clinics, Iowa City, Iowa
Pediatric Fluid and Blood Therapy; Anesthetic Considerations for Pediatric Orthopedic Procedures; Neuroanesthesia; Pediatric Diagnostic and Therapeutic Procedures; Anesthesia for Pediatric Patients with Respiratory Diseases

C. J. Biddle, PhD, CRNA
Associate Professor of Anesthesiology, Dartmouth Medical School, Hanover, New Hampshire
Pediatric Considerations in Airway Management

Eva Bowden, MS, CRNA
Anesthesia Clinical Coordinator, William Beaumont Hospital, Royal Oak, Michigan
Pediatric Diagnostic and Therapeutic Procedures

Michael Boytim, MSN, CRNA
Assistant Director, Kaiser Permanente School of Anesthesia, Pasadena, California
Pediatric Equipment

Michael J. Cosgrove, MS, CRNA
Adjunct Faculty, University of Detroit–Mercy, Detroit, Michigan; Adjunct Faculty, Oakland University, Rochester, Michigan; Certified Registered Nurse Anesthetist, William Beaumont Hospital–Troy, Troy, Michigan
Pediatric Monitoring Guidelines

Joseph P. Cravero, MD
Assistant Professor of Anesthesia and Pediatrics, Dartmouth Medical School, Hanover, New Hampshire
Pediatric Considerations in Airway Management

David Crowninshield, MS, CRNA
Certified Registered Nurse Anesthetist, Kaiser Permanente Los Angeles Medical Center, Los Angeles, California
Pharmacologic Considerations for Pediatric Patients; Pharmacologic Agents

Theresa L. Culpepper, PhD, CRNA
Assistant Professor, Nurse Anesthesia Program, The University of Alabama at Birmingham, Birmingham, Alabama
Postoperative Care; Neonatal Anesthesia

Tammy Dukatz, MSN, CRNA
Didactic and Clinical Instructor, Program of Nurse Anesthesia, Oakland University/William Beaumont Hospital, Royal Oak, Michigan
Resuscitation Guidelines

James P. Embrey, PhD, CRNA
Staff Nurse Anesthetist, Midlothian Anesthesia Associates, Richmond, Virginia
Pediatric Fluid and Blood Therapy

Margaret Faut-Callahan, DNSc, CRNA, FAAN
Professor and Chair, Adult Health Nursing, and Director, Nurse Anesthesia Program, Rush University College of Nursing, Chicago, Illinois
Regional Anesthesia and Pain Management

Pamela Friedman, MS, CRNA
Clinical and Didactic Instructor, Oakland University–Beaumont Graduate Program of Nurse Anesthesia, Rochester, Michigan; Staff Certified Registered Nurse Anesthetist, William Beaumont Hospital, Royal Oak, Michigan
Anesthetic Considerations for Pediatric Orthopedic Procedures

Stanley M. Hall, MD, PhD
Adjunct Professor, Nurse Anesthesiology Graduate Studies, Xavier University of Louisiana, New Orleans, Louisiana; Co-director, Department of Anesthesiology, Children's Hospital, New Orleans, Louisiana
Anesthesia for Pediatric Ear, Nose, Throat, and Maxillofacial Surgery

Claudine N. Hoppen, MSN, CRNA
Guest Lecturer, Wayne State University—Detroit Receiving Program of Nurse Anesthesia, Detroit, Michigan; William Beaumont Hospital–Oakland University Program of Nurse Anesthesia, Royal Oak, Michigan; Certified Registered Nurse Anesthetist, Children's Hospital of Michigan, Detroit, Michigan
Cardiothoracic Surgical Procedures; Anesthesia for Pediatric Patients with Cardiovascular Diseases

Anne Marie Hranchook, MSN
Clinical and Didactic Instructor, Oakland University, Rochester, Michigan; Education Coordinator, Anesthesia Department, William Beaumont Hospital, Royal Oak, Michigan
Anesthesia for Pediatric Urologic Procedures

Mary Karlet, PhD, CRNA
Winston-Salem, North Carolina
Anesthesia for Pediatric Patients with Musculoskeletal System Diseases; Anesthesia for Pediatric Patients with Endocrine System Diseases; Anesthesia for Pediatric Patients with Renal System Diseases

Michael J. Kremer, DNSc, CRNA
Assistant Professor, Adult Health Nursing Faculty, Nurse Anesthesia Program, Rush University College of Nursing; Staff Nurse Anesthetist, Department of Anesthesiology, Rush–Presbyterian–St Luke's Medical Center, Chicago, Illinois
Regional Anesthesia and Pain Management

Ronald J. Manningham, MS, CRNA
Didactic and Clinical Instructor and Senior Review Coordinator, Henry Ford Hospital/University of Detroit–Mercy Graduate Program in Nursing Anesthesiology, Detroit, Michigan
Anesthesia for Pediatric Patients with Respiratory Diseases

Rex A. Marley, MS, CRNA, RRT
Staff Nurse Anesthetist, Poudre Valley Hospital, Fort Collins, Colorado
Preoperative Preparation for the Pediatric Patient; Anesthesia for Pediatric Patients with Respiratory Diseases

Denise Martin-Sheridan, EdD, CRNA
Associate Professor of Anesthesiology and Associate Graduate Director, Albany Medical College Nurse Anesthesiology Program, Albany Medical Center Hospital, Albany, New York
Malignant Hyperthermia

John J. Nagelhout, PhD, CRNA
Director, Kaiser Permanente School of Anesthesia, Pasadena, California
Pharmacologic Considerations for Pediatric Patients; Pharmacologic Agents

Cormac T. O'Sullivan, MSN, CRNA
Associate Program Director, Nurse Anesthesia Program, University of Iowa College of Nursing; Staff Nurse Anesthetist, University of Iowa Hospitals and Clinics, Iowa City, Iowa
Pediatric Fluid and Blood Therapy; Anesthetic Management of the Pediatric Burn Patient

Tim Palmer, MS, CRNA
Clinical and Didactic Instructor, William Beaumont Hospital; Adjunct Clinical and Didactic Faculty, Henry Ford Hospital; William Beaumont Hospital–Oakland University Graduate Program in Nurse Anesthesia, Royal Oak, Michigan; Henry Ford Hospital–University of Detroit Mercy Graduate Program in Nurse Anesthesia, Detroit, Michigan
Anesthesia Considerations for Pediatric General Surgery and Gastrointestinal and Hepatobiliary Disease

Therese M. Pilchak, MS, CRNA
Clinical Coordinator, Oakland University–Beaumont Graduate Program of Nurse Anesthesia, William Beaumont Hospital, Royal Oak, Michigan
Anatomy and Physiology of the Pediatric Population

Brent Sommer, CRNA, MPHA
Assistant Professor, Clinical Coordinator, Graduate Program of Nurse Anesthesia, Samuel Merritt College, Oakland, California; Senior Staff Anesthetist, The Permanente Medical Group, Inc., Kaiser Permanente Medical Care Program, Oakland, California; Alta Bates Medical Center, Berkeley, California
Latex Allergy

Kathy Swendner, MSN, CRNA
Clinical Coordinator, William Beaumont Hospital; Didactic and Clinical Instructor, Oakland University/William Beaumont Hospital Program of Nurse Anesthesia, Royal Oak, Michigan
Anesthesia Care Plans

Karen Zaglaniczny, PhD, CRNA
Director of Graduate Nurse Anesthesia Program and of Perioperative Services, Education and Research, William Beaumont Hospital, Royal Oak, Michigan; Adjunct Associate Professor, Oakland University, Rochester, Michigan
Pediatric Trauma

Foreword

The thought of providing anesthesia care for a child can be quite intimidating for a practitioner with only occasional exposure to pediatric patients. One can imagine a scene involving a pediatric "code blue" with brave clinical providers racing toward the site. Meanwhile, more timid souls try to ease away or blend into the background. Much of the trepidation involving pediatric anesthesia can be eliminated by preparation and experience. A pediatric advanced life support (PALS) course is a great confidence builder.

One of my teachers in a joking mood told me that in anesthesia, you learn from experience and you get experience from bad experiences. Fortunately, I have found that it does not have to be *our* bad experience. All too often we forget the hundreds of uneventful, successful cases we have been involved in and focus only on the rare mishap. This handbook is a compilation based on the vast clinical experience of several anesthesia practitioners. It should not be viewed as a cookbook for specific procedures but rather as helpful hints and background information for greater understanding of specific cases.

Much of the fear of pediatric anesthesia is based on the fact that children can "go bad so quickly." Their precipitous desaturation is due to their rapid metabolism, which can require twice the rate of oxygen consumption of an adult adjusted for weight. Fortunately, children usually rebound just as rapidly upon reestablishing oxygenation.

This handbook is intended as a practical guide to the delivery of anesthesia care to children. It was produced by the combined efforts of physician and nurse anesthesia care providers.

Stanley M. Hall, MD, PhD

Preface

Pediatric anesthesia is a challenging yet rewarding area of clinical practice that requires the integration of specialty knowledge, skills, and abilities. It is essential that the pediatric anesthesia provider have a thorough understanding of normal growth and psychological development, anatomical and physiologic differences with maturation, and the influence of the immature organ systems upon anesthetic pharmacokinetics and pharmacodynamics.

Our goal in the development of the *Clinical Guide to Pediatric Anesthesia* was to assemble a clinically useful reference for pediatric anesthesia care. This reference includes the information necessary for the anesthetic management of children related to the basic principles of common surgical procedures, common pediatric disease, regional anesthesia, immediate postoperative care, and pain management. The appendixes include reference materials for the development of age-appropriate anesthesia care plans, as well as drug administration and resuscitation guidelines. This comprehensive resource is organized in an outline form to facilitate an organized approach to the anesthetic management of the pediatric patient.

Karen Zaglaniczny
John Aker

Acknowledgments

The production and success of this book required the collaborative efforts of many contributors. We wish to recognize each contributor for his or her knowledge and expertise in the field of pediatric anesthesia as well as the extensive review and research for each topic area.

We are also indebted to others who have facilitated the development and realization of this book. These include the staff at W.B. Saunders Company, Maura Connor Murcar, Senior Editor, Victoria Legnini, Assistant Developmental Editor, Joan Sinclair, Production Manager, and Thomas Eoyang, Vice President and Editor-in-Chief of Nursing Books. In addition, Mary Espenschied for her production of this book. We are grateful for the support of the staff at William Beaumont Hospital and the University of Iowa Hospitals and Clinics during this worthwhile endeavor. Finally we would like to thank our professional colleagues, friends, and especially our families for their patient endurance and endless encouragement.

Karen Zaglaniczny
John Aker

Contents

Physiologic and Pharmacologic Principles

I

1

Anatomy and Physiology of the Pediatric Population

Therese M. Pilchak, MS, CRNA

I. Overview

A. The physical appearance of a newborn contrasts sharply with that of a toddler and even more so with that of a school-age child.

B. Differences in both the anatomy and physiology of a pediatric patient must be appreciated and understood to properly assess, plan, and deliver safe anesthesia care.

II. Physical Appearance

A. Physical size is the most dramatic difference in the pediatric patient.

B. Several methods to compare body size can be used, including height and weight or head, chest, and abdominal circumference; however, body surface area (BSA) is the most useful when judging fluid and nutritional requirements since it closely parallels variations in the basal metabolic rate.

C. BSA can be determined using a nomogram (see Fig. 1–1), or it can be crudely estimated using the following formula: BSA $(m^2) = (0.02 \times kg) + 0.40$. This formula is reasonably accurate for average-sized children weighing between 21 and 40 kg.

D. Proportion of body parts.

1. The head of a newborn is large at birth (35 cm in circumference). This exceeds the circumference of the chest, which is relatively small compared to the protuberant abdomen of the newborn.

2. Arms and legs are relatively short and underdeveloped.

3. To appreciate the degree of skeletal growth that occurs throughout childhood, it is helpful to note that the midpoint in length for a neonate is at the level of the umbilicus, whereas in adults the midpoint is at the level of the symphysis pubis.

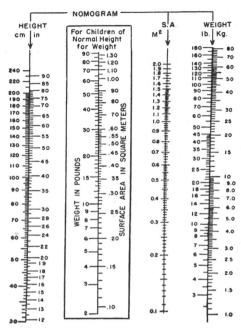

FIGURE 1-1. Nomogram for the determination of body surface area of children and adults. (From Behrman, R.E. [1996]. *Nelson textbook of pediatrics* [15th ed., p. 2079]. Philadelphia: W.B. Saunders.)

III. Musculoskeletal System

A. Bone growth does not occur at the same rates for the long, flat, or short bones of the body.

B. The anatomic landmarks and their relationship to underlying structures vary, depending on age.

C. In the neonate, the imaginary line joining the two iliac crests crosses the S1 vertebral body. In the adult, this line crosses the L5 vertebral body.

D. The sacrum is incompletely fused in infancy, making it relatively easy to enter the spinal canal at all four sacral levels. The sacrum is fused by adulthood.

E. The sacral hiatus is larger and higher in the body in the neonate. After the age of 7 years, caudal anesthesia becomes more difficult because the sacral hiatus dimensions are reduced.

F. At birth the spinal column has only an anterior curvature. The spinous processes have a similar relationship to each other throughout the spinal column as a result.

G. At approximately 3 months, when the infant is gaining the ability to hold the head up, the cervical curvature appears.

H. As walking begins, late in the first year of life, the lumbar curvature also develops.

IV. Central Nervous System

A. The brain of a full-term newborn is approximately one tenth of the body weight.

B. This relatively large brain is in contrast to the adult brain, which makes up only one fiftieth of adult body weight.

C. Brain weight doubles by the age of 6 months and triples by 1 year of age.

D. Neuronal cell development.
   1. Only one fourth of the total number of neuronal cells that exist in an adult are present at birth.
   2. By the age of 12 months, the development of neuronal cells in the cortex and brain stem is nearly complete.
   3. Myelination and development of dendritic processes are not complete until the third year of life.
   4. Primitive infant reflexes such as the Moro or grasp reflexes will disappear as myelination occurs. Checking for the existence of these reflexes is a useful tool when assessing neural development.
   5. The autonomic nervous system is relatively well developed in the newborn.
   6. Parasympathetic innervation to the heart and vasculature is fully functional at birth.
   7. Components of the sympathetic nervous system, such as baroreflexes that are responsible for maintaining heart rate and blood pressure, are functional in an awake newborn.
      a. These reflexes involve the pressor and depressor areas of the vasomotor centers of the medulla.
      b. Animal studies suggest that these reflexes are diminished in anesthetized newborns.

E. Embryogenesis of nerve cells of the spinal cord is completed at age 6 or 7 years.

F. In an embryo, the spinal cord occupies the entire spinal canal. As the axial skeleton grows, the cord and spinal nerves are drawn up into the vertebral canal. At birth, the distal portion of the canal is free of neural tissue.

G. The lower end of the cord is at the level of the L3 vertebral body at birth, and by 1 year of age it is at the level of L1.

H. The dural sac ends at the level of S3–4 in a newborn and is at the S1–2 level at 1 year old.

I. As the vertebral column grows, the spinal nerve roots are drawn into the spinal canal and form the cauda equina.

V. Cardiovascular System

A. Fetal circulation
   1. The placenta receives about 55% of the combined output of the two ventricles pumping in parallel. This blood is carried to the placenta via two umbilical arteries, where it is oxygenated and returned to the fetus via the umbilical vein.
   2. The majority of this blood passes through the ductus venosus to the inferior vena cava, but a small portion is mixed with the portal circulation.
   3. The blood from the inferior vena cava flows through the foramen ovale from the right to the left atrium, bypassing the fetal lungs. This blood is pumped by the left ventricle into the aorta, where it is distributed to branches of the ascending aorta.
   4. Deoxygenated blood from the superior vena cava goes through the right ventricle to the pulmonary artery. Since the pulmonary vascular resistance is so high in the fetus, most of this blood passes into the aorta via the ductus arteriosus.
   5. This poorly saturated blood enters the aorta distal to the innominate and left carotid arteries and is directed peripherally to the umbilical arteries. A portion of this poorly saturated blood perfuses the lower part of the fetus.

B. Circulatory changes after birth
   1. Fetal blood flow no longer travels to the placenta, causing the systemic vascular resistance to approximately double.
   2. Left heart chamber and aortic pressures increase.
   3. With the infant's first cry, the lungs expand and pulmonary vasculature dilates, decreasing pulmonary vascular resistance and right ventricular end-diastolic pressure.
   4. The foramen ovale closes as the left atrial pressure becomes greater than right atrial pressure. A small valve lying over the foramen ovale on the left side of the atrial septum closes, thereby preventing further flow.
   5. Immediately after birth, blood that was diverted from the pulmonary artery into the aorta via the ductus arteriosus begins to flow backward into the pulmonary arteries, probably as a result of decreasing pulmonary pressures and increasing arterial pressures. The muscular walls of the ductus arteriosus constrict markedly a few hours after

birth, and functional closure is attained after 1 to 8 days, preventing all further blood flow from the pulmonary artery to the aorta. Over the next 1 to 4 months, fibrous tissue anatomically occludes the lumen of the ductus arteriosus.

6. The reason for the closure of the ductus is not completely understood but is thought to be related to the increased partial pressure of the blood flowing through the ductus.

7. As blood flow through the umbilical vein ceases immediately after birth, portal blood flow continues to travel through the ductus venosus, with only a small amount traveling to the liver. The muscular walls of the ductus begin to contract shortly after birth and close off the portal circulation pathway. Portal venous pressure then rises, which forces blood through the liver.

C. Persistent fetal circulation
1. Hypercarbia, hypoxia, or acidosis in a newborn can precipitate pulmonary vasoconstriction.
2. Right atrial pressures will exceed left atrial pressures and cause the foramen ovale to open, diverting deoxygenated blood directly to the left side of the heart.
3. Hypoxia can also cause the ductus arteriosus to re-open. This additional right-to-left shunting worsens the hypoxia, which sets up a vicious cycle of elevated pulmonary vascular resistance, increase in right-sided heart pressures, and a condition known as persistent fetal circulation.

D. Myocardium
1. The stroke volume of an infant is relatively fixed because of a stiff myocardium that is less contractile than that of an adult.
2. Increases in preload will have relatively little effect on increasing cardiac output.
3. Cardiac reserve is limited.
4. Small changes in end-diastolic volume result in major changes in the end-diastolic pressure.
5. To increase cardiac output, the heart rate must increase. Heart rate plays a major role in increasing or decreasing cardiac output in infancy.
6. After birth, myofibrils increase in number, diameter, and mass. This allows the development of contractile elements and the development of the thick-walled left ventricle during the first 3 postgestational months.
7. Infants are predisposed to bradycardia. The parasympathetic innervation to the heart is completely developed.

Sympathetic innervation is relatively sparse but functional; therefore vagal tone predominates.

8. The unbalanced parasympathetic tone can also manifest in negative inotropy in infants, making them more likely to develop congestive heart failure.
9. The heart rate of an infant is higher and decreases gradually over the first 5 years of life to near adult levels (see Table 1–1).
10. Cardiac output is higher because of the increased oxygen consumption of infants.
11. Systemic vascular resistance and blood pressure are low.

VI. Respiratory System

A. In addition to an overall smaller size, there are anatomic differences of the pediatric airway compared with that of an adult.

1. The head is large with a short neck. The occiput is the most predominant part of the head, with the face being relatively small.
2. In the supine position, the chin meets the chest at the level of the second rib, making the infant prone to upper airway obstruction during sleep.
3. The tongue is large and occupies the entire mouth and oropharynx.
4. The absence of teeth in the oral cavity further predisposes the infant to upper airway obstruction.
5. Infants in the first few weeks of life must breathe through their nose because of the close approximation of the epiglottis to the soft palate. This permits breathing while feeding. The mouth is used for breathing only when the infant is crying.
6. The pharyngeal airway is made up entirely of soft tissue.
   a. It is easily collapsed by posterior displacement of the mandible, flexion of the neck, or external compression over the hyoid.
   b. The pharyngeal lumen may also collapse with negative pressure generated through inspiratory effort, particularly when muscles that maintain airway structure are depressed or paralyzed.
7. Larynx.
   a. The larynx is funnel shaped, whereas the adult larynx is more cylindric.
   b. The larynx is more cephalad in location when compared to the adult (see Chapter 6 for a complete description).

TABLE 1-1. Circulatory Variables in Infants and Children

Age	Heart Rate (bpm)	Systolic Blood Pressure (mm Hg)	Diastolic Blood Pressure (mm Hg)	Cardiac Index (L/min/m^2)	Oxygen Consumption (ml/kg/min)
Preterm	150 ± 20	50 ± 3	30 ± 3		8 ± 1.4
Term	133 ± 18	73 ± 8	50 ± 8		6 ± 1.0
6 mo	120 ± 20	89 ± 29	60 ± 10	2.5 ± 0.6	5 ± 0.9
1 yr	120 ± 20	96 ± 30	66 ± 25	2.0 ± 0.5	5.2 ± 0.1
2 yr	105 ± 25	99 ± 25	64 ± 25	2.5 ± 0.6	6.4 ± 1.2
5 yr	90 ± 10	94 ± 14	55 ± 9	3.1 ± 0.7	6.0 ± 1.1
12 yr	70 ± 17	109 ± 16	58 ± 9	3.7 ± 0.9	3.3 ± 0.6
Young adult	75 ± 5	122 ± 30	75 ± 20	4.3 ± 1.1	3.4 ± 0.6
				3.7 ± 0.3	

From Katz, J., & Steward, DJ. (1993). *Anesthesia and uncommon pediatric diseases* (2nd ed., p. 5). Philadelphia: W.B. Saunders.

       c. In adults and older children, the larynx lies at the level of C4–6, whereas in infants, the larynx is approximately two vertebral levels higher. The high position of the larynx permits simultaneous swallowing and breathing.

    8. The cricoid cartilage is a complete ring that aids in the prevention of upper airway compression. This is the narrowest part of the pediatric airway, which makes it more susceptible to edema following traumatic intubation or tissue trauma from the insertion of a large endotracheal tube.

    9. The epiglottis is narrower and shorter, and the vocal cords are angled. (The anterior commissure of the vocal cords is more caudad than the posterior commissure.)

B. Anatomic differences of the thorax.

    1. The chest wall is very compliant and deformable.

    2. In the newborn the ribs are horizontally located, which limits the increase in thoracic cross-sectional area with inspiration. Accordingly, the rib cage has a limited contribution to the development of tidal volume.

    3. The diaphragmatic and intercostal muscles are deficient in type I muscle cells.

       a. Type I cells are necessary to perform the repeated exercise associated with respiration.

       b. Factors that increase the work of breathing contribute to fatigue of these muscles, especially in the preterm infant. This fatigue manifests as apnea, which leads to hypoxia, carbon dioxide retention, and respiratory failure.

       c. Type I muscle fiber quantity is similar to adult levels by age 2 years.

    4. The diaphragm consists of the crural and costal diaphragm, whose motor innervation arises from the third, fourth, and fifth cervical roots (the phrenic nerve).

C. Lung development.

    1. Maturation of the lungs is not complete until 8 years of age.

    2. The earliest alveolar/capillary networks are functional at 24 to 26 weeks' gestation.

    3. Alveoli increase in number and size until approximately 8 years of age. Growth after this age manifests only as an increase in airway and alveoli size.

    4. Surfactant, which reduces surface tension at the air-tissue interface of the alveoli and is responsible for preventing alveolar collapse during expiration, first appears at about

20 weeks' gestational age. Production accelerates between weeks 30 and 34.

D. Respiration.

1. Onset of respiration occurs in utero. Breathing movements of the fetus can be detected as early as 11 weeks' gestation.

2. After the twentieth week, the movements become more patterned, and by 36 weeks' gestation, the breathing movements are 30 to 70/min and regular.

3. Several factors come into play at birth to contribute to the respiratory movements becoming strong and rhythmic:

    a. The umbilical cord is clamped.

    b. The infant experiences relative "hyperoxia" as normal ventilation with air commences. This higher degree of oxygenation (compared to the low Po_2 levels of the fetus) maintains continual and rhythmic breathing.

4. Infants have a markedly higher metabolic rate, resulting in a higher respiratory rate (35–40/min in a newborn) and greater degree of alveolar ventilation (see Table 1–2).

TABLE 1–2. Mean Values for Normal Pulmonary Parameters in Normal Neonates and Adults

	Newborn	Adult
Body weight (kg)	3	70
Tidal volume (ml/kg)	6	6
Respiratory rate (bpm)	35	15
Alveolar ventilation (ml/kg/min)	130	60
Oxygen consumption (ml/kg/min)	6.4	3.5
Total lung capacity (ml/kg)	63	86
Functional residual capacity (ml/kg)	30	34
Vital capacity (ml/kg)	35	70
Residual volume (ml/kg)	23	16
Closing capacity (ml/kg)	35	23
Arterial pH	7.38–7.41	7.35–7.45
$Paco_2$	30–35	35–45
Pao_2	60–90	90–100
Sao_2 (%)	95–100	95–100

From Dobbins, P., & Hall, S.M. (1997). Pediatric anesthesia. In Nagelhout, J., & Zaglaniczny, K.L. *Nurse anesthesia* (p. 336). Philadelphia: W.B. Saunders.

$Paco_2$, Partial pressure of arterial carbon dioxide; *Pao_2*, partial pressure of arterial oxygen; *Sao_2*, oxygen saturation.

5. The functional residual capacity (FRC) is similar in terms of ml/kg to that of an adult. In an infant or small child, however, the FRC is not nearly as effective in improving the oxygen reserve or acting as a buffer between pulmonary circulation and inspired gases because of the greater metabolic rate, the increased oxygen consumption, and the high degree of alveolar ventilation that exist.

6. Newborns and infants up to 2 or 3 weeks of age differ from adults in their response to hypoxia.
   a. Initially, the infant will hyperventilate in response to hypoxia.
   b. A sustained decrease in ventilation occurs rapidly thereafter.
   c. Preterm infants placed in a cool environment will not exhibit the transient hyperpnea associated with the newborn response to hypoxia and will exhibit immediate respiratory depression.

7. When 100% oxygen is administered to a newborn, a transient decrease in ventilation followed by sustained hyperventilation is noted.

8. An increased ventilatory rate is noted when infants become hypercapnic. The slope of the CO_2 response curve is not as steep in infants, however, as in older children and adults. This is thought to be because of immature chemosensors for CO_2 and the fact that the chest wall mechanics are immature.

9. Periodic breathing occurs in 78% of full-term neonates, usually during quiet sleep. Central apnea is defined as cessation of breathing lasting 15 seconds or longer. This type of apnea is rare in full-term neonates but quite common in preterm infants. This apnea can be life threatening and can occur up to 41 to 55 weeks after conceptual age in the preterm infant, particularly after surgical procedures and anesthesia.

10. Hemoglobin levels of 19 g/dl are normal in healthy newborns. Most of this hemoglobin is fetal hemoglobin (HbF), which has a greater affinity for oxygen than adult hemoglobin.

11. Oxygen is bound tightly to HbF; therefore cyanosis occurs at a lower Po_2 in a newborn than in an adult.
    a. The P_{50} is approximately 27 mm Hg in an adult and 20 mm Hg in a newborn.
    b. Oxygen delivery at the tissue level is low because HbF reacts poorly with 2,3-DPG.
    c. The Po_2 is 60 to 90 mm Hg in the newborn.

12. HbF rapidly disappears in the first few weeks after birth, with the lowest hemoglobin level (10–11 g/dl) occurring at 2 to 3 months of age (physiologic anemia).
13. Similarly, the P_{50} increases rapidly during this time and in fact exceeds the adult level by 3 months of age. It remains high, and the hemoglobin remains relatively low (11–12 g/dl) until the early teen years.
14. Children have a lower oxygen affinity for hemoglobin; therefore tissue unloading of oxygen is higher. As a result, the lower hemoglobin levels of infants and children are just as efficient as the higher hemoglobin levels of adults in terms of tissue oxygenation.

VII. Renal System

A. Formation of glomeruli occurs at approximately 34 weeks' gestation. Maturation occurs between 34 and 36 weeks' gestation.
B. Full-term infants have the same number of nephrons as adults, but glomeruli are smaller. The renal tubules are not fully grown at birth and may not extend into the medulla.
C. The glomerular filtration rate (GFR) is approximately 30% that of an adult at birth. The high vascular resistance of the newborn and the reduced surface area of the immature glomeruli contribute to this reduced rate. At 5 to 6 months of age glomerular filtration is mature; however, tubular maturation lags behind.
D. Tubular immaturity is manifest by the infant's inability to concentrate the urine. However, sodium conservation is greater in the full-term infant compared to the premature infant.
E. Fluid turnover in an infant is seven times greater than that of an adult. Consequently, altered fluid balance may have significant consequences in terms of organ perfusion and metabolism. These factors coupled with the functional immaturity of the kidney place the infant at risk for the development of dehydration and acidosis.

VIII. Hepatic System

A. The neonatal liver is relatively large compared to that of an adult (4% vs. 2% of total body weight).
B. Enzyme systems exist but have not yet been sensitized or induced; hence they are immature.
C. The neonate must rely on his or her limited supply of stored fats, as well as the hepatic and muscle glycogen stores for

energy in the first few hours of extrauterine life. The gluconeogenesis capability of the neonatal liver is deficient.
  D. The ability of the liver to metabolize drugs increases as the infant matures. The two factors responsible are
    1. Hepatic blood flow increases, delivering more drug to the site.
    2. The enzyme systems become developed and are induced.
  E. Plasma proteins necessary for binding of drugs are lower in term infants and even more so in preterm infants. Greater levels of free drug result.

IX. Gastrointestinal System

  A. The incidence of gastroesophageal reflux is high in infants since the ability to coordinate breathing and swallowing does not fully mature until 4 or 5 months of age.
  B. The gastric pH is in the normal adult range by the second day of life; however, it is alkalotic immediately following delivery.

ADDITIONAL READINGS

Behrman, R.E., & Vaughan, V.C. (1996). *Nelson textbook of pediatrics* (15th ed.). Philadelphia: W.B. Saunders.

Dalens, B. (Ed.). (1995). *Regional anesthesia in infants, children and adolescents.* Baltimore: Williams & Wilkins.

Gray, H. (1977). *Anatomy, descriptive and surgical* (15th ed., revised). New York: Bounty Books.

Gregory, G.A. (1994). *Pediatric anesthesia* (3rd ed.). New York: Churchill Livingstone.

Guyton, A.C. (1995). *Textbook of medical physiology* (8th ed.). Philadelphia: W.B. Saunders.

Katz, J., & Steward, D.J. (1987). *Anesthesia and uncommon diseases.* Philadelphia: W.B. Saunders.

Motoyama, E.K., & Davis, P.J. (Eds.). (1996). *Smith's anesthesia for infants and children* (6th ed.). St. Louis: Mosby.

2

Pharmacologic Considerations for Pediatric Patients

John J. Nagelhout, PhD, CRNA, and
David Crowninshield, MSN, CRNA

I. Introduction

A. The administration of anesthetic drugs and agents to pediatric patients requires careful considerations unique to this population.

B. A child cannot be considered and medicated merely as a small adult.

C. The pharmacodynamics and pharmacokinetics of drugs are quite different in children and play important roles in proper dosing.

1. Pharmacodynamics describes the effects of drugs on the body over time.

2. Pharmacokinetics describes the movement of drugs through the body and is discussed as absorption, distribution, and elimination.

D. Consideration of these guidelines when managing pediatric cases will promote the safe and appropriate administration of drugs.

II. General Principles

A. Uptake

1. The drug's route of administration affects its uptake in pediatrics.

a. The intravenous (IV) route has the fastest onset.

b. The oral and rectal routes have the slowest.

2. Any pathologic processes that may be present in the child can alter the uptake of drugs, including significant cardiac or hepatic disease.

3. Topical agents are more rapidly absorbed in children because of their relatively thin skin layers.

B. Distribution

1. The distribution and effects of a drug are considerably

affected by the rapid growth in body mass and physiologic changes as a child matures.

2. Approximately 85% of the body weight of a premature newborn is composed of body fluids, and 55% to 70% of the body weight of a full-term infant is body fluids.

3. Whereas only 20% of an adult's body weight is composed of extracellular fluid (ECF), an infant's ECF compartment is as much as 40% of total body weight.

4. The concentration and effects of water-soluble agents are affected by the large ECF, resulting in a much greater volume of distribution.

5. The volume of distribution of lipid-soluble agents is smaller in children. As they grow, this compartment proportionally enlarges.

C. Plasma protein binding

1. Plasma protein–bound drugs have a greater pharmacologically active free fraction in infants because of lower levels of serum albumin.

2. The effects and toxicity of an unbound drug can be potentiated by conditions that reduce plasma protein levels, for example, malnutrition and nephrotic syndrome.

3. Endogenous molecules, such as bilirubin, can be displaced by protein-binding drugs or vice versa.

4. Drugs that are weakly protein bound can likewise be displaced by endogenous molecules, leading to higher active free fractions of the agent.

D. Metabolism

1. The metabolism of a drug by a neonate depends on the properties of the agent and the soundness of the enzyme system of the liver.

2. The metabolic pathway of glucuronidation, which makes many agents water soluble to promote renal excretion, is underdeveloped in neonates. Consequently, normal pediatric doses should not be given until the infant has reached the age of 1 month.

3. Maternal use of some medications during late pregnancy may cause hepatic enzyme induction in the fetus, enabling the newborn to more quickly metabolize agents.

4. Older children may have enhanced hepatic enzyme activity and are able to metabolize some agents more quickly.

5. Medications such as phenobarbital can also cause hepatic enzyme induction. As a result, greater doses and more frequent redosing may be necessary.

E. Excretion
 1. The rate of renal excretion of an agent depends on glomerular filtration, active tubular secretion, and passive tubular reabsorption.
 2. The dosages and effects of drugs that are excreted by the kidneys, such as pancuronium (Pavulon) and digoxin, can be markedly affected by immature renal development or renal impairment.
 3. The possibility of accumulation and even toxicity exists if the child cannot excrete the drug, and dosages may need to be reduced accordingly.
 4. The kidneys of the infant receive a lower percentage of the cardiac output and have a higher resistance to blood flow than those of an adult.
 5. The immature development of the glomerular and tubular elements and small, undeveloped loops of Henle affect the renal excretion of drugs in infants.
 6. An infant's glomerular filtration rate does not reach that of an adult until about 3 to 5 months of age.
 7. This decreased glomerular filtration rate can delay the elimination of renally excreted agents.
 8. The tubular secretion rate of an adult is only attained after the age of 7 to 12 months. Until this time, the infant has a reduced capability to reabsorb filtered substances such as glucose and to concentrate urine, and the proximal tubules have a decreased ability to secrete organic acids.

F. Calculating and monitoring pediatric dosages
 1. Only body weight (mg/kg) or body surface area (mg/m^2) should be used to determine proper drug dosages in pediatrics.
 2. Although a precise weight should always be used to calculate any drug dosages, a rough estimate of a child's weight may be obtained with the following formula based on the age in years:

$$\text{Average weight (kg)} = (\text{Age} \times 2) + 9$$

 3. In premature and full-term infants, use only body weight (mg/kg) to calculate correct doses.
 4. Careful monitoring of the patient is required to assess the effects of drug doses and the need for any subsequent redosing. All dosages should be titrated to effect.

III. Routes of Administration

A. Oral medications
 1. If administering a preoperative medication orally to an

infant, give it in liquid form to ensure rapid absorption. Always use a syringe to measure the dose to guarantee accuracy.

2. The infant's head should be held up to prevent aspiration and the chin pressed down to avert choking.

3. Do not coax a toddler to take a preoperative oral drug by describing it as "candy," even if it has a sweet, agreeable taste.

4. If a route of administration other than the oral route is required for a preoperative agent, try to explain to toddlers how you are going to give the medication. Use the parents in obtaining the child's cooperation.

B. Intramuscular (IM) injections
   1. If a drug cannot be given by the IV route, an IM injection can be given to provide swift absorption.
   2. Administer IM injections in the gluteus medius muscle or the ventrogluteal region in children older than 2 years of age.
   3. For those children younger than 2 years, use the area of the vastus lateralis muscle.
   4. If administering an IM injection to an awake child, explain in simple words that the child will understand that the medication will help him or her and that the injection may sting.
   5. For safety, restrain the child firmly if needed, remembering to praise and soothe the child afterward.

C. IV infusions
   1. Ensure the IV insertion site is well protected.
      a. The use of a peripheral site is preferred in infants because veins in the extremities are readily accessed.
      b. However, since the child will likely be actively moving in the postoperative area, care must be taken to firmly secure the insertion site and tubing.
      c. In certain cases, a vein of the scalp in the temporal region may be used if necessary. The risk of dislodgment is unlikely, but this site can potentially lead to transient blemishing of the head from the catheter, hematomas, or the infiltration of fluids. Although these are usually benign complications, they can be quite distressing to some parents.
      d. The insertion site must be well protected and secured to prevent infiltration or dislodgment of the catheter. A pediatric arm board, padded to protect the skin, is useful to secure the IV catheter.

    e. All tubing connections should be firmly attached and secured. The roller clamp should be placed out of the child's reach, particularly in the postoperative area.

    f. A child should be restrained only if it is an absolutely necessity.

2. Monitor infusion rates and fluid balance.

    a. Carefully monitor fluid balance in children. Use of a Buretrol helps prevent accidental volume overload in infants.

    b. Use standard formulas for fluid requirements, and vigilantly supervise IV flow rates and the child's vital signs and condition. The margin for error can be extremely slight in maintaining the proper fluid balance in neonates and infants.

3. Dilutions.

    a. To prevent the risk of central nervous system (CNS) hemorrhage in infants, hyperosmolar drugs, such as sodium bicarbonate, should be diluted to at least half-strength to avoid excessive alterations in serum osmolarity.

IV. Inhalational Agents

A. The effect of general inhalation anesthetics on children is similar to adults with a few important differences.

1. Pediatric patients undergo a more rapid induction and recovery from volatile agents because of their high alveolar and minute ventilation, low functional residual capacity, and large vessel-rich organ group.

2. The minimum alveolar concentration (MAC) of inhalational agents is the highest in infants, followed by children, neonates, and adults.

3. MAC of the inhalational agents decreases approximately 25% when nitrous oxide is used.

4. In neonates and infants the potent inhalation agents readily depress the myocardium and blood pressure because of immature compensatory mechanisms.

B. Characteristics of the commonly used agents.

1. Desflurane is a fluorinated methyl ether that is identical to isoflurane with the exception of fluorine for the chlorine on the alpha-ethyl carbon.

    a. It has a blood gas coefficient of 0.42, which allows for a rapid induction, alteration of anesthetic depth, and emergence.

  b. Problems associated with its use are the pungent odor, respiratory tract irritation (breath-holding apnea, laryngospasm), and emergence delirium.
  c. Because of the pungent odor it is not ideal for inhalation induction.
  d. The emergence delirium can be attenuated with the administration of preemptive analgesics and sedatives.
  e. MAC: children, 6% to 10%; infants (6–12 months), 9%; neonates, 9.2%
 2. Halothane is a halogenated hydrocarbon and is commonly used in pediatric patients.
  a. It is well tolerated by pediatric patients for inhalation induction.
  b. Because of its pharmacologic characteristics (blood gas coefficient of 2.3), a slow uptake and elimination are produced.
  c. Contraindicated in patients with hepatic dysfunction.
  d. Myocardial depression is dose dependent with resultant hypotension and bradycardia.
  e. Myocardial sensitivity to catecholamines can occur, and caution is advised when epinephrine is used for the surgical procedure.
  f. MAC: induction, 1% to 4%; maintenance, 0.5% to 1.5%
  g. MAC: neonates, 0.87%; infants, 1.2%
 3. Isoflurane is an inhalation agent that provides a relatively rapid induction and emergence.
  a. Because of the pungent odor and potential airway irritant effects, it is not ideal for inhalation induction in the pediatric population.
  b. It has a blood gas coefficient of 1.4 and has a moderate uptake and elimination.
  c. Dose-related decreases in systemic vascular resistance and increases in heart rate can be seen.
  d. MAC: neonates, 1.6%; infants, 1.6%; children, 1.6%
 4. Nitrous oxide is frequently used as an adjunct for induction and maintenance of general anesthesia.
  a. When used with the inhalation agents it reduces the MAC.
  b. It has a blood gas coefficient of 0.46 and extremely rapid uptake and elimination.
  c. Caution is advised for procedures (i.e., ear, bowel) in which diffusion into air-filled cavities is a concern.
 5. Sevoflurane is fluorinated methyl isopropyl ether that has become popular for inhalation induction in the pediatric population.

a. Because of its pharmacologic properties (blood gas co-efficient of 0.6) a rapid induction and emergence occur.

b. It has a pleasant odor and is used for induction without any respiratory irritation.

c. Controversy exists regarding the metabolism of sevo-flurane and is related to the potential renal effects of inorganic fluoride and chemical instability with absorbents.

d. A concentration-dependent elevation in serum fluoride levels can be produced with the metabolism of sevo-flurane. These levels decline rapidly with discontinuation of the agent. Extensive clinical investigations have not revealed evidence of renal dysfunction.

e. A chemical interaction between sevoflurane and soda lime or Baralyme occurs that can produce several compounds. One of these, compound A, has been shown to be nephrotoxic in rats, and the clinical significance in humans has not been elucidated. Associated factors for the increased production of compound A include the use of low fresh gas flows, increased absorber temperature from rebreathing, and the selection of Baralyme.

f. Dose-dependent cardiovascular depression occurs, and dysrhythmias are uncommon.

g. MAC: 2% to 3%

V. Intravenous Agents

A. Pediatric patients exhibit resistance to IV induction agents and typically require higher doses than those needed for adults.

B. Induction agents.

1. Thiopental is an ultra–short acting barbiturate that produces a smooth induction in the pediatric population.

   a. The barbiturate mechanism of action is related to the postsynaptic augmentation of gamma–aminobutyric acid (GABA)–mediated inhibition.

   b. It is contraindicated in children with porphyria.

   c. Neonatal dose: 3 to 4 mg/kg

   d. Infant dose (1–6 months): 5 to 7 mg/kg

   e. Children: 5 to 6 mg/kg

2. Methohexital is a rapid-acting barbiturate with a shorter duration of action than thiopental.

   a. Clinical effects are similar to thiopental.

   b. There is a higher incidence of involuntary muscle movements, hiccups, and pain on injection associated with its use.

      c. It is contraindicated in children with porphyria.

      d. Dose: 1.5 to 3 mg/kg

3. Propofol is a rapid-acting, short-duration alkyl phenol that produces its effects through GABA-mimetic action.

      a. Pharmacologic characteristics include a rapid redistribution and metabolism because of its high metabolic clearance, large volume of distribution, high protein binding, and short half-life.

      b. Clinical uses include bolus or infusion techniques of administration for sedation, induction, and maintenance of anesthesia.

      c. It has antiemetic, antipruritic, and anxiolytic properties.

      d. Dose-dependent decreases in blood pressure and heart rate can occur.

      e. Side effects include pain on injection, anaphylactic reactions, and involuntary movements.

      f. Dose: 2 to 3 mg/kg

4. Etomidate is a carboxylated imidazole derivative that has a rapid onset and recovery.

      a. As an induction agent, it is most commonly used in patients with significant cardiac or respiratory diseases. Etomidate has minimal hemodynamic and respiratory depressant effects.

      b. It has no intrinsic analgesic properties.

      c. Common side effects are myoclonic movements, pain on injection, and increased incidence of nausea and vomiting.

      d. Dose: 0.3 to 0.4 mg/kg

5. Ketamine is a nonbarbiturate cyclohexamine derivative that has profound analgesic effects.

      a. It produces a rapid loss of consciousness and stimulates the cardiovascular system with a resultant increase in heart rate and blood pressure.

      b. Respiratory effects include dose-dependent depression of airway reflexes, bronchodilation, and increased pharyngeal and tracheobronchial secretions. The increased secretions may produce coughing, gagging, and laryngospasm.

      c. Side effects can include hallucinations, bad dreams, and excitement on emergence. The incidence and severity of emergence reactions may be decreased with the administration of a benzodiazepine, such as midazolam.

      d. It is contraindicated in patients with increased intracranial pressure.

    e. Ketamine can be used as an IM injection in the pre-operative area to facilitate cooperation in children and also in burn patients.

    f. Dose: IV, 2 mg/kg; IM, 5 to 6 mg/kg

C. Benzodiazepines.

  1. Diazepam has a slow onset and prolonged duration of action.

    a. It is used primarily as a premedicant or for sedation.

    b. Dose: IV, 0.05 to 0.2 mg/kg; PO, 0.1 to 0.5 mg/kg

  2. Midazolam is a water-soluble, short-acting agent that has a half-life of 2 to 4 hours.

    a. It may cause respiratory depression, especially in combination with narcotics.

    b. Uses include premedication and sedation.

    c. Dose: IV, 0.01 to 0.02 mg/kg; nasal, 0.2 to 0.3 mg/kg; PO, 0.3 to 0.5 mg/kg

    d. When administered orally, mix with flavored syrup to offset bitter taste.

VI. Narcotic Agonists

A. Pediatric patients can be very sensitive to the respiratory depressant effects of narcotics.

B. Careful titration of these agents is warranted, especially when administered IV.

C. Characteristics of the commonly used agents.

  1. Fentanyl is a synthetic mu-receptor agent that is 75 to 125 times more potent than morphine.

    a. It is short acting and has minimal hemodynamic effects.

    b. Side effects include itchy nose, nausea, and vomiting.

    c. Dose: 1 to 5 µg/kg IV

    d. Oral transmucosal fentanyl (Oralet): 5 to 15 µg/kg

  2. Sufentanil is a synthetic mu-receptor agonist that is 5 to 10 times more potent than fentanyl.

    a. It has a greater degree of respiratory depression and may cause chest wall rigidity, laryngospasm, and apnea.

    b. Dose-related bradycardia and hypotension could occur.

    c. Dose: 0.1 to 0.5 µg/kg

  3. Alfentanil is one-fifth to one-tenth less potent than fentanyl and has a faster onset of action and shorter duration of action.

    a. It can cause respiratory depression, nausea, and vomiting.

    b. Dose: 8 to 20 µg/kg for induction; 3 to 10 µg/kg for maintenance

4. Remifentanil is an ultra–short acting agent that is rapidly hydrolyzed by specific esterases in the blood.
   a. It is a potent respiratory depressant and may cause chest wall rigidity and apnea, especially with rapid bolus administration.
   b. Careful IV titration is strongly advised with appropriate monitoring and resuscitative equipment nearby.
   c. Consideration of postoperative analgesic requirements is essential when remifentanil is administered for intraoperative analgesia.
   d. It can cause nausea and vomiting.
   e. Dose: infusion only, 0.5 to 1 µg/kg/min for induction; maintenance, 0.05 to 0.8 µg/kg/min
5. Morphine is a long-acting narcotic agonist with a duration of action of 1.5 to 3 hours.
   a. It is a potent respiratory depressant and may cause histamine release.
   b. Other side effects include pruritus, nausea, and vomiting.
   c. Dose: 0.05 to 0.2 mg/kg IV; 0.1 to 0.2 mg/kg IM or SQ
6. Meperidine is a synthetic agonist with a duration of action of 2 to 4 hours.
   a. It is a potent respiratory depressant.
   b. Other side effects include pruritus, nausea, and vomiting.
   c. Dose: 0.5 to 1 mg/kg IV; 1 to 2 mg/kg IM

VII. Muscle Relaxants

A. Pediatric patients, especially neonates and infants, have a larger volume of distribution for water-soluble drugs, such as the muscle relaxants.
B. Therefore increased doses of these drugs are required to produce paralysis.
C. Depolarizing muscle relaxant.
   1. Succinylcholine is an ultra–short acting agent that is metabolized by plasma cholinesterase.
   2. Its use in pediatric patients is controversial and related to the clinical problems associated with administration.
   3. Conduction abnormalities can be seen, with bradycardia the most common.
   4. Pretreatment with atropine is recommended by some practitioners.
   5. Other potential problems include hyperkalemia, and it is a known triggering agent for malignant hyperthermia (MH).

6. It is contraindicated in patients with muscular dystrophies, burns, neurologic disease, and familial history of MH.
7. Dose: 1 to 2 mg/kg IV; 2 to 4 mg/kg IM

D. Nondepolarizing muscle relaxants (NDMRs).
   1. Mivacurium is a short-acting NDMR that is metabolized by plasma cholinesterase.
      a. Histamine release can occur and is related to the dose administered and speed of injection. Clinical symptoms include flushing and hypotension.
      b. Dose: 0.1 to 0.2 mg/kg IV over 5 to 10 seconds; 0.2 to 0.3 mg/kg intubation; 10 to 20 µg/kg/min infusion
   2. Atracurium is an intermediate-acting benzylisoquinolinium derivative metabolized by Hofmann elimination and ester hydrolysis.
      a. Histamine release can occur and is related to the dose administered and speed of injection. Clinical symptoms include flushing and hypotension.
      b. Dose
         (1) 1 month to 2 years: 0.3 to 0.4 mg/kg, maintenance 0.08 to 0.1 mg/kg
         (2) Older than 2 years: 0.4 to 0.5 mg/kg, maintenance 0.08 to 0.1 mg/kg
   3. Cis-atracurium is an intermediate-acting benzylisoquinolinium derivative that is metabolized primarily through Hofmann elimination.
      a. It is devoid of histamine effects and related cardiovascular changes that can be seen with atracurium.
      b. Dose: children 2 to 12 years, 0.1 mg/kg IV
   4. Rocuronium is an intermediate-acting monoquaternary steroidal NDMR that has a rapid onset of action.
      a. It has a favorable cardiovascular profile and is metabolized by the liver.
      b. Because of its rapid onset of action, it is used to facilitate intubation for rapid sequence inductions.
      c. Dose: 0.6 to 1 mg/kg IV for intubation; 0.08 to 0.12 mg/kg for maintenance
   5. Vecuronium is an intermediate-acting monoquaternary steroidal NDMR that has favorable cardiovascular characteristics.
      a. It is metabolized by the liver.
      b. Dose: 0.07 to 0.2 mg/kg IV; 0.8 to 1 µg/kg/min infusion

6. Pancuronium is a long-acting NDMR.
   a. Tachycardia and hypertension can occur and are related to the dose administered and speed of injection.
   b. It is excreted by the kidneys.
   c. Dose: 0.08 to 0.15 mg/kg IV
E. Anticholinesterase agents.
   1. The use of anticholinesterase agents in pediatric patients depends on the drug and dose administered.
   2. Routine reversal is not advocated and should be guided by clinical judgment.
   3. Administration of an anticholinergic agent is required to avoid the significant cardiac effects associated with the anticholinesterase agents.
      a. Atropine: 0.015 mg/kg IV
      b. Glycopyrrolate: 0.01 mg/kg IV
   4. Neostigmine: 0.05 to 0.07 mg/kg IV
   5. Edrophonium: 0.5 mg/kg; may repeat for total dose of 1 mg/kg

ADDITIONAL READINGS

Dobbins, P., & Hall S.M. (1997). Pediatric anesthesia. In Nagelhout, J., & Zaglaniczny, K. *Nurse anesthesia*. Philadelphia: W.B. Saunders.

Gregory, G.A. (1997). *Pediatric anesthesia* (3rd ed.). New York: Churchill Livingstone.

Motoyama, G.K., & Davis P.J. (1996). *Smith's anesthesia for infant and children* (6th ed.). St. Louis: Mosby.

Yaffee, S.J., & Aranda J.V. (1992). *Pediatric pharmacology: therapeutic principles in practice* (2nd ed.). Philadelphia: W.B. Saunders.

Preparation of the Pediatric Patient

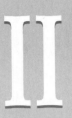

3

Preoperative Preparation for the Pediatric Patient

Rex A. Marley, MS, CRNA, RRT

I. Introduction

A. Efficiently conducting the process of patient assessment, laboratory testing, and readying the patient for surgery is a major challenge for anesthesia providers that entails collaboration among the medical facility, anesthesia and surgical staffs, primary care physicians, and occasionally specialists.

B. No consensus has been reached on how best to properly assess and prepare the patient for surgery. Specific objectives of preoperative assessment and preparation of the pediatric patient include

1. To optimize patient care, satisfaction, and comfort

2. To minimize perioperative morbidity and mortality by accurately assessing factors that influence the risk of anesthesia or that might alter the planned anesthetic technique

3. To minimize surgical delays or preventable cancellations on the day of surgery

4. To determine appropriate postoperative disposition of the patient regarding whether the patient and procedure are best managed on an ambulatory, inpatient, or intensive care basis

5. To evaluate the patient's health status, thus determining which preoperative investigations and specialty consultations are required

6. To formulate a plan of the most appropriate perianesthetic care and postoperative supportive patient care

7. To communicate patient management issues effectively between care providers

8. To ensure time-efficient and cost-effective patient evaluation

C. The *preanesthesia assessment clinic* has been shown to be the most comprehensive and cost-effective method for preoperative evaluation and preparation. When appropriately established, this "one-stop shopping" enables the patient to accomplish the required appointments (e.g., registration, physical examination, diagnostic testing) in an efficient, convenient single visit.

D. Optimal preoperative evaluation and preparation for anesthesia and surgery should take place sufficiently in advance of the proposed operation to allow ample time for necessary risk assessment, preoperative testing, and specialty consultations.

E. The patient with complex medical conditions should be evaluated at least 1 week before the scheduled procedure.

F. Preoperative assessment on the day of surgery means a greater risk of last-minute discovery (i.e., inappropriate fasting; suspected difficult airway) that may result in surgical postponement or cancellation.

II. Preoperative Assessment

A. Preoperative evaluation focuses on obtaining information about the surgical candidate to determine the patient's condition for surgery and to implement appropriate strategies to optimize his or her condition for the upcoming surgery.

B. A thorough medical history and physical assessment serve as the foundation of an organized approach to further patient workup and consultation. The preoperative assessment is not intended to be a universal health screening and is not cost effective if patients are assessed for medical problems that do not alter plans for anesthetic management.

C. Medical history: A medical history and review of systems are elicited to gather information from the patient or parents and other data sources regarding pertinent preoperative conditions (see Table 3–1). The level of detail in eliciting the medical history depends on the patient's physical status, the availability of information, and the time available to conduct the patient assessment before surgery.

   1. The patient interview should include the parents since the majority of children are not capable of giving a medical history.

   2. Current and past medical records should be reviewed, including laboratory and diagnostic test results and physical examination. Prior anesthesia records should be examined for complications, response to anesthesia, and postoperative course before meeting with the patient and family when possible.

   3. Appropriate growth and development, as compared with norms and percentiles for age and gender, should be evaluated. Failure to meet expected growth parameters can

TABLE 3–1. Components of the Patient's Medical History

SURGICAL ILLNESS
What surgical procedure is the child having?
What other surgeries and hospitalizations has the child had?

COEXISTING MEDICAL ILLNESS
Has the child had any serious illnesses other than the condition for which surgery is indicated?
Does the child feel sick?

ANESTHETIC HISTORY
Has the child ever had an anesthetic before?
Has the child or any blood relatives ever had a problem with any type of anesthesia (e.g., prolonged paralysis, malignant hyperthermia)?

SOCIAL HISTORY
Is the child exposed to passive smoking?

REVIEW OF SYSTEMS
Birth and Developmental History
Was the child's delivery premature or at term?
Did the child experience any neonatal complications?
Did the child have a history of low heart rate (bradycardia) or periods of low or absent respirations (apnea)?
Is there any history of sudden infant death syndrome in your family?

Heart Disease
Have you been told that your child has a heart murmur?

Pulmonary Problems
Has the child ever required supplemental oxygen therapy?
Has the child ever had pneumonia, bronchitis, or asthma?
Has the child had a recent cough or cold?
Does the child ever wheeze?

Bleeding Disorders
Does the child bleed and bruise easily or have any problems with blood clotting?
Has the child been evaluated for sickle cell anemia?

Liver Disease (Jaundice, Hepatitis)
Has the child ever had any jaundice or liver problems?

Kidney, Urinary, or Bladder Problems
Has the child ever had any kidney problems?

Gastrointestinal Problems (Hiatal Hernia, Bowel Problems)
Does the child have gastric acid reflux or hiatal hernia?
Has the child recently experienced diarrhea?

Seizures
Does the child have any neurologic problems, such as seizures?

Table continued on following page

TABLE 3–1. Components of the Patient's Medical History
Continued

Obstetric History (Children of Childbearing Age)
Could you be pregnant?

Airway Problems
Did the child have a history of difficult intubation with previous anesthesia, trouble opening the mouth, or loose teeth?

Exercise Tolerance
Does the child have any physical limitations?
Does the child get short of breath or "turn blue" during normal activities?

Other Concerns
Does the child have any problems with the thyroid or adrenal glands?
Does the child have diabetes?
Is there objection to receiving blood products under any circumstances?

MEDICATIONS
What medications has the child taken in the past 3 months (including dose and schedule)?
Has the child taken any steroid (e.g., prednisone) within the past year?

INGESTION OF FOOD OR DRINK
Elicit just before anesthesia to assess potential risk of pulmonary aspiration.

ALLERGIES
Please list drugs, foods (e.g., eggs), and environmental items (e.g., latex) to which the child is allergic or has had a bad reaction.

From Cassidy, J., & Marley, R.A. (1996). Preoperative assessment of the ambulatory patient. *Journal of Perianesthesia Nursing,* 11(5), 334–343.

indicate a prenatal pathologic condition or major systemic illness.
4. Developmentally delayed infants, as evaluated through age-related markers, may have associated neurologic or neuromuscular disease.
D. Physical examination: The objective of the preoperative physical examination is to recognize, evaluate, and record physical findings consistent with conditions relevant to the anticipated procedure and anesthetic technique (see Table 3–2).
E. Laboratory testing: Routine preoperative diagnostic testing should be based on (1) an established need from findings of an abnormal medical history or physical examination or (2) its impact on perioperative care. The use of testing protocols (typically governed by hospital or state policy) offers a standardized and timely approach to diagnostic assessment.

Mandatory diagnostic screening without specific indications is neither cost effective nor predictive of postoperative complications and is no longer acceptable in clinical practice. Conditions and systemic disorders in which preoperative laboratory screening is appropriate are listed in Table 3–3.

TABLE 3–2. Components of the Physical Examination

PATIENT DEMOGRAPHICS
Age (postconceptual age if appropriate), height, weight

VITAL SIGNS
Blood pressure (both arms if indicated), resting pulse, respiratory rate, oxyhemoglobin saturation on room air, body temperature

GENERAL
Observation of body habitus and general physical appearance (i.e., color, nutrition, hydration)

HEAD AND NECK
Airway assessment, dental conditions, tongue size, oral opening size, maxillary/mandibular shape, thyromental distance, Mallampati classification, oral lesions, cervical spine motion, tracheal deviation, cervical masses
Fontanelle
Craniofacial dysmorphisms (nose, mouth, jaw)

SKIN
Jaundice, cyanosis, nutritional abnormalities, dehydration, turgor, pallor

PRECORDIUM
Cardiac auscultation for regularity of rate and rhythm, and presence of murmurs, gallops, and rubs

LUNGS
Auscultation for equal bilateral breath sounds, wheezing, rhonchi, rales
Observation for use of accessory muscles

ABDOMEN
Distention, masses, ascites

EXTREMITIES
Muscle wasting or weakness, mobility for age, bruising, clubbing, cyanosis, cutaneous infection, edema, sensation, skin texture

NEUROLOGIC
Baseline mental status, cranial nerve function, cognition, peripheral sensorimotor function, gait, muscle strength

EYES
Abnormal movement, strabismus, pupillary size and reactivity

From Cassidy, J., & Marley, R.A. (1996). Preoperative assessment of the ambulatory patient. *Journal of Perianesthesia Nursing*, 11(5), 334–343.

TABLE 3–3. Indications for Laboratory Testing

COMPLETE BLOOD COUNT
Hematologic disorder
Vascular procedure
Chemotherapy
Unknown sickle cell syndrome status

HEMOGLOBIN/HEMATOCRIT
<6 months of age (<1 year if born premature)
Hematologic malignancy
Recent radiation or chemotherapy
Renal disease
Anticoagulant therapy
Procedure with moderate to high blood loss potential
Coexisting systemic disorders (e.g., cystic fibrosis, prematurity, severe malnutrition, renal failure, liver disease, congenital heart disease)

WHITE BLOOD CELL COUNT
Leukemia and lymphomas
Recent radiation or chemotherapy
Suspected infection that would lead to cancellation of surgery
Aplastic anemia
Hypersplenism
Autoimmune collagen vascular disease

BLOOD GLUCOSE LEVEL
Diabetes mellitus
Current corticosteroid use
History of hypoglycemia
Adrenal disease
Cystic fibrosis

SERUM CHEMISTRY
Renal disease
Adrenal or thyroid disease
Chemotherapy
Pituitary or hypothalamic disease
Body fluid loss or shifts (e.g., dehydration, bowel prep)
CNS disease

Potassium
Digoxin therapy
Diuretic therapy

CREATININE AND BUN
Cardiovascular disease (e.g., hypertension)
Renal disease
Adrenal disease
Diabetes mellitus
Diuretic therapy
Digoxin therapy

TABLE 3-3. Indications for Laboratory Testing *Continued*

CREATININE AND BUN *Continued*
Body fluid loss or shifts (e.g., dehydration, bowel prep)
Procedure requiring radiocontrast

LIVER FUNCTION TESTS
Hepatic disease
Exposure to hepatitis
Therapy with hepatotoxic agents

COAGULATION STUDIES
Prothrombin Time (PT) and Partial Thromboplastin Time (PTT)
Leukemia
Hepatic disease
Bleeding disorder
Anticoagulant therapy
Severe malnutrition or malabsorption

Platelet Count and Bleeding Time
Bleeding disorder
Abnormal hemorrhage, purpura, easy bruisability

URINALYSIS
Not indicated as a routine screening test

PREGNANCY
Possibility of pregnancy

SERUM MEDICATION LEVELS
Monitor for medications (i.e., theophylline, phenytoin [Dilantin], carbamazepine [Tegretol]) if the patient exhibits signs of ineffective therapy, potential drug side effects, or poor drug compliance or has recently changed
medication therapy without documentation of the drug level

ELECTROCARDIOGRAM
History of previously unevaluated pathologic-sounding murmur or palpi-
tation
Family history reveals possibility of inherited prolonged QT syndrome
History of moderate to severe sleep apnea or those with chronic anatomic
airway obstruction (e.g., Pierre Robin syndrome) may be at risk for right
heart strain)

CHEST RADIOGRAPH
Suspected intrathoracic pathologic condition (e.g., tumors, vascular ring)
History of congenital heart disease
History of prematurity associated with residual bronchopulmonary dys-
plasia
Severe obstructive sleep apnea (may have cardiomegaly)
Down's syndrome (may have asymptomatic subluxation of the atlantoaxial
junction)

From Cassidy, J., & Marley, R.A. (1996). Preoperative assessment of the ambulatory patient. *Journal of Perianesthesia Nursing*, 11(5), 334–343.

III. The Child At Risk

The following clinical conditions deserve consideration when assessing the pediatric patient for anesthesia and surgery.

A. Heart murmur: Cardiac murmurs are a common finding during the physical assessment of children, and most are innocent. If there is a history of a heart murmur or a new murmur is identified, a full medical history, including the timing of onset and any associated signs and symptoms, should first be obtained and reviewed with the child's pediatrician.

   1. Heart murmurs are categorized as innocent or pathologic; and proper identification is important. Auscultation of heart sounds is the most efficient method to assess murmurs. If the child is completely asymptomatic, as with innocent murmurs, it is unlikely that the murmur is due to an impairment that will pose an anesthetic problem; thus specialist referral is not warranted. Pathologic murmurs, often detected in early childhood, may be due to complex congenital malformations or heart disease and have accompanying physical dysfunction. If the patient is symptomatic, it is important to establish the degree of physiologic compromise or hemodynamic effects.

   2. Signs and symptoms of pathologic murmurs may include atypical vital signs (e.g., a heart rate of 50 bpm, a blood pressure of 140/90 in a school-age child), cyanosis, dyspnea, orthopnea, tachypnea, tachycardia, diaphoresis, difficulty feeding, failure to thrive, fatigue, hepatomegaly, rales, syncope, chest pain, or abnormal pulses.

   3. If proper history and physical examination determine the murmur to be innocent, neither further investigation nor referral is indicated. Pathologic murmurs, or any questionable murmurs, require further preoperative diagnostic evaluation (i.e., chest radiograph; electrocardiogram [ECG]; cardiac catheterization; echocardiogram) as determined by consultation with a specialist. The specialist's description of the nature and severity of the cardiac defect, along with perioperative care recommendations, is indispensable. All children with congenital heart disease must have a preoperative hemoglobin or hematocrit measurement to evaluate anemia or polycythemia.

   4. Prophylactic antibiotics should be administered to the child with a suspected or proven congenital cardiac defect, including patients who have had surgery to correct congenital cardiac defects. In 1997 the American Heart

Association updated its recommendations for the appropriate administration of antibiotics for the prevention of subacute bacterial endocarditis.

B. Sickle cell disease: Patients with the sickle cell trait are unlikely to develop perioperative sickling crisis, but those with sickle cell disease are at risk for multiple organ vasoocclusive crisis.

1. All black children presenting for anesthesia should be evaluated for sickle cell disease if they have not been previously screened (hemoglobin electrophoresis is the benchmark standard test).

2. Determine the extent of major organ involvement secondary to vasoocclusive events: pulmonary (chest pain, dyspnea on exertion, fever, wheezing, prolonged expiratory phase, recent or recurrent respiratory infection, orthopnea, paroxysmal nocturnal dyspnea, recent cough), neurologic (seizures, strokes, subarachnoid hemorrhage, focal neurologic findings), or cardiac problems (murmur, ankle edema, palpitations, exercise tolerance, neck vein distention, heart size) and renal (change in urine color, hematuria, nocturia, dysuria, infections) or hepatic (right upper quadrant pain, jaundice, hepatitis, change in stool color, hepatosplenomegaly) disease.

3. The need for preoperative transfusion of erythrocytes is controversial and depends on the existing degree of anemia, which is typical among sickle cell disease patients, and the magnitude of the surgical procedure. In general, sickle cell disease patients who have a hemoglobin <10 g/dl will require simple transfusion with fresh banked blood to bring the hemoglobin >10 g/dl, which will increase the oxygen-carrying capacity and is just as effective in preventing perioperative complications as exchange transfusions.

4. A complete blood count (CBC) with platelet and reticulocyte count, SMA-18, and urinalysis should be performed on patients with sickle cell disease. Patients with recurrent sickle cell crisis may have preexisting pulmonary hypertension secondary to pulmonary infarcts, cardiomyopathy, and respiratory symptoms (i.e., wheezing, chest syndrome) and should have an ECG and chest radiograph (heart size, atelectasis) testing. Depending on the degree of respiratory involvement, arterial blood gas analysis and pulmonary function testing might be indicated.

5. Risk factors that can exacerbate a sickle cell crisis include

stress, acidosis, hypercarbia, hypothermia, and hypovolemia. Goals to minimize these risk factors include
  a. Ensuring adequate hydration by minimizing the fasting interval and initiating early intravenous (IV) fluid therapy
  b. Correcting coexisting infection (treat with appropriate antibiotics)
  c. Judicious use of opioid and sedative premedication (to prevent respiratory and cardiovascular depression resulting in hypoxia and increased blood viscosity)
  d. Assessing requirements for analgesic medication (patients with crisis may have chronic dependence on analgesic agents)
  e. Avoiding hypothermia
  f. Ensuring adequate oxygenation (monitor; supplemental oxygen therapy to keep oxyhemoglobin saturation by pulse oximetry [Spo_2] >90%)
C. Cystic fibrosis: The main clinical manifestations include obstructive pulmonary disease, pancreatic insufficiency, abnormally high sweat electrolyte concentrations, nasal polyps, and opacification of sinuses.
  1. Evaluate for acute pulmonary infection and need for appropriate antibiotic therapy along with respiratory therapy procedures (i.e., chest physical therapy, postural drainage). Optimize pulmonary function status; consider regional technique when appropriate. Patients are commonly taking beta-adrenergic bronchodilators, corticosteroids, and mucolytic agents, which should be continued.
  2. Assess nutritional status because malnutrition may be severe in these infants. Nutritional consultation may indicate need for parenteral nutrition or supplemental enteral nutrition preoperatively. Patient may be receiving pancreatase enzyme replacement therapy.
D. Asthma.
  1. Obtain a thorough history of frequency of attacks, their severity (was endotracheal intubation required?), time from last attack, when the patient was last hospitalized or treated in the emergency room for asthma, what triggers an attack, and what works for treating acute exacerbations of the patient's asthma.
  2. Patients considered at greater risk if history is suggestive of
    a. Frequent nocturnal awakenings from asthma

   b. Frequent or continuous systemic corticosteroid need
   c. Recent hospitalizations or emergency room (ER) visits for asthma
   d. Prior perioperative complications from asthma
   e. A large volume of sputum production
   f. Coexistent cardiovascular disease
3. Children with asthma should be under optimal medical management before receiving anesthesia. If the patient has a persistent cough, wheezing, or tachypnea on the day surgery is scheduled, it is best to reschedule surgery.
4. Utilization of diagnostic tests is based on the clinician's assessment of the severity of the disease and magnitude of the operative procedure. Indications for obtaining an ECG are rare in children; however, an ECG is indicated if right ventricular hypertrophy is suspected because it generally implies long-standing insufficient therapy. A chest radiograph is only considered if the child may have an acute infiltrative process (i.e., pneumonia) or if a recent change in the child's physical status suggests deterioration has occurred. Arterial blood gases are usually only indicated when signs of chronic respiratory insufficiency (e.g., hypoxia, hypercarbia) are suspected or when a child with acute asthma requires emergency surgery. If age appropriate, spirometric evaluation consisting of a peak expiratory flow rate (PEFR) should be done the morning of surgery if active disease is suspected and compared with the patient's best value in recent weeks: 80% to 100% of baseline = normal, 50% to 80% of baseline = moderate exacerbation, and <50% of baseline = severe episode indicating the need for delay of surgery and more intensive therapy.
5. All medications should be continued up to and including the day of surgery. Prophylactic beta-adrenergic metered dose inhalers should be used on the morning of surgery and accompany the patient to the operating room. Oral medications (e.g., theophylline) may be taken with a sip (1–2 oz) of water up to 1 to 2 hours before surgery. Therapeutic serum theophylline levels (10–20 μg/ml) should be confirmed if utilized. Supplemental stress doses of corticosteroids may be appropriate if the patient has recently been taking corticosteroids. Antianxiety premedication should be considered since the psychologic triggers (e.g., anxiety) are well known.

6. Ensure adequate hydration (i.e., minimize the fasting interval) to reduce airway desiccation and to improve mobilization of secretions.

7. If signs and symptoms of infection are present, surgery may be postponed while antibiotic therapy, based on sputum Gram stain and cultures, is given.

E. Upper respiratory tract infections (URTI): Children with URTI, particularly those younger than 1 year of age, have an increased risk (twofold to sevenfold increase) of respiratory-related adverse events intraoperatively and postoperatively (i.e., bronchospasm, laryngospasm, hypoxemia, atelectasis, croup, stridor).

1. Signs and symptoms of URTI include sore throat; inflamed and reddened nasopharyngeal and oropharyngeal mucosa; sneezing; rhinorrhea (clear secretions) or mucopurulent nasal secretions; nasal congestion, including watery eyes; malaise; bulging, tender eardrums with associated inflammation; nonproductive cough; fever 37.5°C to 38.5°C (>38°C associated with lower respiratory tract involvement); laryngitis/tonsillitis; viral ulcers in the oropharynx; WBC count >12,000/mm^3 with a left shift. Positive chest findings, such as pulmonary congestion or rales, are usually associated with lower respiratory tract involvement.

2. Each case should be reviewed individually and the decision to operate made based on the urgency of the surgery, the duration and complexity of the surgery, and the need for instrumentation of the airway. It is important to obtain a specific history to distinguish a patient's chronic state from an acute, superimposed infectious process, which has predictive value for morbidity. If the parents state the child typically has a cold or chronic runny nose (clear rhinorrhea) and the child is in his or her optimal state (afebrile, without respiratory distress), then he or she may be considered for short elective procedures. If the child has a productive cough from lower respiratory tract involvement or an infectious-appearing, runny nose, then elective surgery should be postponed. However, it may be necessary to schedule children who have chronic URTIs for procedures such as myringotomy with ventilation tube placement or tonsillectomies, since URTIs are frequently associated with these conditions. Exercise caution when proceeding with children <5 years of age (consider canceling for children <1 year old) since risks increase. If the child is >1 year of age with resolving URTI, it is

reasonable to proceed with minor procedures not requiring endotracheal intubation (intubation with URTI increases the risk elevenfold).

3. Infectious nasopharyngitis (without lower respiratory tract involvement) requires cancellation of the surgery for about 2 weeks. If the child exhibits signs and symptoms of lower respiratory tract involvement, it is prudent to postpone an elective surgical procedure for 4 to 6 weeks, which is the time necessary to minimize airway hyperactivity.

4. Laboratory testing should consist of a CBC, including differential. Nasal or throat cultures may be obtained if signs of an infectious process are observed. A chest radiograph is not warranted, especially if chest sounds are clear. Pulmonary function tests and arterial blood gas analysis likewise will rarely offer any useful information.

F. Prematurity: The premature infant, defined as 37 weeks' or less gestational age at birth, is susceptible for the development of certain conditions: anemia, pulmonary aspiration with feeding secondary to immature gag reflex, intraventricular hemorrhage, perioperative apneic spells and bradycardic episodes, and chronic respiratory dysfunction secondary to respiratory failure at birth requiring mechanical ventilation and supplemental oxygen therapy. Expremature infants less than 55 to 60 weeks' postconceptual age (gestational age plus postnatal age) are at greatest risk of postoperative complications.

1. Determine the prematurity status (postconceptual [time from conception to the present time] and gestational [time from conception to birth] ages at birth).

2. Extremely premature infants (24 to 26 weeks' gestational age) and former preterm infants (risk markedly diminishes at >43 weeks' postconceptual age) are known to be at higher risk for postoperative apnea than are full-term infants. Anemia (hematocrit <30%) is a risk factor for postoperative apnea even for the >43 weeks' postconceptual aged infant.

3. Evaluate for residual respiratory dysfunction. The former preterm infant may also have mild bronchopulmonary dysplasia or extensive disease with chronic hypoxemia and hypercarbia, tracheomalacia, or bronchomalacia and increased pulmonary vascular resistance with cor pulmonale. A child who (a) required mechanical ventilation or long-term supplemental oxygen therapy following birth, (b) requires bronchodilator therapy, and (c) has

recurrent pulmonary infections is at high risk for residual pulmonary disease. Subglottic stenosis may be suspected in the infant who required prolonged endotracheal intubation.

4. Continue medications (i.e., diuretics, bronchodilators, corticosteroids) commonly required to manage bronchopulmonary dysplasia.

5. Laboratory testing should include, at minimum, a determination of hematocrit, since anemia is associated with postoperative apnea. Pulmonary function testing may be suitable for the older, cooperative child to quantitate the extent of pulmonary disease. Arterial blood gas analysis is indicated to quantitate suspected hypoxemia or hypercarbia.

6. Physical examination should look for significant pulmonary pathologic findings and include observation of the child for nasal flaring, the respiratory rate, evidence of retractions, use of accessory muscles, prolongation of inspiration or exhalation, or expiratory grunting. Cardiovascular dysfunction may result from pulmonary pathologic findings, leading to right ventricular hypertrophy with increased pulmonary artery pressures and pulmonary vascular resistance.

G. Seizure disorder.

1. Medical history should include the type and frequency of seizures, seizure medication, and whether the seizure disorder is under optimal control.

2. Anticonvulsants, unless contraindicated, should be administered on schedule with water (1 or 2 oz) until 1 to 2 hours before surgery. Serum levels (e.g., phenytoin [Dilantin]) may be indicated to determine adequacy of treatment.

H. Diabetes.

1. Medical history should include the child's age at the onset of diabetes, insulin requirements, dietary habits, and frequency of hypoglycemic or hyperglycemic episodes.

2. It is best to schedule surgery as early in the day as possible to minimize the fasting period.

3. Just before surgery, the diabetic child requiring insulin or oral hypoglycemic agents should have a blood glucose value checked. Depending on the type and length of surgery, and the lability of diabetes, serum glucose levels will be checked intraoperatively and in the postanesthesia care unit (PACU) at 2- to 4-hour intervals.

4. Several different regimens are used to treat diabetic children undergoing surgery and anesthesia. A common approach is to administer a fraction (often one half to two

thirds) of the child's usual morning dose of intermediate or long-acting insulin.

5. The fasting child who is receiving insulin should have IV access established with a crystalloid solution containing 5% glucose.

6. Consultation with the physician responsible for managing the patient's diabetes is helpful in determining an acceptable range of serum glucose and when and what type of insulin therapy may be appropriate.

7. The diabetic patient should be screened for renal disease, including electrolytes, blood urea nitrogen (BUN), and creatinine, if not checked by the pediatrician.

IV. Fasting Considerations

A. The risk of perioperative pulmonary aspiration of gastric contents that results in morbidity or mortality is relatively low. Recommendations for withholding oral feeding before elective surgery have recently become much more liberal.

B. When studies were conducted challenging the traditional fasting times (7 hours or more) for clear liquids, it appears that a reduced fasting interval does not increase the risk of pulmonary aspiration in normal, healthy children.

C. Modest amounts of clear liquids orally 2 to 3 hours preoperatively when compared with the conventional fasting interval of 7 hours or "after midnight" are acceptable and have been shown to lower residual gastric volume (stimulation of the gastric emptying reflex) and raise gastric pH in a majority of patients. Acceptable clear fluids include water, apple juice, clear juice drinks, clear gelatin, clear broth, ice popsicles, or Pedialyte.

D. Children at increased risk for pulmonary aspiration and not suitable for a shortened fasting interval include patients with morbid obesity, renal failure, hepatic dysfunction, ascites, neurologic dysfunction including head injury or increased intracranial pressure, depressed level of consciousness, cerebral palsy, atypical pain or trauma, drug overdose, difficult airway, prior esophageal surgery or dysfunction, gastrointestinal obstruction, emergency surgery, anorexia nervosa, esophageal motility disorders, diabetes mellitus, delayed gastric emptying, and lack of coordination of swallowing and respiration.

E. Prolonged fasting, especially in children, can be quite distressing in addition to causing physiologic alterations. Periods of long preoperative fasting have been shown to contribute to hypovolemia, hypoglycemia (in smaller children), and discomfort-related thirst. When the fasting interval is minimized, children are reported to be less irritable, thirsty, and hungry and more comfortable; have fewer headaches; and generally tolerate the preoperative phase better than children who have fasted for longer periods of time.

F. Current fasting guidelines for healthy children presenting for elective surgery
   1. No chewing gum or candy after midnight
   2. Clear liquids up to 2 hours before surgery
   3. Breast milk until 4 hours before surgery
   4. No infant formula, nonhuman milk, or light meal for at least 6 hours before surgery
   5. Prescribed medications (e.g., premedication) administered with a sip of water or prescribed liquid mixture

V. Premedication

A. Uses of preoperative medication.
   1. To decrease patient anxiety and fear
   2. To facilitate smooth induction and emergence from anesthesia
   3. To supplement anesthesia and reduce the need for general anesthetic agents
   4. To reduce the volume and acidity of gastric contents
   5. To provide a more pleasant stay in the PACU
B. The ideal premedicant should be available in a form readily accepted by the child, should be absolutely dependable with rapid, reliable onset and offset, and should not produce undesirable side effects.
C. Pharmacologic premedication in preparing the child for surgery should not become routine; rather, it should be reserved on an individual basis for the child who is extremely apprehensive.
   1. The oral route is the most acceptable and appropriate route of administering premedication to children. Oral midazolam, 0.5 to 0.75 mg/kg, for pediatric use has gained widespread acceptance, with sedation occurring within 20 minutes and lasting nearly 60 minutes. Midazolam has a bitter taste (IV formulation contains benzyl alcohol) and must be mixed with a small amount (<20 ml) of liquid (i.e., flavored syrup, soda, juice) to mask the taste. Acetaminophen (with or without codeine) elixir effectively masks the taste of midazolam and affords postoperative analgesia.
   2. Since the introduction of oral midazolam, intramuscular premedication has become less popular. However, in the rare child who cannot or refuses to swallow a liquid,

intramuscular injection of premedication may be the route of choice. As a premedicant, intramuscular ketamine in a dose of 3 to 5 mg/kg continues to remain popular for very uncooperative children who refuse both an oral premedicant and a mask induction. It has a reliable and fast onset, producing amnesia and intense analgesia within 5 minutes. Because ketamine causes a marked increase in secretions, which may precipitate laryngospasm, an antisialagogue drug is often coadministered. Emergence delirium, nightmares, and vomiting can be seen with ketamine; they can be reduced by the addition of a benzodiazepine.

3. If IV access is required before the induction of anesthesia, midazolam is easily titrated to effect, up to 0.2 mg/kg in increments of 0.03 to 0.05 mg/kg. Topical anesthesia, such as EMLA (eutectic mixture of local anesthetics) Cream, is effective in reducing or eliminating the discomfort associated with IV cannula placement. EMLA cream is composed of prilocaine and lidocaine and must be applied to the skin under a clear adhesive dressing and left in place at least 45 to 60 minutes in the older child before venipuncture.

ADDITIONAL READINGS

Cassidy, J., & Marley, R.A. (1996). Preoperative assessment of the ambulatory patient. *Journal of Perianesthesia Nursing,* 11(5), 334–343.

Hamid, R.K.A. (1998). Pediatric premedication. In Lake, C.L., Rice, L.J., & Sperry, R.J. (Eds.). *Advances in Anesthesia* (Vol. 15, pp. 227–289). St. Louis: Mosby–Year Book.

Means, L.J., Ferrari, L.R., Fisher, Q.A., et al. (1996). Evaluation and preparation of pediatric patients undergoing anesthesia. *Pediatrics,* 98(3), 502–508.

Pandit, U.A., & Pandit, S.K. (1997). Fasting before and after ambulatory surgery. *Journal of Perianesthesia Nursing,* 12(3), 181–187.

Rasmussen, G.E. (1997). The preoperative evaluation of the pediatric patient. *Pediatric Annals,* 26, 455–460.

4

Pediatric Equipment

Michael Boytim, MSN, CRNA

The equipment used in pediatric anesthesia is selected based on the proposed procedure and the weight and age of the patient. All equipment should be functional and readily available before the start of the procedure.

I. Airway Apparatus
A. Masks
   1. The available anesthesia masks for various pediatric patients are shown in Figure 4–1
   2. To provide a correct fit
      a. The apex of the mask rests on the nasal bridge between the eyes
      b. The base of the mask rests in the crease between the lower lip and chin
B. Airways
   1. Types
      a. Oral
         (1) Poorly tolerated in awake or lightly anesthetized patients
         (2) Proper size: flange at lip, distal tip at angle of mandible
         (3) Sizes for the various age ranges
            (a) Preterm infant: size 000 or 00; 3.5 to 4.5 cm
            (b) Age <3 months: size 0; 5.5 cm
            (c) Ages 3 to 12 months: size 1; 6.0 cm
            (d) Ages 1 to 5 years: size 2; 7.0 cm
            (e) Age >5 years: size 3; 8.0 cm
         (4) The currently available oral airways are shown in Figure 4–2A
      b. Nasal
         (1) Better tolerated in awake patients than oral airways
         (2) Not frequently placed in pediatric patients because of adenoidal hypertrophy, which peaks between 2 and 6 years of age
         (3) Can cause bleeding

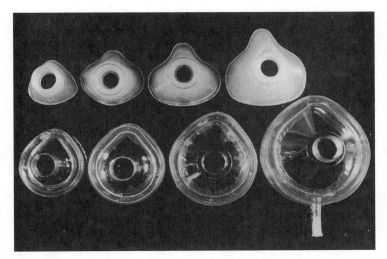

FIGURE 4–1. Types of pediatric anesthesia face masks. *Top row,* Rendell-Baker-Soucek masks, which
- have the least amount of dead space
- have a low profile: permit surgical access to face, i.e., probing of lacrimal ducts
- require practice to maintain airtight fit
- are transparent

Bottom row, masks with pneumatic cushion (bubble masks), which
- have more dead space
- provide effective seal for positive pressure ventilation
- are easier to maintain an airtight fit; are transparent

       (4) Small internal diameter, which can increase the work of breathing
       (5) To determine the proper size the flange is placed at the tip of the nose and the distal tip at the angle of the mandible.
       (6) The various sizes are shown in Figure 4–2*B*
   C. Laryngeal mask airway (LMA)
     1. Suitable for short surgical or diagnostic procedures
     2. May be useful in maintaining an airway in children with previous history of difficult intubation
     3. Low ventilatory resistance
     4. Ability to cough or cry on awakening
     5. Not recommended for positive pressure ventilation
     6. Contraindicated in patients at risk for gastric aspiration
     7. Sizes listed in Table 4–1

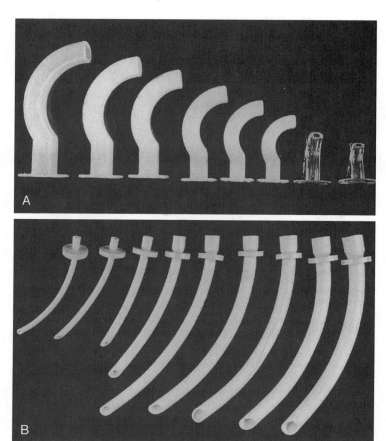

FIGURE 4–2. **A,** Oral airways. Sizes range from neonate *(right)* to adolescent *(left).* **B,** Nasal airways. Sizes range from infant *(left)* to adolescent *(right).*

TABLE 4–1. Laryngeal Mask Airway Sizes

Size	Pediatric Use
1	Neonates and infants up to 5 kg; cuff volume up to 4 ml
1.5	Infants 5–10 kg; cuff volume up to 7 ml
2	Infants and children 10–20 kg; cuff volume up to 10 ml
2.5	Children 20–30 kg; cuff volume up to 14 ml
3	Children >30 kg; cuff volume up to 20 ml

8. Insertion technique
    a. Same as in the adult
    b. May use intravenous (IV) or inhalation induction

II. Endotracheal Intubation Equipment

A. Endotracheal (ET) tubes (see Fig. 4–3): The recommended ET tube sizes are listed in Figure 4–3 legend. Guidelines for selection of ET tube size include
    1. There is no perfect formula for estimating sizes.
    2. The most appropriate size should
        a. Be confirmed by testing the airway pressure at which gas audibly escapes around the tube
        b. Allow for leak at 20 to 25 cm H_2O airway pressure
    3. If there is a leak at >30 cm H_2O pressure, change ET tube to smaller size to decrease the risk of postextubation croup.
    4. If leak at <15 cm H_2O pressure, change ET tube to a larger size to decrease the risk of aspiration and decreased ability to effectively ventilate.
    5. Cuffed ET tube rarely necessary in children <8 years of age.
    6. If cuffed ET tube needed, the calculated tube size (internal diameter [ID]) should be decreased by 0.5 mm.
    7. Cuffed ET tubes are available starting at 3.0 mm ID.
    8. ET tubes 0.5 mm ID larger and smaller than calculated tube size should be immediately available in the room.
    9. The methods to determine the depth of insertion are listed in Figure 4–3 legend.
        a. Oral RAE
            (1) Used in ear, nose, and throat (ENT) and head and neck procedures.
            (2) The distal tip lies nearer to carina than in conventional ETT.
            (3) The two Murphy eyes allow continuous ventilation should bronchial migration occur.
            (4) Always use a left precordial stethoscope to detect bronchial migration.
        b. Nasal RAE: used in surgery involving mouth, mandible, or face
        c. The greatest disadvantage of both types of RAE tubes is the fixed flexion point. Since the flexion point of the tube is taped at the lip or nares, the tip may be too long or short in some patients
B. Laryngoscope blades and handles
    1. Laryngoscope blades are available in an assortment of sizes and styles (see Fig. 4–4).

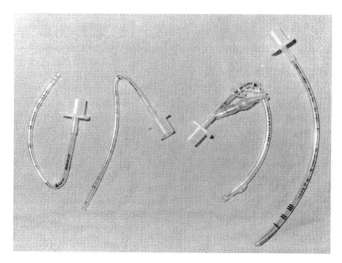

FIGURE 4–3. Common pediatric endotracheal tubes. From left, uncuffed oral RAE, uncuffed nasal RAE, cuffed oral RAE, and uncuffed straight ET tube.

RECOMMENDED ET TUBE SIZES FOR INFANTS/CHILDREN*

Age	Sizes (ID)
Premature	
<1000 g	2.5
>1000 g	3.0
Neonate to 3 months	3.0
3–9 mo	3.5
9–18 mo	4.0
≥2 y	16 + age (y) divided by 4

METHODS FOR DEPTH OF INSERTION OF ET TUBES†

1. 7 cm at lip for a 1 kg child; 1 additional cm/kg up to 4 kg

kg	cm at lip
1	7
2	8
3	9
4	10

   4 kg to age 1 year: 10 cm at lip

   Age 1 year: (age divided by 2) + 12

2. Three times the internal diameter; for example, insert no. 4.0 ET tube to 12 cm

3. When double black line on the uncuffed ET tube passes through vocal cords, tip is proximal to carina

*From Motoyama, E.K., & Davis, P.L. (1996). *Smith's anesthesia for infants and children* (ed. 6). St. Louis: Mosby.

†From Ehrenwerth, J., & Eisenkraft, J.B. (1993). *Anesthesia equipment: Principles and applications* (6th ed.). St. Louis: Mosby.

2. The straight blade is the most commonly used.
    a. Miller blade: facilitates lift of epiglottis, improving visualization
    b. Wis-Hippel or Robertshaw: has a wide flange that engages tongue to left to facilitate passage of ET tube (see Fig. 4–4C)
3. The curved blade (Macintosh), sizes 0, 1, 2, may also be used.

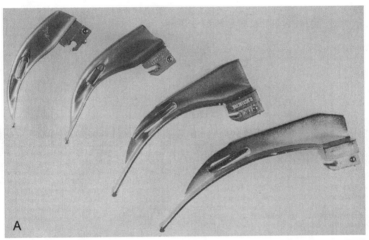

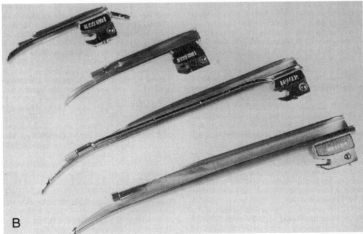

FIGURE 4–4. Pediatric laryngoscope blades. **A,** Macintosh blades. **B,** Miller blades. *Figure continued on following page*

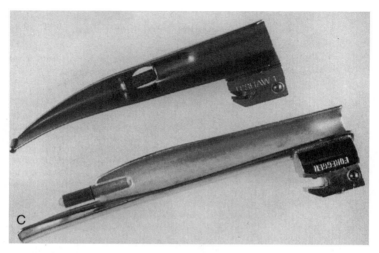

FIGURE 4–4 *Continued.* **C,** Robertshaw blade *(top)* and Flagg blade *(bottom).* Following are recommended ages for using various blades:

Macintosh 1	Ages 1–2 y
Macintosh 2	Ages 3–5 y
Miller 0	Neonate
Miller 1	Ages 1–2 y
Miller 2	Age >3 y
Wis-Hippel 1	Ages 1–2 y
Wis-Hippel 1.5	Ages 3–4 y

   4. Pediatric laryngoscope handles are shown in Figure 4–5. They are less cumbersome and of lighter weight than standard handles.

III. Anesthesia Machine and Appendages
   A. Anesthesia machine
      1. Pediatric patients can effectively be anesthetized with standard adult machine.
      2. The machine should have the capability of delivering air.
      3. Many neonates require F_{IO_2} approaching that of room air to prevent retinopathy of prematurity.
      4. For types of surgeries where N_2O is contraindicated (i.e., bowel), allow air to decrease the F_{IO_2} in absence of N_2O.
      5. The air/O_2 blending ratios and the formula for calculation of the desired percent of oxygen by mixing air and oxygen are listed in Table 4–2.

B. Pediatric circuits
   1. The characteristics of an ideal pediatric breathing system are listed in Table 4–3.
   2. The most commonly used circuits are the Mapleson D, Mapleson F (Jackson-Reese), Bain, and circle systems.
   3. Mapleson D and Mapleson F (see Fig. 4–6).
      a. Modifications of the T-piece system
      b. Advantages: low dead space, low resistance to breathing (valveless), lightweight
      c. Disadvantages: heat and moisture loss, no scavenge, high fresh gas flows to produce desirable $Paco_2$
      d. Difficult to predict fresh gas flows and minute ventilation to produce desired $Paco_2$ levels in spontaneous versus controlled ventilation
      e. Factors affecting CO_2 elimination in Mapleson systems: fresh gas flow, minute ventilation, CO_2 production, expiratory pattern (spontaneous vs. controlled ventilation)
      f. Table 4–4 lists the fresh gas flow requirements

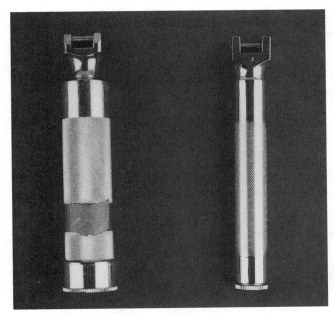

FIGURE 4–5. Laryngoscope handles. Pediatric handle *(right)* is thinner than adult handle.

TABLE 4–2. Air/O_2 Blending Ratios and Calculation for Selecting Desired O_2 Percent

Blending Ratios Air/O_2 (L/min)*	% O_2
10/0.5	24
9/1	28
8/1	30
5/1	35
3/1	40
1.7/1	50
1/1	60
0.6/1	70
0.3/1	80

CALCULATION FOR SELECTING DESIRED PERCENT O_2, MIXING AIR AND O_2
1. 100 – Desired % O_2 = Air (L/min)
2. Desired % O_2 – 20 = O_2 (L/min)
3. Air (L/min) divided by O_2 (L/min) = Ratio of air/O_2 on flowmeter

For example, to obtain 34% O_2
1. 100 – 34 = 66
2. 34 – 20 = 14
3. 66 ÷ 14 = 4.7 L/min
Run 4.7 L/min air and 1 L/min O_2 on flowmeters

*For example, to obtain 28% O_2, set the air flowmeter at 9 L and the O_2 flowmeter at 1 L.

      g. The use of capnography allows detection of rebreathing CO_2 to adjust fresh gas flows
    4. Bain circuit (coaxial) (see Fig. 4–6)
      a. Advantages: low dead space, valveless, conserves heat because of counterwarming of inspired gases

TABLE 4–3. Characteristics of an Ideal Pediatric Anesthesia Breathing System

Low dead space
Low resistance
Lightweight and compact
Low compression volume
Easily humidified
Easily scavenged
Suitable for both controlled and spontaneous ventilation
Economy of fresh gas flow

From Ehrenwerth, J., & Eisenkraft, J.B. (1993). *Anesthesia equipment: Principles and application.* St. Louis: Mosby.

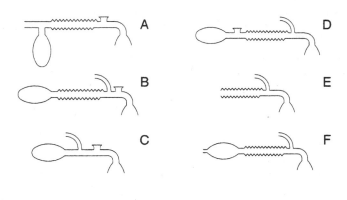

BAIN SYSTEM - BASED
ON MAPLESON "D"

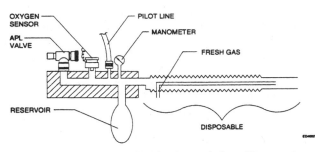

FIGURE 4-6. Mapleson's classification of breathing systems. (From Cicman, J., Himmelwright, C., Skibo, V., & Yoder, J. [1993]. *Operating principles of NARKOMED anesthesia systems.* Telford, PA: North American Dräger, 4–28.)

TABLE 4–4. Fresh Gas Flow (FGF) Requirements in the Mapleson System

SPONTANEOUS VENTILATION

Mask Anesthesia ≤30 kg: FGF = 4 × [1000 + (100 × kg)]
>30 kg: FGF = 4 × [2000 + (50 × kg)]

Intubated ≤30 kg: FGF = 3 × [1000 + (100 × kg)]
>30 kg: FGF = 3 × [2000 + (50 × kg)]

CONTROLLED VENTILATION

10–30 kg: 1000 ml + 100 ml/kg
>30 kg: 2000 ml + 50 ml/kg

Adapted from Ehrenwerth, J., & Eisenkraft, J.B. (1993). *Anesthesia equipment: Principles and application.* St. Louis: Mosby.

TABLE 4–5. Flow Calculations for the Bain Circuit

PATIENTS ≤50 kg
N_2O flow = 2.5 L/min
O_2 flow = 1 L/min
Tidal volume = 10 ml/kg
Respiratory rate = 12–14/min

PATIENTS >50 kg
N_2O flow = 50 ml/kg
O_2 flow = 20 ml/kg
Tidal volume = 10 ml/kg
Respiratory rate = 12–14/min

       b. Disadvantages: requires high fresh gas flows and special setup; rupture of fresh gas inner tube results in rebreathing

       c. Table 4–5 lists the flow calculations for the Bain circuit

       d. The **Pethick test for the Bain circuit,** which follows, is used to assess patency of the inspiratory portion of the circuit:

          (1) Close pop-off valve.

          (2) Obstruct patient end of breathing circuit.

          (3) Fill reservoir bag.

          (4) Flush O_2 valve.

          (5) If inner tube is intact, the reservoir bag will collapse.

    5. Pediatric circle system (see Fig. 4–7)

       a. Incorporates same components as adult circle

       b. Modified to decrease dead space and resistance to breathing

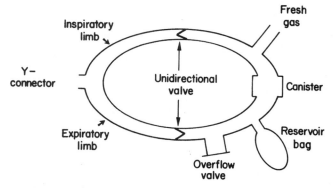

FIGURE 4–7. Components of the circle system and their usual arrangement. (From Gregory, G.A. [ed.]. [1994]. *Pediatric anesthesia* [3rd ed.]. New York: Churchill Livingstone.)

   c. Shorter, more narrow caliber delivery tubes
   d. Smaller reservoir bag (see Fig. 4–8)
      (1) 0.5 L: newborn
      (2) 1 L: ages 1 to 3 years
      (3) 2 L: ages 3 to 5 years
      (4) 3 L: age >5 years
   e. Advantages: conserves heat, humidity, and anesthetic agent; decreases environmental pollution; standard equipment on most anesthetic machines
   f. Disadvantages: possible resistance to breathing in unidirectional valves and absorber; high compliance in tubing with controlled ventilation
   g. Resistance to breathing: slightly higher than Mapleson or Bain systems; however, no significant difference in adequacy of ventilation
   h. Compliance of delivery tubing
      (1) Great importance during controlled mechanical ventilation

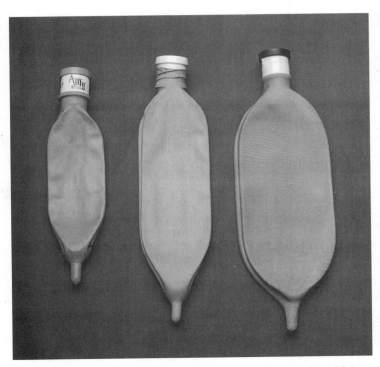

FIGURE 4–8. Reservoir bags: 1 L *(left)*, 2 L *(middle)*, and 3 L *(right)*.

  (2) Large portion of tidal volume may be lost to the highly compliant tubing

  (3) Discrepancy possible between the tidal volume desired and what is actually being delivered (called compression – amount of volume lost to compliance of the circuit)

  (4) Close monitoring of capnography, oximetry, peak airway pressure, exhaled tidal volume, and breath sounds

 i. Figure 4–7 shows the components of the circle system

C. Anesthesia ventilators

 1. Nearly any adult ventilator can be used in pediatrics; must adjust tidal volume, respiratory rate, inspiratory/expiratory (I/E) time, and fresh gas flows.

 2. Before placement of patient on ventilator, preset respiratory rate, tidal volume, I/E ratio; gradually increase tidal volume until desired peak airway pressure and tidal volume are reached.

 3. Whenever any readjustment is made, chest movement, breath sounds, peak airway pressures, and capnography or oximetry must be reevaluated.

D. Humidifiers

 1. Heating/humidifying gases: decreases atelectasis, prevents heat and energy loss, improves mucociliary clearance

 2. Types of anesthesia humidifiers

  a. Passive (heat moisture exchanger [HME])

   (1) Allows rebreathing of endogenous heat and moisture

   (2) Simplest method of conserving heat

   (3) Placed between endotracheal tube and circuit

   (4) Provides approximately 100% relative humidity after 80 minutes

   (5) New pediatric HMEs provide low dead space and minimal resistance

  b. Active (heated humidifier)

   (1) Provides 100% relative humidity almost immediately

   (2) Potential disadvantages: costly and cumbersome; disconnections can occur, leading to a significant compressible volume and causing tracheal burns and overhydration

IV. Miscellaneous

A. Suction apparatus

 1. Sizes

    a. 6.5 French: neonates
    b. 8 to 14 French: age >1 year
B. Intravenous equipment
  1. Catheters (recommended sizes)
    a. 24 gauge: neonates
    b. 22 gauge: ages 1 to 5 years
    c. 20 gauge: age >5 years
  2. Size of infusion bottle: should not exceed patient's estimated fluid deficit
  3. Microdrip infusion set with volume limiting device: neonate to age 10 years
  4. A standard adult infusion set (macrodrip): age >10 years
  5. Air bubbles should be purged from all infusion sets before use
  6. Syringe pumps can be used for accurate delivery of dextrose in the neonate or vasoactive drugs in the hemodynamically unstable patient
  7. Neonates to 1 year old: terminate line with a T-connector
  8. Use a three-way stopcock in cases where blood or colloid may be necessary (see Fig. 4–9)
C. Warming devices
  1. Overhead radiant heat warmer
    a. Employed during anesthesia preparation before and

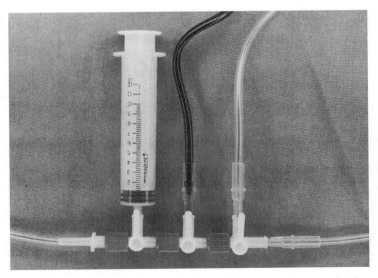

FIGURE 4–9. Three-way stopcock allows precise amounts of colloids or blood products to be administered.

including induction, during surgical preparation, and after drapes are removed at end of procedure
  b. Warmed to a maximal skin temperature of 37°C
  c. Must be at least 3 feet away from patient
2. Warming blanket
  a. Circulating H_2O mattress: only effective in children <10 kg
  b. Fluid temperature not to exceed 39°C
  c. One or two layers of sheets between patient and blanket; each additional sheet decreases heat transfer 20%
3. Forced air warmer: most effective units direct flow toward areas with major blood vessels (chest, axilla, abdomen, groin).
4. Wrapping of head decreases heat loss 70%.

ADDITIONAL READINGS

Brain, A., et al. (1996). *Laryngeal mask airway—instructional manual.* The Laryngeal Mask Company Limited.

Coté, C.J., Ryan, J.F., Todres, I.D., & Goudsouzian, N.G. (Eds.). (1993). *A practice of anesthesia for infants and children* (2nd ed., Chap. 28). Philadelphia: W.B. Saunders.

Ehrenwerth, J., & Eisenkraft, J.B. (1993). *Anesthesia equipment principles and applications* (Chap. 26). St. Louis: Mosby.

Gregory, G.A. (Ed.). (1994). *Pediatric anesthesia* (3rd ed., Chap. 8). New York: Churchill Livingstone.

Motoyama, E.K., & Davis, P.L. (1996). *Smith's anesthesia for infants and children* (6th ed., Chap. 8). St. Louis: Mosby.

5

Pediatric Monitoring Guidelines

Michael J. Cosgrove, MS, CRNA

I. Introduction

  A. Preventable anesthetic mishaps are frequently associated with human error. Appropriate vigilance and monitoring on the part of the anesthetist result in fewer clinical mishaps.

  B. Anesthesia has gradually evolved from a practice with few monitors into a specialty that uses sophisticated monitoring instruments.

  C. Monitoring devices cannot replace the assessment of clinical signs; however, they have proven to be quite sensitive at detecting adverse events.

  D. Children are more likely than adults to sustain a serious complication resulting from anesthesia. Such complications are often linked to either the cardiovascular or the respiratory system.

  E. Vigilance and monitoring practices are at times compromised in this high-risk population because of technical limitations or because of the cost of pediatric monitoring equipment.

  F. Clinicians must be capable of delivering anesthesia as safely as possible, and the advent of monitoring instruments has contributed to the decline in morbidity and mortality associated with anesthesia.

  G. The information derived from monitors should augment the information that the anesthetist collects clinically, not replace vigilance on the part of the anesthetist.

II. Basic Monitoring Standards

  A. In 1986 the Harvard Medical School published standards for monitoring during anesthesia (see box, pp. 62–64). These guidelines constitute the minimum monitoring accepted by the Department of Anesthesia at Harvard and are widely accepted as a standard of anesthesia practice.

  B. The American Association of Nurse Anesthetists (AANA) has developed "Standards of Nurse Anesthesia Practice," which include a monitoring standard (see box, p. 64).

  C. When practiced consistently, monitoring standards should

The Harvard Medical School Standards for Anesthesia Monitoring Practice

These standards apply for any administration of anesthesia involving department of anesthesia personnel and are specifically referable to preplanned anesthetics administered in designated anesthetizing locations (specific exclusion: administration of epidural analgesia for labor or pain management). In emergency circumstances in any location, immediate life support measures of whatever appropriate nature come first, with attention turning to the measures described in these standards as soon as possible and practical. These are minimal standards that may be exceeded at any time based on the judgment of the involved anesthesia personnel. These standards encourage high-quality patient care, but observing them cannot guarantee any specific patient outcome. These standards are subject to revision from time to time, as warranted by the evolution of technology and practice.

ANESTHESIOLOGIST'S OR NURSE ANESTHETIST'S PRESENCE IN OPERATION ROOM

For all anesthetics initiated by or involving a member of the department of anesthesia, an attending or resident anesthesiologist or nurse anesthetist shall be present in the room throughout the conduct of all general anesthetics, regional anesthetics, and monitored intravenous anesthetics. An exception is made when there is a direct known hazard, e.g., radiation, to the anesthesiologist or nurse anesthetist, in which some provision for monitoring the patient must be made.

BLOOD PRESSURE AND HEART RATE

Every patient receiving general anesthesia, regional anesthesia, or managed intravenous anesthesia shall have arterial blood pressure and heart rate measured at least every 5 minutes, where not clinically impractical.*

*Under extenuating circumstances, the attending anesthesiologist may waive this requirement after so stating (including the reasons) in a note in the patient's chart.

†Equivalence is to be defined by the chief of the individual hospital department after submission to a review by the department heads, Department of Anesthesia, Harvard Medical School, Boston.

From Eichhorn, J.H., Cooper, J.B., Cullen, D.J., et al. (1986). Standards for patient monitoring during anesthesia at Harvard Medical School. *Journal of the American Medical Association*, 256, 1017–1020. Copyright 1986, American Medical Association.

The Harvard Medical School Standards for Anesthesia Monitoring Practice *Continued*

ELECTROCARDIOGRAM
Every patient shall have the electrocardiogram continuously displayed from the induction or institution of anesthesia until preparing to leave the anesthetizing location, where not clinically impractical.*

CONTINUOUS MONITORING
During every administration of general anesthesia, the anesthetist shall employ methods of continuously monitoring the patient's ventilation and circulation. The methods shall include, for ventilation and circulation each, at least one of the following or the equivalent.†

For Ventilation. Palpation or observation of the reservoir breathing bag, auscultation of breath sounds, monitoring of respiratory gases such as end-tidal carbon dioxide, or monitoring of expiratory gas flow. Monitoring end-tidal carbon dioxide is an emerging standard and is strongly preferred.

For Circulation. Palpation of a pulse, auscultation of heart sounds, monitoring of a tracing of intra-arterial pressure, pulse plethysmography/oximetry, or ultrasound peripheral pulse monitoring.

It is recognized that brief interruptions of the continuous monitoring may be unavoidable.

BREATHING SYSTEM DISCONNECTION MONITORING
When ventilation is controlled by an automatic mechanical ventilator, there shall be in continuous use a device that is capable of detecting disconnection of any component of the breathing system. The device must give an audible signal when its alarm threshold is exceeded. (It is recognized that there are certain rare or unusual circumstances in which such a device may fail to detect a disconnection.)

OXYGEN ANALYZER
During every administration of general anesthesia using an anesthesia machine, the concentration of oxygen in the patient breathing system will be measured by a functioning oxygen analyzer with a low concentration limit alarm in use. This device must conform to the American National Standards Institute No. Z.79.10 standard.*

Box continued on following page

The Harvard Medical School Standards for Anesthesia Monitoring Practice *Continued*

ABILITY TO MEASURE TEMPERATURE

During every administration of general anesthesia, there shall be readily available a means to measure the patient's temperature.

Rationale. A means of temperature measurement must be available as a potential aid in the diagnosis and treatment of suspected or actual intraoperative hypothermia and malignant hyperthermia. The measurement/monitoring of temperature during every general anesthetic is not specifically mandated because of the potential risks of such monitoring and because of the likelihood of other physical signs giving earlier indication of the development of malignant hyperthermia.

AANA Standard V

AANA Standard V states "Monitor the patient's physiologic condition as appropriate for the type of anesthesia and specific patient needs."

A. Monitor ventilation continuously. Verify intubation of the trachea by auscultation, chest excursion, and confirmation of carbon dioxide in the expired gas. Continuously monitor end-tidal carbon dioxide during controlled or assisted ventilation. Use spirometry and ventilation pressure monitors.

B. Monitor oxygenation continuously by clinical observation, pulse oximetry, and if indicated, arterial blood gas analysis.

C. Monitor cardiovascular status continuously via electrocardiogram and heart sounds. Record blood pressure and heart rate at least every 5 minutes.

D. Monitor body temperature continuously on all pediatric patients receiving general anesthesia and when indicated, on all other patients.

E. Monitor neuromuscular function and status when neuromuscular blocking agents are administered.

F. Monitor and assess patient positioning and protective measures at frequent intervals. (Adopted November 6, 1997 and became effective April 6, 1998.)

From American Association of Nurse Anesthetists. (1996). *Scope and standards for nurse anesthesia practice.* Park Ridge, IL: AANA. Used with permission.

initiate the similar use of equipment and thinking patterns by anesthesia providers in such a way that decreases the incidence of anesthesia-related mishaps.

D. These monitoring guidelines emphasize the need to monitor ventilation, oxygenation, cardiovascular status, body temperature, and neuromuscular function and status on a consistent basis.

E. Vigilance is paramount, and nothing should distract the anesthetist from clinical observation of the patient, including observation, auscultation, and palpation.

III. Monitoring Guidelines

A. Ventilation

1. Auscultation: A properly positioned stethoscope (precordial, esophageal) gives valuable insight into a child's cardiac and respiratory status.

2. Inspection of ventilation: Valuable clinical information can be gained from observing the child's ventilation, including respiratory rate, chest motion, abdominal motion, rhythmicity of ventilation cycle, and inspiratory circuit airway pressure.

3. Measurement of exhaled gas flow and analysis of respiratory gases.

   a. Capnometry: measurement of carbon dioxide (CO_2) at the patient's airway during a ventilatory cycle

   b. Capnography: graphic representation of the CO_2 waveform

   c. Spirometry: measurement of the quantity of air taken into and exhaled from the lungs; useful for detecting airway disconnections and elevated inspiratory airway pressures

B. Monitoring oxygenation

1. Observation of skin and blood color is unreliable for assessment of oxygenation because cyanosis is a late-occurring sign that requires near-normal hemoglobin levels.

2. Oxygen analyzer: When located within the inspiratory limb of a gas delivery system this instrument identifies the oxygen level being administered.

3. Pulse oximetry: Assesses the ratio of absorbency of oxyhemoglobin versus deoxyhemoglobin in a vascular bed. During pediatric anesthesia pulse oximetry monitoring is invaluable and can decrease the incidence and duration of desaturation episodes.

C. Monitoring circulation
  1. Clinical monitoring
     a. Auscultation: Heart sounds give a qualitative assessment of cardiac function.
     b. Palpation: Pulse gives a qualitative assessment of circulation.
  2. Monitoring technology
     a. Electrocardiography (ECG): Surface ECG monitors the heart's electrical activity and rhythm and aids in assessing patient's heart rate and diagnosing dysrhythmias.
     b. Noninvasive blood pressure measurement: Appropriate-fitting blood pressure cuff is necessary for correct recording. Use the largest cuff that can be placed on the upper arm without encroaching on the child's axilla or antecubital fossa.
     c. Pulse oximetry: The oximeter will detect complete loss of peripheral pulse but not major pulse decreases.
D. Monitoring temperature.
  1. Available to aid in the identification and treatment of hypothermia and malignant hyperthermia
  2. Iatrogenic hypothermia: body heat loss via radiation, conduction, convection, and evaporation
  3. Intraoperative hyperthermia
     a. Associated with aggressive heating with a warming blanket, fluid warmer, airway humidifier, and room temperature
     b. Malignant hyperthermia (MH) is a genetic muscle disorder that manifests when the patient is administered particular anesthetic drugs

IV. Additional Monitoring Guidelines

A. The proliferation of new technologies in the area of monitoring provides the anesthetist with additional information measured by machines
B. The variables measured by such equipment must build on the information gathered from the direct observation of a patient
C. Invasive monitors of the respiratory system
  1. Intravascular oxygen electrode: small-gauge catheters inserted through the umbilical artery that have an O_2 electrode at the tip. Current-generation intravascular electrodes provide a useful guide to oxygen therapy.
  2. Intravascular saturation monitor: fiberoptic catheter that measures the hemoglobin saturation within the walls of major arteries or veins. Use of a pulmonary artery sat-

uration catheter provides useful information in certain patients.

D. Invasive monitors of the cardiovascular system
  1. Direct measurement systemic arterial monitoring
     a. A 22- or 24-gauge catheter may be used for peripheral artery cannulation in infants and young children.
     b. In older children a 20-gauge catheter can be inserted.
  2. Monitoring of central venous pressure (CVP)
     a. Every insertion site that is used in adults may be used in children.
     b. The small vascular lumen can make cannulation difficult.
     c. Blood loss occurring during insertion must be monitored carefully.
     d. The normal values for CVP in children are similar to adult measurements (2–6 mm Hg).
     e. Catheter sizes range from 2.5 to 10 French, and insertion lengths vary with age.
  3. Monitoring of pulmonary artery pressure
     a. May be placed in any site used for CVP insertion.
     b. In infants and small children (<15 kg) the femoral veins are preferable because of the size of the introducer sheath.
     c. The value and validity of the data are controversial and vary according to age, disease state, and intracardiac communications.
  4. Intraoperative transesophageal echocardiography
     a. Provides anatomic and functional information, including flow within the heart in infants as small as 3 kg
E. Monitoring urine output
  1. Observing the composition and production of urine reflects the adequacy of cardiovascular performance and renal function.
  2. Urine output is a valuable measurement to monitor the volume status in children.
  3. Indicated in procedures where large fluid shifts are anticipated or when the potential for blood loss is expected.
  4. Neonates produce 0.5 to 5 ml/h; therefore urine output alone is not a sensitive indicator of volume status.
  5. Infants and children produce urine at approximately 0.5 to 1 ml/kg/h when renal perfusion is not impaired.
F. Neurophysiologic monitoring
  1. Nervous system monitors provide information necessary for the assessment of the central nervous system

2. Intraoperative neurophysiologic monitoring can be useful in the early detection of altered neurologic function, in quantitating the depth of anesthesia, and in evaluating the degree of neuromuscular blockade
3. Electroencephalogram (EEG)
   a. Measures the cortical function and activity levels
   b. Recordings can reflect changes in cortical functioning related to hypoxia or to pharmacologic manipulation
4. Somatosensory evoked potentials (SSEPs)
   a. Measure the activity of the large ascending nerve fibers of peripheral nerves.
   b. Monitoring during spine surgery allows cord injury to be recognized.
   c. Recordings can reflect changes in cortical functioning related to hypoxia or to pharmacologic manipulation.
5. Visual evoked potentials (VEPs)
   a. Measure the functional integrity of the visual system in the vicinity of the optic nerves
6. Brainstem auditory evoked potentials (BAEPs)
   a. Useful in measuring the functional integrity of the auditory system along the eighth cranial nerve
7. Electromyogram (EMG)
   a. Measures the integrity of descending activity in the spinal cord by producing electrical activity in muscle fibers below the skin
   b. Neuromuscular blocking agents should be avoided for this monitoring technique
8. Near-infrared spectroscopy (NIRS)
   a. Noninvasive technique useful in monitoring cerebral and cardiac oxidative metabolism
9. Bispectral analysis (BIS)
   a. A significant predictor of anesthetic depth and a predictor of patient response to surgical stimulation
10. Neuromuscular blockade function
    a. The recovery of neuromuscular function from the effects of neuromuscular blocking agents may be assessed in children by evaluating the electrical stimulation of a motor nerve.

ADDITIONAL READINGS

American Association of Nurse Anesthetists (1996). *AANA professional practice manual: standards for nurse anesthesia practice.* Park Ridge, IL: AANA.
Eichhorn, J.H., Cooper, J.B., Cullen, D.J., et al. (1986). Standards for patient

monitoring during anesthesia at Harvard Medical School. *Journal of the American Medical Association, 256,* 1017–1020.

Kirby, R.R., & Gravenstein, N. (1994). *Clinical anesthesia practice.* Philadelphia: W.B. Saunders.

Lake, C.L. (1990). *Clinical monitoring.* Philadelphia: W.B. Saunders.

Longnecker, D.E., Tinker, J.H., & Morgan, G.E. (1998). *Principles and practice in anesthesiology* (vol. 1). St. Louis: Mosby.

Motoyama, E.K., & Davis, P.J. (1996). *Smith's anesthesia for infants and children* (6th ed.). St. Louis: Mosby.

6

Pediatric Considerations in Airway Management

Joseph P. Cravero, MD, and C.J. Biddle, PhD, CRNA

I. Introduction

A. No responsibility facing the anesthesia provider is more formidable than maintaining a patent airway. Experienced practitioners recognize that any change in a patient's state of alertness—ranging from unconsciousness to semiconsciousness—can lead to asphyxia from obstruction of the upper airway. Because of anatomic, physiologic, and technical issues, airway management in the pediatric patient can prove particularly challenging. This chapter focuses on pediatric airway–related management issues.

B. Normally the awake patient's airway is easily maintained no matter what position the head or neck is in and irrespective of whether one is standing, sitting, supine, prone, or even hanging upside down. Airway patency under such a wide variety of postural stressors is an active mechanism that principally involves muscles attached to the hyoid bone and thyroid cartilages. In addition, there is a complex and coordinated set of reflex relationships among these muscles, the upper airway receptors, and even the lungs.

C. The larynx has a wide variety of receptors that react to stretch, gas flow, and muscle movement. Lung stretch receptor reflexes, central and carotid body chemoreceptor reflexes, and central nervous system (CNS) arousal mechanisms all influence airway integrity by influencing airway muscle activity and therefore airway resistance.

D. The hyoid bone is horseshoe shaped and can be moved in virtually any direction by the action of the extrinsic pharyngeal muscles (movement in a caudal direction is somewhat restricted). The epiglottis hangs from the posterior aspect of the hyoid bone much like a lid on a child's lunch box. The thyroepiglottic ligament acts as a hinge with the hyoepiglottic ligament acting as a lever for the lid.

II. The Normal Pediatric Airway

  A. Differences between adult and pediatric airway anatomy and physiology

    1. The infant larynx is located more cephalad than the adult (C3–4 interspace). The adult position at C5 is achieved by 6 years of age.

    2. The epiglottis is U-shaped, short, stiff, and more closely attached to the thyroid cartilage.

    3. The infant tongue is significantly larger relative to the mouth and depresses the epiglottis because of the position of the hyoid bone.

    4. The narrowest part of the infant airway is the cricoid ring—not at the glottis itself.

    5. The infant head (especially the occiput) is larger relative to the shoulders and body.

    6. The distance between the mandible and the thyroid cartilage and hyoid cartilage is about half that of the adult.

  B. Importance of anatomic differences in patient management

    1. The size of the tongue and the position of the epiglottis and hyoid can make mask ventilation more difficult than in the normal adult. Often a relatively neutral head position without extreme chin lift is more helpful than the exaggerated head tilt and jaw thrust required by adult patients. Appropriate pediatric oral airways and nasal airways are crucial for maintaining patency and must be present before giving sedation or beginning the intubation sequence.

    2. The larger head and occiput of the child lead to an "automatic sniffing position" when the neck is slightly extended. Proper alignment of the pharynx, epiglottis, and larynx is achieved without placing pillows or support under the head. For neonates a support under the shoulders may enhance the visualization of the cords.

    3. The anatomy of the epiglottis and position of the larynx make the use of a straight laryngoscope blade placed in the vallecula an ideal strategy.

    4. There is a relative increase in the size of soft tissue structures (i.e., tongue) in the oral pharynx when compared to the size of the mouth. In addition, there is a smaller potential space (submental distance) for displacement of these structures when direct laryngoscopy is attempted. The combination of these factors makes the pediatric airway appear anterior even in the "normal" patient. Patients who have difficulty opening their mouth

or who have an unusual facies will present a challenge to viewing the glottis.

5. The pediatric airway is narrowest (and round in shape) below the cords at the level of the cricoid cartilage.
   a. This anatomy allows uncuffed tubes to be used in patients <8 years old.
   b. The size of the tube may be selected by matching the size of the fifth digit or using the following formula: $(age + 16)/4$.
   c. For small neonates and infants, the depth of insertion can be closely estimated by using the 1,2,3,4/7,8,9,10 rule. That is, a 1 kg neonate requires insertion to 7 cm for midtracheal positioning, a 2 kg neonate to 8 cm, and so on.
   d. Position will always need to be confirmed by breath sounds.
6. After confirming placement of the endotracheal (ET) tube in young children one should listen over the mouth for the presence of an air leak and at what pressure this occurs.
   a. Generally, an air leak at a pressure *less* than 8 cm of water will not allow effective ventilation with positive pressure; a larger tube should be placed.
   b. An air leak that only occurs at *more* than 40 cm of water has been associated with postextubation airway edema and in most cases should be changed to a smaller tube.
7. Laryngeal mask airways (LMAs) are widely used in routine airway management for pediatric anesthesia. (See Table 4–1 for a list of sizes.)
   a. Although this area is evolving, the LMA is gaining wide acceptance for shorter procedures, especially outpatient procedures involving the inguinal region and legs.
   b. The device comes in various sizes for children and is easily placed after some training.
   c. Generally the device is placed after general anesthesia and intravenous (IV) access have been accomplished.
   d. The child is allowed to breathe spontaneously for the duration of the procedure, and the device is removed on awakening just as an ET tube would be.

III. Normal Physiologic Differences Between Children and Adults

A. Infants have more than twice the oxygen consumption of adults.
B. Functional residual capacity is smaller than adults.

C. Gastric emptying time is generally shorter in children than in adults.

D. Hypoxia in infants quickly results in bradycardia rather than tachycardia seen in adults.

E. Bradycardia is accompanied by poor cardiac output and acidosis.

F. Depending on the initial condition of the child, the time from apnea to cardiovascular collapse is generally much shorter in children than in adults.

G. Clinical importance of the physiology of children in airway management.

    1. The combination of greater oxygen consumption and a smaller functional residual capacity in infants and children results in a much shorter interval from the loss of ventilation to oxygen desaturation.

        a. Preparation for airway management must be complete.

        b. Before inducing anesthesia, the provider must be sure to have appropriately sized working laryngoscopes, oral airways, LMAs, and ET tubes immediately available.

        c. Several airways of each type in multiple sizes should be prepared to allow quick adjustment of fit should this be required.

    2. A shorter gastric emptying time in children allows shorter NPO guideline times.

        a. Although these guidelines are not universal, most practitioners allow solid foods up to 8 hours before induction.

        b. Milk and clear liquids are allowed up to 4 hours and 2 hours, respectively, before anesthesia.

    3. Bradycardia can occur quickly and is associated with a marked decline in cardiac output; airway patency must be treated as the highest priority. This is one of the reasons many practitioners include atropine, 0.01 mg/kg, with other induction medications before intubating infants.

IV. Normal Psychologic Differences Between Children and Adults

A. The age and developmental status of a child will influence his or her ability to understand all the aspects of the anesthesia and surgical experience.

    1. In general, children past the age of 8 months of age are anxious about strangers, especially those in hospital attire. They are also profoundly needle phobic.

    2. Because of the psychologic (and physical) trauma of

placing IV catheters in awake pediatric patients, induction of anesthesia in normal pediatric patients is most often accomplished with nonpungent inhaled potent agents (sevoflurane or halothane) plus nitrous oxide.

3. Spontaneous ventilation is maintained to avoid anesthetic overdose while IV access is obtained.

4. Airway management with an ET tube or laryngeal mask airway can then safely be accomplished.

5. Recent studies have documented that preinduction medication with oral midazolam, 0.50 to 0.75 mg/kg, can decrease the psychologic trauma associated with inhaled induction in a wide variety of pediatric patients.

6. Allowing parents to accompany pediatric patients to the operating room for the induction process has also been associated with less stressful mask inductions.

7. Obviously each patient and parent should be evaluated with respect to the appropriateness of each of these techniques.

V. Pathologic Issues in Pediatric Airway Management

A. With the above considerations in mind, it is not surprising to find that even though the incidence of truly difficult airways in infants and children is relatively low, without proper technique and planning even the normal child may have an airway problem. A difficult pediatric airway can be the result of a disease process, trauma, or congenital anomaly that should be evident from even a brief history and physical examination.

1. Look for indications of airway pathologic conditions (see Table 6–1).

2. Pathologic conditions that result in any of the following (small mouth, large tongue, inability to extend the neck, mobile obstructions within the trachea, infectious distortions of the airway) should raise major concern.

3. Time spent in carefully evaluating the airway, and meticulously developing an airway management approach will go far in ensuring success, minimizing risk, and avoiding catastrophe.

B. Sleep apnea and sudden infant death syndrome (SIDS) research: relevance to anesthesia.

1. Incorrectly, SIDS was first attributed to accidental suffocation by mothers who slept with their newborns. As far back as 1940 the focus of explanation for SIDS had moved toward phenomena associated with bed clothing and sleep position of the infant.

TABLE 6–1. Pediatric Airway Pathologic Conditions

NASOPHARYNX
Choanal atresia
Foreign body
Trauma
Adenoidal hypertrophy
Tumors

TONGUE
Hemangiomas
Angioedema
Down's syndrome
Lacerations
Beckwith-Wiedemann syndrome
Mucopolysaccharidosis
Cystic hygroma

MANDIBLE AND MAXILLA
Pierre Robin syndrome
Treacher Collins syndrome
Goldenhar's syndrome
Fractures
Neck burns
Juvenile rheumatoid arthritis with limited jaw movement

PHARYNX AND LARYNX
Laryngeal web
Laryngeal stenosis
Laryngomalacia
Foreign body
Postintubation croup
Epiglottitis
Peritonsillar abscess
Retropharyngeal abscess
Laryngeal papillomatosis
Arnold-Chiari malformation

2. Recently several large studies have shown an increased incidence of SIDS in infants who sleep in the prone position. Thoughtful and open-minded analysis of the data generated in these studies may prove to be very relevant to understanding airway compromise and intervention in the operating room.

3. For example, to fully understand what is going on in persons with sleep-disordered breathing, one must examine not only the mechanism by which hypoxemia and hypercarbia originate (e.g., apnea, airway obstruction, rebreathing of exhaled gas) but also the nature of (or

absence of) the resuscitative response (e.g., waking up, gasping, recovering the airway).

4. Numerous papers in the literature demonstrate a high incidence of arterial hemoglobin desaturation in children recovering from anesthesia and surgery. When preexisting factors are controlled for, it becomes clear that the use of opioids and airway obstruction are the primary mechanisms involved.

5. Everyday experience shows that gravity has a relatively unimportant influence on the tongue in airway obstruction—this is seen, for example, by the frequent need to maintain head extension or jaw thrust even in patients lying on their side who are going under or recovering from general anesthesia.

6. Similarly, in patients who are lying supine and who have an oral pharyngeal airway in place, it is not uncommon to have to apply the same extension and thrust maneuvers even though the artificial airway might be expected to provide a good airway.

7. In the early 1960s investigators demonstrated that an airway was maintained in conscious babies, despite changes in posture or deliberate movement of pharyngeal structures, even when the tongue was forcefully pushed backward. They concluded that it was the relative position of the mandible and hyoid bone that was critically important and that these were maintained because of traction on the hyoid bone by the submandibular muscles.

C. Clinical management: emphasis on the difficult pediatric airway.

1. Obviously, the identification of a patient whose airway may prove difficult and who requires anesthesia necessitates the presence of all available skilled personnel and equipment. The formulation of a plan, making sure that all those who are present understand it, may avoid needless wasting of time and potentially fatal mistakes.

2. Remember the dictum, "a breathing patient is a living patient." Because ventilation with a bag and mask may be difficult, awake intubations are absolutely appropriate for pediatric patients with suspected difficult airways (especially neonates and young infants).

   a. However, obtaining any level of cooperation with an awake pediatric patient under these circumstances can be difficult.

   b. More often, careful induction of anesthesia with a potent inhalational agent, keeping the patient breathing

spontaneously and intubating or placing an LMA after an appropriate level of anesthesia has been reached, is the preferred approach.
3. Awake intubations may be aided by the following:
  a. Atropine (given either orally or intravenously) results in drying of secretions for easier visualization of the glottis and better absorption of local anesthetics
  b. Local anesthesia to the airway. This may include
    (1) Lidocaine jelly sucked off a finger or tongue depressor
    (2) 4% Lidocaine solution nebulized and inhaled or sprayed on the airway (for larger children)
    (3) 2% Lidocaine jelly–covered nasal airways with 4% lidocaine solution dripped through the lumen (Remember that the maximum dose of lidocaine is 5 mg/kg and this will limit the total volume that can be used for these purposes.)
  c. Sedation
    (1) Slowly titrated IV sedation with an agent associated with anxiolysis and amnesia (midazolam) may aid intubation in the child who requires awake intubation.
    (2) A small dose of opiate will decrease the stress associated with airway manipulation.
    (3) Ketamine should be used with extreme caution. Manipulation of the airway with ketamine sedation can easily lead to laryngospasm.
    (4) As a general rule, avoid IV induction of general anesthesia in the pediatric patient suspected of having a difficult airway.
  d. Swaddling the child in a blanket maximizes control and minimizes extraneous movement
4. If induction of anesthesia with muscle relaxation is deemed absolutely necessary, all airway equipment and personnel to aid in a surgical airway must be present before administering these drugs. Cricoid pressure (Sellick maneuver) should be considered and will aid in preventing aspiration of stomach contents and facilitating visualization of the larynx.
5. When IV agents are used in pediatric difficult airway situations, only short-acting or easily reversible agents should be used. In this way, if ventilation is difficult and intubation is impossible at least the patient can breathe spontaneously again in a relatively short time.
D. Special technique for intubation: The following is a brief

description of special techniques for emergency intubation of pediatric patients with suspected difficult airway problems. Many other techniques exist, and more detail on each of these techniques is available in the additional readings.

1. "Awake look"
   a. This is a common anesthesia technique for patients who may have a challenging airway.
   b. One may lightly sedate a child, use local anesthesia on the oral pharynx, and then place a laryngoscope to attempt to visualize the glottis (not advised for suspected epiglottitis).
   c. If the glottis is easily visualized, the child may receive muscle relaxation and sedation to aid in placing the ET tube.
   d. If the visualization of the glottis is difficult, an alternative method of intubation will be needed.
2. Blind nasotracheal intubation
   a. For spontaneously breathing patients with very large tongues or other oral obstructing lesions, this technique is ideal.
   b. Success is greatest when local anesthesia is applied via nasal airways as mentioned above. If the patient is not obtunded, sedation may be required.
   c. A standard ET tube (or Endotrol trigger type of tube) may be prepared either with a stylet in place or may be "preformed" and placed on ice for several minutes to keep its shape better.
   d. Using the left nostril is preferred because the bevel of the endotracheal tube is less likely to hang up in the vallecula or vocal cords.
   e. The procedure is then similar to that used with adult patients: listening for maximum breath sounds, using a CO_2 detector or whistle device to detect when the tube is at the glottic opening.
   f. Because of the shape of the pediatric airway this technique is a little more difficult with children than adults even when cooperation is excellent.
   g. Contraindications to nasotracheal intubation include facial fractures, coagulopathy, nasal polyps, and obstructing lymphoid tissue.
3. Light wand or lighted stylet
   a. A stylet with a bright light at the tip can be useful for "blind" intubations in which direct visualization of the glottis is impossible. Recently light wands have been

developed that have a diameter of just 2.5 mm, making them useful for pediatric patients.

b. The light wand is placed in the ET tube and curved to the expected shape of the airway.

c. The ET tube can then be placed either through the mouth or nose. A bright pink glow is observed just below the thyroid cartilage when the tip of the tube is positioned at the glottic opening and threaded into the trachea.

d. Although it is safest to use the light wand on a breathing patient it is helpful in the apneic patient as well, as long as one moves quickly and the patient has been given sufficient oxygen before any attempt.

e. Practice is required before consistent success is attained, but this instrument has been shown to be useful in cases where rapid intubation of a difficult airway is required.

4. Flexible fiberoptic bronchoscope (FFB)

a. The FFB has revolutionized the management of the difficult airway in both children and adults. Good training and familiarization with this particular equipment are crucial to success.

b. In general the FFB is easiest to use on spontaneously breathing patients who have received topical anesthesia to the airway.

c. It can be useful in the obtunded or relaxed patient, but special airways and positioning are required to displace the tongue and raise the epiglottis off the posterior pharynx.

d. Pediatric-size scopes are now readily available and may be placed orally or nasally.

e. Although many strategies exist, for the emergency patient the ET tube is initially loaded on the FFB and held near the proximal end of the scope. The FFB is then threaded around or through an oral airway and into the trachea. The ET tube can then be passed over the scope and into position.

5. The Bullard laryngoscope

a. The Bullard laryngoscope is another type of fiberoptic laryngoscope that uses a radically curved blade attached to a fixed fiberoptic viewing scope to allow visualization of the glottis.

b. The ET tube is loaded onto an attached stylet and guided through the cords under visualization through

the scope. This scope is preferred by some practitioners in trauma cases because it is not obscured as easily by blood.
- c. Hints for use in the pediatric patient
  - (1) Preintubation atropine
  - (2) Liberal use of topical lidocaine
  - (3) Sedation
  - (4) Oxygen flow through the accessory port during intubation: increases Fio_2 and blows secretions off the optics
  - (5) Lowering the bed and standing on stools so that the only bend in the scope is in the posterior pharynx
  - (6) Increased ease of threading flexible reinforced ET tubes in the trachea rather than conventional tubes
6. The laryngeal mask airway (LMA)
   - a. The LMA consists of a masklike device with an inflatable cuff that fits directly over the perimeter of the larynx connected to a wide-bore tube that is attached to the anesthesia circuit.
   - b. This device represents a watershed in airway management in anesthesia and is finding broad application in the area of emergency airway management.
   - c. The LMA comes in several sizes: 1 (neonates, infants), 2 (toddlers, young children), 3 (older children, small adults). (Half sizes are available.)
   - d. The American Society of Anesthesiologists' difficult airway algorithm recommends the use of the LMA for those obtunded, apneic patients who are difficult or impossible to ventilate and difficult to intubate. It therefore represents an alternative to the immediate use of a surgical airway in many cases.
   - e. Placement of the airway is not difficult but requires some training. Studies and experience indicate that ascending the learning curve for successful placement is quite rapid.
   - f. To place the device, the inflatable cuff is deflated and the device is lubricated. It is then inserted into the posterior area of the pharynx and over the larynx. The cuff is inflated and ventilation confirmed. Once ventilation has been established, the trachea may be intubated blindly through the LMA, or an FFB may be placed through the LMA with the ET tube placed over it. An intubating LMA has recently been introduced for adults. At this time there is no such instrument for children.

g. Studies concerning the use of the LMA for emergency airway management in children are just now appearing, but there is no doubt its use will expand greatly in the near future.

7. Needle-catheter cricothyroidotomy
   a. When all the above techniques fail or are not available, the placement of a 14-gauge IV catheter through the cricothyroid membrane may be life saving. After placement, the needle is removed and the catheter can be attached to a high-pressure jet ventilator (part of most difficult airway carts).
   b. O_2 from the ventilator, 20 bursts/min, will provide oxygenation and ventilation for 30 to 40 minutes before CO_2 accumulation becomes excessive.
   c. Alternatively the catheter may be attached to a 3 ml syringe with the plunger removed. This in turn is attached to the adapter for a 7.0 ET tube and ventilated with any type of ventilation bag.
   d. Unfortunately the air flows generated by this arrangement allow only a brief period before hypoxia and hypercarbia set in.
   e. This technique is only a stopgap measure and must be accompanied by immediate moves toward definitive airway management.

VI. Summary and Recommendations

A. The many studies employing pulse oximetry in the intraoperative and postoperative period now show that hypoxemia can occur with astonishing suddenness even in otherwise healthy patients. Airway dysfunction occurs so frequently in patients receiving even small doses of anesthetic drugs that it should be presumed to be present rather than discounted. The following general recommendations should be kept in mind:

1. Recognize that airway obstruction is likely to occur in anyone given an anesthetic drug and that pediatric patients are especially susceptible to airway obstruction.
2. If difficulty with the airway is anticipated, be prepared for alternative methods of securing the airway; consider awake, sedated intubation approaches, and ensure that help is immediately available.
3. Maintain a high index of suspicion. That is, assume that all patients have some degree of airway dysfunction even if they appear to be breathing satisfactorily. Otherwise, even subtle dysfunction may lead to disaster should the airway

be "challenged," such as when the patient vomits, needs to cough out accumulating secretions, falls back to sleep, or becomes anxious because of fear or pain.

4. Pediatric patients who have received muscle relaxants should remain intubated until adequate minute ventilation, sufficient muscle strength, and reflex control have returned. The ability to sustain a head lift for at least 5 seconds and the ability to stick out the tongue for a similar period of time are good clinical tests that can be readily performed at the bedside. Alternatively, the ability to flex the legs at the hip joints has been associated with adequate muscle strength for airway maintenance in babies.

B. Patients with a recognized difficult airway

1. If a difficult airway is suspected based on clinical examination or history, alert all available personnel who may be of help. Have all equipment and drugs immediately available.

2. With the child breathing spontaneously, administer atropine and topical anesthesia and proceed with an awake look to evaluate the airway. If the glottis is not visible, consider an alternative method, such as blind nasotracheal intubation, light wand intubation, or fiberoptic intubation.

3. Proceed with induction of anesthesia using careful inhalation of a nonpungent, potent agent and maintaining spontaneous respirations.

4. If the child must have IV sedation and relaxation, be fully prepared to take over the airway. Maintain the Sellick maneuver, and proceed with standard laryngoscopy, light wand, or fiberoptic intubation as your expertise allows. Consider use of the LMA if intubation is impossible and the patient is difficult to ventilate with a face mask. Remember that intubation through this device is possible.

ADDITIONAL READINGS

Coté, C.J., & Todres, I.D. (1993). The pediatric airway. In Ryan J.F., Coté, C.J., Todres, I.D., & Goudsouzian, N.G. (Eds.). *A practice of anesthesia for infants and children* (2nd ed). Philadelphia: W.B. Saunders.

Patil, V., Stehling, L., & Zauder, H. (1983). *Fiberoptic endoscopy in anesthesia.* Chicago: Year Book Medical Publishers.

Riazi, J. (1996). The difficult pediatric airway. In Benumof, J. (Ed.). *Airway management principles and practice.* Chicago: Mosby–Year Book.

7

Pediatric Fluid and Blood Therapy

John Aker, MS, CRNA, Cormac T. O'Sullivan, MSN, CRNA, and
James P. Embrey, PhD, CRNA

I. Introduction

A. A discussion of the administration of intravenous (IV) fluids in pediatric patients is warranted because caloric expenditure is twice as great as in adult patients, and the physiologic tolerance for states of dehydration is less well tolerated in the infant than in the adult patient.

B. A minimal amount of fluids and electrolytes is generally required to ensure normal growth and development. In addition, fluid homeostasis is altered during the preoperative period from prolonged fasting and intraoperatively via the influences of anesthesia and surgical trauma.

C. Preoperative oral fluid abstinence in combination with inhalation and IV anesthetic agents alters preload and afterload, resulting in peripheral vasodilation and some degree of myocardial depression. These changes in autonomic tone decrease systemic blood pressure and ultimately end-organ blood flow. These agents also modify the neuroendocrine control of fluid and electrolyte balance.

D. Surgical trauma impacts fluid balance, the degree to which depends on the invasiveness and duration of the surgical procedure. Intracavitary procedures (e.g., intraabdominal or intrathoracic procedures) are associated with greater blood loss, third-space fluid losses, and evaporative fluid losses.

E. Consequently, the pediatric patient requires attentive perioperative management of fluids and electrolytes to maintain physiologic balance and attenuate the cardiovascular changes induced by anesthetic agents.

F. Purposes of perioperative IV therapy.

1. To reestablish a hydrated state following the NPO period

2. To replace fluid and electrolyte losses incurred with operative blood loss, evaporative fluid losses, and third-space fluid losses that follow surgical trauma

3. Following are the **perioperative factors that modify fluid and electrolyte balance:**

a. Oral fluid abstinence results in preoperative dehydration.
b. Cold surgical theater increases basal caloric and water requirements.
c. Increases of core temperature of 1°C increase caloric expenditure 12% to 14%.
d. Insensible fluid losses occur via the inhalation of cold, dry, nonhumidified anesthetic gases.
e. Inhalation agents (sevoflurane, desflurane, isoflurane, enflurane) produce peripheral vasodilation and myocardial depression (halothane), reducing glomerular filtration and renal blood flow.
f. Decreased renal blood flow causes release of renin.
g. Renin stimulates release of aldosterone, increasing renal retention of sodium and water.
h. Iatrogenic hyperventilation will produce hypokalemia.
i. Morphine and halothane increase antidiuretic hormone (ADH) release from the posterior pituitary, increasing renal retention of sodium and water.
j. The stress of anesthesia and surgery results in induced hyperglycemia.
k. Insulin utilization is decreased.

II. Physiology of Pediatric Fluid Distribution

A. Water is a medium that freely diffuses across cell membranes and is essential for metabolic reactions and the transport of cellular nutrients and substrates.
B. The individual child's daily water requirement is that amount that would result in no changes in body weight.
C. Satisfactory hydration can be estimated by measuring the urine volume, which should be >1 ml/kg/h.
D. Since water flows from an area of high solute concentration to low solute concentration, body fluid compartments are consequently regulated by the osmotic balance determined by the number of particles (the presence of sodium) in each fluid compartment.
E. Disorders that may alter the amount of hourly urine production:
   1. Renal disease
   2. Cardiac disease
   3. Inappropriate antidiuretic hormone secretion
   4. Diabetes mellitus
   5. Diuretic agents
F. Total body water (TBW), expressed in liters, is deter-

mined as a percentage of total body weight (1 L of water weighs 1 kg).

G. TBW steadily decreases with increasing age and varies according to gender and body habitus.

H. TBW is distributed into two primary fluid compartments: the intracellular (ICF) compartment and the extracellular (ECF) compartment.

I. Aging is accompanied by a decrease of the relative fluid compartment volumes of TBW and ECF during the first year of life, followed by additional decreases in ECF later in childhood. These developmental changes in TBW composition are accompanied by changes in sodium content.

   1. Following birth, naturesis and diuresis reduce the extracellular compartment volume with accompanying decreases in sodium and chloride content.

   2. The kidney is stimulated to conserve sodium and water following the reduction of ECF volume.

J. The changes in TBW, ICF, and ECF compartments during stages of human maturation are listed in Table 7–1.

III. Pediatric Intravenous Fluid Requirements

A. Maintenance fluid calculation

   1. The most widely accepted method for determining IV fluid requirements is based on patient weight. This determination ignores important factors, such as varied metabolic rates, caloric intake, patient core temperature, the ratio of body surface area to weight, and ongoing fluid losses (e.g., nasogastric suction).

   2. The proposed hourly maintenance fluid is determined using the 4-2-1 formula (see p. 86).

B. Preoperative fluid deficit calculation and replacement

   1. This fluid deficit is calculated by determining the hourly maintenance fluid rate (i.e., the 4-2-1 formula) and multiplying this rate by the number of hours the child

TABLE 7–1. Fluid Compartment Volumes

	Premature Infant	Infant	Child	Adult
Total body water (TBW)	80%–90%	75%	65%–70%	55%–60%
Extracellular fluid (ECF)	50%–60%	40%	30%	20%
Intracellular fluid (ICF)	60%	35%	40%	40%

Hourly Maintenance Fluid Determination

1. For the *first 10 kg of body weight,* 4 ml of crystalloid IV (e.g., lactated Ringer's) solution is administered for each kilogram of body weight per hour.

   Example: The hourly maintenance fluid requirement for a child weighing 10 kg is calculated as 10 kg × 4 ml/kg/h = 40 ml/h.

2. Children *weighing >10 kg through 20 kg* would receive an additional 2 ml of crystalloid IV fluid for each kilogram of body weight >10 kg: 11 kg through 20 kg = 40 ml/h + 2 ml/kg/h for each kilogram >10 kg.

   Example: The hourly maintenance fluid requirement of a child weighing 14 kg is calculated as follows:
   10 kg × 4 ml/kg/h = 40 ml/h, plus
   4 kg × 2 ml/kg/h = 8 ml/h
   Total fluid requirement = 48 ml/h

3. Children *weighing >20 kg* would receive an additional 1 ml of crystalloid IV fluid for each kilogram of body weight >20 kg: >20 kg = 60 ml/h + 1 ml/kg/h for each kilogram >20 kg.

   Example: The hourly maintenance fluid requirement of a child weighing 24 kg is calculated as follows:
   10 kg × 4 ml/kg/h = 40 ml, plus
   10 kg × 2 ml/kg/h = 20 ml, plus
   4 kg × 1 ml/kg/h = 4 ml/h
   Total fluid requirement = 64 ml/h

---

has been without IV or oral intake. For example, the preoperative fluid deficit of an 8 kg child who has been NPO for 6 hours is determined as follows:

$$Maintenance\ fluid = 8\ kg \times 4\ ml/kg/h = 32\ ml/h$$

$$Preoperative\ fluid\ deficit = 6\ h \times 32\ ml/h = 192\ ml$$

2. The calculated fluid deficit is replaced as follows:
   a. One half of the deficit is replaced the first intraoperative hour, with the remainder divided in half and replaced in the subsequent 2 hours.
   b. The IV fluid administration for the 8 kg child in the above example is shown in Table 7–2.

TABLE 7–2. IV Fluid Administration for an 8 kg Child

	Surgical Hour 1	Surgical Hour 2	Surgical Hour 3
Maintenance fluid (ml/h)	32	32	32
Deficit (ml/h) (192 ml total)	96	48	48
Hourly fluid total (ml/h)	128	80	80

IV. Third-Space Fluid Losses

A. IV fluid administration (in addition to maintenance and deficit fluid calculation) is necessary to replace insensible fluid losses and third-space loss of fluid caused by surgical trauma.

B. Lactated Ringer's solution, 0.9% normal saline, and Plasma-lyte are recommended for the replacement of insensible and third-space fluid losses.

C. Expected third-space fluid losses can be categorized as minimal surgical trauma, moderate surgical trauma, or major surgical trauma.

1. Insensible losses = 1–2 ml/kg/h
2. Minimal surgical trauma = 3–4 ml/kg/h
3. Moderate surgical trauma = 5–6 ml/kg/h
4. Major surgical trauma = 7–8 ml/kg/h

V. TBW Deficit Assessment and Replacement

A. A deficit of TBW can be estimated via a physical examination of the child. The general appearance of the child changes as the degree of TBW deficit increases.

B. Mild dehydration (<5% of body weight) is difficult to determine but may be identified clinically as dry mouth, malaise, and decreased urine output; it may be accompanied by a clinical history of vomiting or diarrhea. Blood pressure remains in the normal range, and capillary refill is less than 2 seconds, demonstrating acceptable perfusion.

C. The pediatric patient with moderate dehydration (5%–10% decrease of body weight) presents clinically with lethargy, loss of appetite, thick mucus, dry mucous membranes, and oliguria; the eyes may be sunken in the orbits. Infants up to 6 months of age with an open anterior fontanelle may have a visible depression. Capillary refill is increased up to 3 seconds, and although blood pressure is normal, tachycardia (>100 bpm) will be noted.

D. The pediatric patient with severe dehydration (>10% loss of body weight) presents clinically with hypotension (<60 mm

Hg systolic), tachycardia (up to 150 bpm), mottled cool skin, capillary refill >3 seconds, and anuria. A delay in treatment leads to a high mortality.

E. Replacement of deficit fluid.

   1. Fluid deficit can be determined by knowing the change in body weight: a loss of 1 g of body weight equals a loss of 1 ml of TBW. If body weight is not known, the previous clinical signs and symptoms of dehydration can be utilized. For example, clinical signs reflective of a moderate dehydration (up to 10% of body weight) in a 10 kg patient equal a TBW deficit of 1000 ml.

   2. Initial deficit replacement is carried out with an isotonic crystalloid solution (0.9% normal saline; lactated Ringer's if nonconcurrent hyperkalemia). In general, approximately 10 ml of crystalloid solution per kilogram of body weight is necessary to replace each 1% loss of body weight. An initial bolus of the selected fluid, 10 to 20 ml/kg, is administered over 10 to 30 minutes. Caution should be exercised in administering repeated fluid boluses rapidly because heart failure could occur.

   3. Children with severe dehydration may require additional fluid boluses of 10 to 20 ml/kg, with continuous assessment of blood pressure, heart rate, and urine output.

   4. Following hemodynamic stabilization, the remainder of the fluid deficit (calculated fluid deficit – bolus crystalloid administration) can be replaced over an 8- to 10-hour period.

   5. Maintenance fluid requirements should not be ignored during this period. The calculated maintenance fluid must also be provided.

VI. Electrolyte Abnormalities

A. General requirements

   1. In general, sodium, potassium, and chloride, 1 to 3 mEq/kg of body weight, are required each day.

   2. Infants have a higher extracellular fluid volume and hence have a higher sodium requirement than children or adults. Mineral replacement (calcium, magnesium, phosphorus) is rarely needed except in children who have poor dietary intake or who are chronically ill.

B. Hyponatremia

   1. A plasma Na^+ <135 mEq/L that develops from an excess of TBW

   2. Etiology

a. Drug induced (prostaglandin, morphine, barbiturates, nonsteroidal antiinflammatory agents)
b. Endocrine disease (glucocorticoid deficiency, myxedema, syndrome of inappropriate ADH secretion, hypothyroidism)
c. Renal disease (obstructive uropathy, nephrolithiasis, acute and chronic renal failure, postobstructive diuresis, nephrotic syndrome, ileus, pancreatitis)
d. Central nervous system disease (syndrome of inappropriate ADH secretion, head injury)
e. Gastrointestinal dysfunction (vomiting, diarrhea, cirrhosis, ileus)

3. Signs and symptoms
   a. Anorexia, headache, irritability, personality changes, muscle weakness with depressed deep tendon reflexes
   b. Nausea and vomiting, hypothermia, convulsions, and death in individuals when the serum sodium <120 mEq/L

4. Sodium maintenance
   a. Serum Na^+ should be ≥125 mEq/L.
   b. General treatment for correction is with isotonic solutions.
   c. Serum Na^+ may be corrected with the administration of hypertonic saline (e.g., 3% normal saline) but should be accomplished under close observation and direction from a pediatrician to avoid overcorrection and the development of central pontine myelinitis.
   d. Sodium required can be calculated as follows: $(NaD - NaA) \times Body\ weight\ (kg) \times 0.6 = mEq$, where NaD = desired concentration of sodium and NaA = actual concentration of sodium.

C. Hypernatremia
   1. Develops when the plasma sodium exceeds 145 mEq/L
   2. Individuals with existing hypernatremia have disorders of intravascular volume, and management may require monitoring central venous pressure and invasive monitoring of arterial pressure
   3. Etiology
      a. Inadequate water replacement (fever, use of radiant warmers)
      b. Water loss in excess of sodium loss (vomiting, diarrhea, profuse sweating, hyperosmolar coma)
      c. Excess sodium intake (administration of sodium bicarbonate, ingestion of NaCl tablets)

d. Excess glucocorticoid (Cushing's syndrome), excess mineralocorticoid (hyperaldosteronism)
e. Endocrine disease (hypothalamic/pituitary disease, diabetes insipidus)
f. Renal disease (chronic renal failure, polycystic kidney disease, obstructive uropathy, nephritis)
g. Drug induced (inhalation agent, methoxyflurane, lithium carbonate, amphotericin B)

4. Signs and symptoms
   a. Central nervous system is most affected by loss of intracellular water content, producing clinical symptoms that include thirst, lethargy, confusion, seizures, hyperreflexia, coma, and death.
   b. If hypernatremia develops because of hypovolemia, clinical signs and symptoms include hypotension, tachycardia, dry oral mucous membranes, and decreased skin turgor.

5. Correction of hypernatremia
   a. Accomplished over 24 to 48 hours with isotonic or hypotonic solutions under close observation and direction from a pediatrician.
   b. Administration of hypotonic fluids to lower plasma Na^+ may produce cerebral edema, which may tear bridging veins, producing intracranial hemorrhage and death.
   c. Replacement of free water is accomplished following the calculation of the TBW deficit: Water deficit (L) = 0.6 (weight in kg) × [(serum sodium/140) − 1)].

D. Hypochloremia
   1. Deficiency develops with excess intake of chloride or when chloride loss exceeds intake.
   2. Etiology.
      a. Chronic vomiting, diarrhea, or gastric suctioning (pyloric stenosis)
      b. Excess loss of chloride (Bartter's syndrome, defective reabsorption of chloride in ascending thick loop of Henle)
      c. Long-term diuretic therapy (treatment of infants with congenital heart disease)
   3. Signs and symptoms.
      a. ECF volume depletion with decreased glomerular filtration.
      b. Tubular reabsorption of sodium occurs with binding to bicarbonate rather than chloride, resulting in metabolic alkalosis.

    c. Volume contraction of ECF produces renin release, increased aldosterone secretion, with tubular absorption of Na^+, secretion of K^+ and H^+, and increased degree of metabolic alkalosis.

  4. Correction of hypochloremia will follow the correction of the underlying etiology (administration of excess normal saline), seeking a positive chloride balance of 2 to 8 mEq/d.

E. Hypokalemia

  1. Hypokalemia is defined as a plasma potassium level <3.5 mEq/L developing as a result of a renal depletion or transcellular shifts of potassium without renal losses such as may occur in metabolic alkalosis or following insulin or beta-adrenergic administration

  2. A decrease in the extracellular plasma concentration of 0.3 mEq/L results in an intracellular deficit of approximately 100 mEq/L

  3. Etiology

    a. Transcellular shifts (alkalosis, insulin administration, beta-adrenergic administration)

    b. Nutrition (inadequate K^+ intake; daily intake = 0.5–2 mEq/kg/d)

  4. Signs and symptoms

    a. Hypokalemia alters the electrical forces across the cell membrane, reducing the resting potential and hyperpolarizing the cell membrane.

    b. Laboratory evaluation assesses the extracellular concentration (3.5–5.5 mEq/L), whereas the majority of K^+ is intracellular (145–155 mEq/L).

    c. Electrocardiogram (ECG) changes include increases in T wave amplitude, the appearance of a U wave, and increases in the QT interval, P wave amplitude, and QRS duration.

    d. Dysrhythmias associated with hypokalemia include atrial fibrillation, premature ventricular contraction, supraventricular tachycardia, junctional tachycardia, and type I second-degree block.

  5. Correction of hypokalemia

    a. Replacement of K^+.

    b. Before initiating treatment, the urine output should be at least 0.5 ml/kg/h. The total amount of K^+ to be replaced is as follows: Weight $\times (C_D - C_M) \times 0.3 = $ mEq required, where $C_D =$ serum concentration desired and $C_M =$ serum concentration measured.

    c. Infusion rates should not exceed 0.5 mEq/kg/h.

F. Hyperkalemia
1. Plasma concentrations of potassium that exceed 5.5 mEq/L. The kidney plays a major role in preventing acute increases in plasma potassium with ongoing renal secretion
2. Accordingly, disease states that decrease urine production produce increases in plasma potassium
3. Etiology
   a. False elevations: hemolysis following blood draw, leukocytosis
   b. Transcellular shifts (succinylcholine administration; digitalis intoxication; acidosis; hyperkalemic periodic paralysis; cellular injury that follows burns, crushing tissue injuries, ischemic extremities)
   c. Supplemental potassium administration (oral or IV K^+ replacement, administration of old banked blood, or administration of K^+ in some medications [e.g., Pen VK])
   d. Decreased renal excretion (acute and chronic renal failure, Addison's disease, administration of potassium-sparing diuretics)
4. Signs and symptoms
   a. Like hypokalemia, hyperkalemia alters membrane electrical activity.
   b. Extracellular K^+ (normally 3.5–5.5 mEq/L) is increased, changing the intracellular/extracellular ratio, slowing depolarization and conduction velocity (specifically myocardial conduction).
   c. Alterations in cardiac conduction generally occur when the plasma potassium meets or exceeds 6.5 to 7 mEq/L.
   d. Characteristic ECG changes include symmetric, peaking T waves and QRS and PR interval widening with the rhythm changing to a sinusoidal pattern followed by ventricular tachycardia and fibrillation.
   e. Alterations in membrane activity affect skeletal muscles as well, resulting in muscle weakness, flaccid paralysis, and paresthesias of the lower extremities.
5. Treatment of hyperkalemia
   a. Predicated on the presence of cardiac instability.
   b. Chronic hyperkalemia is effectively treated with the oral or rectal administration of sodium polystyrene sulfonate (Kayexalate) (1–2 g/kg/d in four divided doses). Kayexalate, 1 g/kg, lowers the plasma K^+ by approximately 1 mEq/L.

    c. Acute hyperkalemia, which may follow succinylcholine administration to a trauma patient, can be managed with hyperventilation; sodium bicarbonate, 1 or 2 mEq/kg; IV calcium chloride, 5 to 10 mg/kg; or 25 g of glucose with 10 to 15 units of regular insulin.

    d. The elimination of potassium can also be facilitated with peritoneal dialysis and hemodialysis.

VII. IV Fluid Selection

A. IV maintenance fluid is chosen after evaluating the child's current physical condition and laboratory results (if available) and assessing the ongoing surgical trauma and concurrent third-space and blood losses

B. Consideration must be given to the requirement for free water and electrolytes. Lactated Ringer's, an isotonic solution with an osmolarity between 280 and 310 mOsm/L, is excellent for replacing fluid and electrolyte losses

C. Water requirements

    1. Daily insensible water loss in the neonate and child occurs from evaporation from the skin (sweating, radiant therapy, radiant heaters), respiration (hyperventilation), urination, and the gastrointestinal tract (vomiting, gastrointestinal suctioning).

    2. Total insensible water loss equals 60 to 100 ml/kg/d.

    3. The indiscriminant administration of free water (D_5W) is not recommended because of the possibility of water intoxication and iatrogenic hyponatremia. D_5W is distributed throughout all fluid compartments, and continued administration may lead to increasing TBW and dilutional hyponatremia.

D. Crystalloid IV solutions

    1. Crystalloid fluids contain water, various concentrations of electrolytes, and possibly varying concentrations of glucose.

    2. These solutions move freely between the intravascular and interstitial fluid compartments.

    3. These fluids are inexpensive, nonallergenic, and acceptable for the replacement of preoperative, intraoperative, and postoperative isotonic fluid deficits.

    4. Table 7–3 illustrates the composition and commonly used osmolarity of popular IV solutions.

E. Colloid IV fluids

    1. Colloid IV fluids (e.g., albumin, hetastarch, dextran) contain large-molecular-weight particles (protein or glu-

TABLE 7–3. Popular Intravenous Crystalloid Solutions

	Na$^+$	Cl$^-$	K$^+$	Ca^{2+}	Lactate	Sugar (mg/ml)	mOsm/L
			(mEq/L)				
HYPOTONIC SOLUTIONS							
0.45% Normal saline	77	77	—	—	—	—	154
5% Dextrose in water	—	—	—	—	—	50	252
ISOTONIC SOLUTIONS							
0.9% Normal saline	154	154	—	—	—	—	308
Lactated Ringer's	130	109	4	3	28	—	274
Ringer's	130	109	4	3	—	—	246
Plasmalyte A	140	98	5	—	—	—	243
HYPERTONIC SOLUTIONS							
5% Sodium chloride	855	855	—	—	—	—	1710
7.5% Sodium chloride	1283	1283	—	—	—	—	2566

From Aker, J. (1995). The selection and administration of intravenous fluids. *Current Reviews for Perianesthesia Nursing, 17,* 61–68.

cose polymers) impenetrable to the semipermeable membrane that separates the intravascular and interstitial fluid compartments.

2. These protein molecules create an osmotic force (colloid osmotic pressure) that acts to recruit water into the intravascular fluid compartment.

3. Colloid solutions are preferentially distributed to the intravascular fluid compartment and remain for a longer time than crystalloid solutions.

4. Colloid IV solutions should not be administered indiscriminantly because of expense (more expensive than crystalloid solutions) and because protein and glucose constituents may be antigenic, producing allergic reactions during administration; coagulopathies may develop following administration (particularly noted with dextran); and osmotic diuresis may be produced, further decreasing intravascular volume.

5. Table 7–4 lists the popular IV colloid solutions and their characteristics.

F. Glucose administration

1. Historically a 5% glucose IV solution was administered to all pediatric patients to prevent intraoperative hypoglycemia, provide free water (replace insensible water loss), conserve protein, and prevent ketosis.

2. Children receiving 5% dextrose infusions intraoperatively consistently develop hyperglycemia.

3. Surgical stress elicits a neuroendocrine response, increasing plasma glucose; thus healthy pediatric patients rarely become hypoglycemic intraoperatively.

TABLE 7–4. Popular Intravenous Colloid Solutions

Agent	Average Molecular Weight (daltons)	Colloid Osmotic Pressure (mm Hg)	H$_2$O Binding (ml) per Gram of Fluid
ALBUMIN			
5%	69,000	20	18
25%	69,000	100	18
HETASTARCH			
6%	450,000	30	20
DEXTRANS			
10% Dextran 40	40,000	70	25
6% Dextran 70	70,000	60	25

From Aker, J. (1995). The selection and administration of intravenous fluids. *Current Reviews for Perianesthesia Nursing, 17,* 61–68.

4. Critically ill infants and those <10 kg may develop hypoglycemia with prolonged fasting.
5. Hypoxic or ischemic neurologic events with concurrent glucose administration have been shown to worsen neurologic outcome in animals.
6. Hypoglycemia may develop in special clinical circumstances (persons with type I diabetes who have received preoperative insulin; children receiving glucose-based parenteral nutrition at risk for rebound hypoglycemia when abruptly discontinued). Administer a piggyback infusion of D_5W intraoperatively, and monitor plasma glucose concentration.

VIII. Fluid Management of the Premature Infant

A. Glomerular filtration is 15% to 30% of adult values at birth, reaching adult values at 1 year.
B. Immature renal tubular function limits ability to excrete sodium and fluid. Inability to concentrate urine and inability to reabsorb sodium result in excretion of dilute urine.
C. Infants <6 months of age benefit from maintenance fluids of 0.9% normal saline or 5% dextrose in 0.45% normal saline at the calculated maintenance rate.
D. Infants >6 months of age and healthy children may be managed with lactated Ringer's solution.

IX. Volume-Limiting Infusion Devices

A. Control of the amount of administered fluid is as important as selecting the correct fluid.
B. Fluid overload is minimized with the use of volume-limiting devices such as minidrip or Buretrol administration set (60 drops/ml). When using the Buretrol set, only 1 hour of maintenance fluid is placed into the chamber.
C. Infusion pumps infuse a specific rate of fluid over a specified period. These devices limit the ability to rapidly administer fluid boluses or drugs.
D. Syringe pumps function as infusion pumps but are limited by the size of the syringe that will fit into the pump.
E. Rapid infusion devices must be used with caution if at all in children because a relative fluid overload may occur.
F. Venous air embolism may occur when the infusion tubing is not properly purged.
1. Venous air embolism will produce increased alveolar dead space, carbon dioxide retention, ventilation-

perfusion mismatch, hypoxemia, and pulmonary hypertension.
   2. If air passes to the arterial side of circulation through a probe-patent foramen ovale, atrial or ventricular septal defect, myocardial or cerebral infarction may result (paradoxical embolism).
   3. A large air embolism may produce an air lock in the superior vena cava or right atrium followed by marked reductions in cardiac output and blood pressure.

X. Establishing Venous Access

   A. Anesthetic induction in the majority of pediatric patients is accomplished by inhaling an anesthetic vapor. IV access is obtained in the anesthetized child.
   B. Indications for IV access.
      1. Surgical procedures in excess of 30 to 60 minutes
      2. Surgical procedures with high incidence of postoperative nausea and vomiting (e.g., strabismus surgery, orchiopexy, otoplasty, dental rehabilitation)
      3. Surgical procedures with significant blood loss (e.g., tonsillectomy, craniotomy, thoracotomy)
      4. Prolonged preoperative oral fluid abstinence
      5. Pediatric patients who develop significant cardiovascular depression after induction with inhalation anesthetics
      6. Need for perioperative administration of IV medications (e.g., prophylactic antibiotics, analgesics)
   C. Preferred sites of IV access include the dorsum of the hand, the saphenous vein, and the radial vein.
   D. The site chosen will depend on the location of the operative field.
   E. Topical local anesthetic creams.
      1. If IV access is required for anesthetic induction, the topical local anesthetic cream EMLA (eutectic mixture of prilocaine and lidocaine) may be applied at least 30 to 45 minutes before venipuncture in young children and up to 60 minutes before venipuncture in older children.
      2. The cream is provided to the parent and applied over potential IV sites marked with an ink pen by the anesthetist.

XI. Considerations for Blood Therapy Replacement

   A. Virtually all surgical procedures are associated with some blood loss
   B. The intraoperative administration of blood and blood

products is undertaken to maintain acceptable oxygen-carrying capacity

C. Determination of intraoperative blood loss
1. Because pediatric patients have relatively small intravascular volume compared to adult patients, vigilance and accurate assessment of intraoperative blood loss are fundamental to intraoperative care.
2. Up to one half of surgical blood loss may be contained in surgical sponges, drapes, and towels.
3. Subjective estimates of blood loss (examining the sponges) is grossly inaccurate.
4. To accurately calculate blood lost, sponges, drapes, and towels should be weighed. The weight of the blood-soaked item is subtracted from the weight of the dry item. Every 1 g of weight equals 1 ml of blood loss.
5. Approximately 25% of surgical blood loss is contained within suction canisters. For small neonates and infants, suction traps may be placed in line to enhance the accuracy of blood loss determination. The subtraction of the amount of irrigation from the total contained within the suction canister equals the blood loss.
6. Ongoing surgical blood loss can be gauged by the patient's physiologic response. Moderate to severe decreases in intravascular volume produce tachycardia, hypotension, narrowed pulse pressure, low to ceasing urine output, decreased central venous pressure, pallor, and slowed capillary refill.
7. In neonates and infants who have heart rate–dependent cardiac output, a sudden decrease in blood pressure indicates significant intravascular volume depletion.

D. Estimation of circulating blood volume
1. The following references may be used to estimate pediatric blood volume:
   a. Premature newborn: 90 to 100 ml/kg
   b. Full-term newborn: 80 to 90 ml/kg
   c. Age 3 months to 3 years: 75 to 80 ml/kg
   d. Age 3 to 6 years: 70 to 75 ml/kg
   e. Age >6 years: 65 to 70 ml/kg
2. Example: A 6-month-old infant weighing 7 kg would have an estimated blood volume of 7 kg × 75 ml/kg = 525 ml.

E. Calculation of allowable blood loss
1. The following simple formula may be used to estimate allowable blood loss (ABL):

$$ABL = EBV \times [H_O - H_L]/[H_A]$$

where EBV = estimated blood volume, H_O = the original hematocrit, H_L = the lowest acceptable hematocrit, and H_A = the average hematocrit, or $[H_O + H_L]/2$.

2. Using the above example, for the 6-month-old infant weighing 7 kg with a hematocrit of 35% and selecting the lowest acceptable hematocrit of 25%:

$$ABL = 525 \times [35 - 25]/[35 + 25]/2 = 174 \text{ ml}$$

3. This 174 ml blood loss may be managed accordingly:
   a. Administer 2 to 3 ml of lactated Ringer's or normal saline for each 1 ml of blood loss.
   b. Blood loss that is less than the calculated allowable blood loss may be replaced with colloid (1 ml of hydroxyethylstarch or 5% albumin) for every 1 ml of blood loss.
   c. Whole blood replacement: 1 ml for each 1 ml of blood loss.
   d. Packed red cell replacement: 0.5 ml for each 1 ml of blood loss.
F. Acceptable hematocrit
   1. Historically, a hemoglobin level of 10 g/L or a hematocrit level of 30% triggered the administration of blood before elective anesthesia and surgery.
   2. This "transfusion trigger" has been redefined in light of the risks of blood-borne pathogen transmission. In 1988 the National Institutes of Health attempted to define a transfusion trigger.
   3. The committee concluded that there was no single defining hemoglobin value but rather that each patient must be considered individually based on his or her unique physiology.
   4. In general, healthy patients with hemoglobin values of 10 g/L or more rarely require red cell transfusion.
   5. Children with normal cardiovascular function can tolerate lower hematocrits and compensate by increasing cardiac output if a higher inspired oxygen concentration is provided to improve oxygen delivery.
   6. The anesthetist must consider the numerous complex biochemical, hemodynamic, and respiratory effects of each patient with ongoing blood loss.
   7. No published studies at this time define optimal and safe

lower limits for hemoglobin concentration and oxygen delivery in critically ill children.

G. Transfusion equipment

1. Before blood component therapy, the proper equipment (filters, infusion devices, blood warming devices) should be obtained and tested.

2. Blood filters.

   a. Standard blood infusion sets contain filters between 170 and 200 μm.

   b. Microaggregate filters (20–40 μm) are sometimes placed between the blood dispensing bag and infusion device, but no studies prove these filters are better than standard 170 μm filters in blood sets.

   c. Filters are never used for platelet infusion.

3. Electronic infusion devices (syringe pumps or piston-driven infusion pumps) should be approved by the manufacturer for the infusion of blood and/or blood products. An excessive infusion rate can produce red cell lysis and damage to blood components.

4. Blood warming devices.

   a. Blood is usually warmed before transfusion. The American Association of Blood Banks has published standards for blood warming devices. Blood warmers must have a visible thermometer and an audible warning indicating heating >42°C.

   b. Adult transfusion heating devices (in-line water baths, or counter-current heating with water through large-bore tubing) are sometimes cumbersome for the small blood volumes transfused in the pediatric patient. However, the blood can be drawn through the infusion tubing by syringe, and then the measured quantity of blood can be administered to the child. The anesthetist should recall that warmed blood encourages bacteria present in the unit to multiply. Warmed blood cannot be returned to the blood bank.

   c. Warming volumes of blood for transfusion is important but can be hazardous. Warming methods include leaving the blood in a room-temperature environment allowing ambient warming, running infusion tubing through a water bath, or using an approved blood warmer. Hazardous methods include the placement of blood in a hot water basin (blood contained in a measured syringe may be contaminated), placing the unit between bags of heated IV solutions (will likely produce overheating), or placement of the blood between the heating blanket. The anesthetist must remember that overheating blood may produce hemolysis.

XII. Blood Component Therapy

A. More than one half of all transfusions are administered during the perioperative period

B. The determination of the patient's correct blood type is important in avoiding fatal reactions with the transfusion of incompatible blood. Table 7–5 lists the blood groups and the associated antibodies

C. The decision to administer blood or blood components depends on the clinical situation, because some patients may require transfusion who do not meet these general guidelines.

D. General guidelines for the transfusion of red blood cells
1. Low preoperative hemoglobin levels as determined for each patient
2. Expected large intraoperative blood loss
3. Intraoperative blood loss exceeding 15% to 20% of the estimated blood volume
4. Clinical evidence of inadequate oxygen delivery

E. Pediatric blood transfusion uses small volumes of blood, and use of adult units may be wasteful. The blood bank can dispense small aliquots of blood for transfusion in a variety of ways:
1. Blood from an assigned donor unit can be given in a calibrated syringe, or a small quantity of blood (50–100 ml) can be put into transfer bags.
2. The blood bank will issue the needed blood from the same donor unit to minimize the exposure from multiple blood donors.

F. Whole blood
1. One unit of whole blood contains 450 ml of blood in 60 to 65 ml of CPDA-1 anticoagulant preservative.

TABLE 7–5. Blood Groups and Their Associated Antibodies

Blood Type	Antigen	Plasma Antibody	Whites	Blacks
A	A	Anti-B	40%	27%
B	B	Anti-A	11%	20%
AB	AB	None	4%	5%
O	None	Anti-A, anti-B	45%	49%
Rh	Rh (D)	None	85%	

2. Whole blood (hematocrit of 40%) accounts for less than 20% of all transfused blood. It is generally used for treatment of hemorrhagic shock. The majority of whole blood is broken down into various components.

G. Packed red blood cell administration

1. Packed red blood cells (hematocrit 70%) account for >50% of all blood transfused because the demand for blood components has required the breakdown of whole blood units.

2. Red blood cells are preserved in 250 to 300 ml of citrated solution or are frozen, with a hematocrit of 70%.

3. The frozen preservation decreases the chance of post-transfusion viral infection and eliminates the transfusion of potassium or citrate.

4. Blood must be administered through a filtered infusion device.

5. Blood should not be diluted before administration to the pediatric patient because this may produce hypervolemia.

6. Blood selected for neonatal transfusion is preferentially irradiated (to prevent graft-versus-host disease) and ideally is preserved before transfusion in the frozen state, or less than 1 week since collection, to preserve red cell 2,3-diphosphoglycerate (DPG) levels.

7. Hemoglobin will increase 1 g/dl with infusion of packed red cells, 3 ml/kg, whereas hematocrit will increase 10% with infusion of 10 ml/kg.

H. Fresh frozen plasma

1. Prepared from single donor units and used as a source of factors V and VIII

2. Prepared as a 250 ml volume with 200 ml of preservative

I. Cryoprecipitate

1. Delivered from the blood bank in 10 to 20 ml volumes

2. Transfused in the treatment of hemophilia A; contains von Willebrand's factor, factor XIII, and fibrinogen

J. Platelets

1. Used in the leukemic patient with thrombocytopenia secondary to chemotherapy, anaplastic anemia, and dilutional thrombocytopenia following massive transfusion.

2. One unit of platelets is administered for every 10 kg of body weight; each unit increases the platelet count 5000 to 10,000/mm^3.

3. Platelets should *never* be filtered during administration.

K. Techniques to minimize blood transfusion

1. Less volume required (1 ml for every 1 ml of blood loss) because of increased oncotic pressure and remains within the vascular space for a longer period than crystalloid solutions. Recall that dextrans may produce coagulopathies as evidenced by increased prothrombin time (PT) and partial thromboplastin time (PTT).

2. Isovolemic hemodilution is the removal of blood with the simultaneous administration of a non–hemoglobin containing solution. Removal immediately before a surgical intervention is termed *acute normovolemic hemodilution (ANH)*. A predetermined volume of blood is removed based on the patient's blood volume and starting hematocrit; and a target, euvolemic hemoglobin concentration is achieved. Blood loss occurring during the subsequent surgical manipulation is diluted, and fewer red cells are lost per milliliter of shed blood.

3. Intraoperative hypotension is a technique that decreases intraoperative blood loss. Hypotension may be produced by a variety of agents, including sodium nitroprusside, nitroglycerin, esmolol, or other combinations of alpha- and beta-adrenergic blockade. Arterial blood pressure monitoring is generally required.

4. Autologous transfusion is infrequently used in small children, but it is a viable option for an adolescent who is scheduled to undergo a surgical procedure with moderate to significant blood loss (e.g., correction of scoliosis). Contraindications include concurrent anemia, bacteremia, or viral infectious process (human immunodeficiency virus [HIV]).

5. Directed blood donation is selection by the patient's guardians of an individual to donate blood before the surgical procedure. No data indicate that directed donation has less blood-borne pathogen transmission risk than blood from the general blood supply.

6. Intraoperative blood salvaging is a technique in which blood lost during the procedure is suctioned into a device that is designed to collect, wash, and prepare the red blood cells for reinfusion. Intraoperative blood salvaging is not suitable for patients with an infectious or septic process, when the patient has a known malignancy, or when there has been fecal contamination of the operative field. This technique is infrequently used in pediatric surgical procedures.

L. Emergency transfusion
   1. The urgent need to replace blood loss may require the use

of uncrossmatched blood. Red blood cells should be used rather than whole blood. In this situation, the following approach may be helpful:

    a. *Type specific, partially crossmatched:* This source of red cells is suitable in emergencies. A partial crossmatch is completed by adding the plasma of the recipient to the erythrocytes of the donor and observing for agglutination. The procedure requires 5 to 10 minutes and minimizes hemolytic reactions caused by ABO incompatibility.

    b. *Type specific, uncrossmatched:* This source of ABO-specific red blood cells is probably safe in the majority of children who have not had a previous blood transfusion.

    c. *O, Rh negative, uncrossmatched:* Type O red blood cells lack the A and B antigens. Therefore the erythrocytes are not hemolyzed by the anti-A and anti-B antibodies present in the recipient plasma. Type O blood is thus designated as the universal donor. The plasma of type O does not contain antibodies capable of destroying type A or B erythrocytes. Uncrossmatched, type O, Rh-negative cells should be administered rather than type O, Rh-negative whole blood. The infusion of red cells minimizes the amount of transfused donor plasma that may contain dangerous antibodies.

M. Transfusion reactions

    1. Transfusion reactions may be categorized as immune/hemolytic or nonimmune in origin

    2. Allergic reactions

        a. Allergic reactions in appropriately typed and cross-matched patients occur in approximately 3% of patients.

        b. Incompatible plasma proteins may be responsible.

        c. Signs and symptoms include pruritus, erythema, urticaria, and increased core body temperature. Bronchospasm and laryngospasm may also develop.

        d. Treatment is symptomatic but may include diphenhydramine (Benadryl; 0.5–1.0 mg/kg) with the discontinuation of the transfusion. Future transfusions are carried out with leukocyte-poor (washed) red blood cells to remove the donor plasma.

    3. Febrile reactions

        a. Febrile reactions are the most common nonhemolytic transfusion reactions, accounting for 0.5% to 1.0% of all transfusion reactions.

    b. Core body temperature increases within 4 hours of the transfusion and generally does not exceed 38°C. Fever may also occur during hemolytic transfusion reactions. Fever occurs as pyrogenic substances are released from the red blood cells.

    c. Headache, nausea and vomiting, and chest or back pain may accompany the temperature elevation.

    d. Slow infusion and the administration of an antipyretic have been successful.

    e. Small doses of IV meperidine (12.5 mg) will attenuate shivering that accompanies the reaction.

4. Hemolytic reactions

    a. Acute hemolytic reactions develop when antibodies in the plasma of the recipient interact with antigens on the red cell membrane of the donor erythrocytes. They are the most serious reactions and are avoided with properly performed crossmatching and meticulous attention to clerical details.

    b. Signs and symptoms in the conscious individual include lumbar and substernal chest pain, fever with or without shivering, restlessness, nausea and vomiting, skin flushing, and hypotension.

    c. Complement activation results in intravascular hemorrhage, increased capillary permeability, hemoglobinuria, oliguria progressing to anuria, and acute renal failure.

    d. Treatment

       (1) Immediately discontinue the transfusion.

       (2) Required laboratory evaluation includes type and crossmatch, coagulation profile, platelet count, and a sample of blood and urine to be sent to the laboratory along with the offending unit of blood.

       (3) Renal function is maintained with liberal fluid administration with concurrent mannitol. IV furosemide (Lasix) will be required if fluid and mannitol do not maintain acceptable urinary output. Hypotension should be promptly treated to prevent decreased urinary output.

5. Delayed hemolytic reactions

    a. Antibody in the plasma of the recipient is responsible for the reaction but is insufficient to produce immediate hemolysis.

    b. A positive indirect Coombs' test suggests the presence of recipient antibodies.

   c. Symptoms include a slowly decreasing hematocrit in the postoperative period with the appearance of jaundice within 14 days after blood transfusion.
   d. Treatment is supportive in nature.
6. Infectious disease
   a. The risk of acquisition of HIV is 1:450,000 per unit transfused.
   b. Hepatitis B: Accounts for 2% of cases of posttransfusion hepatitis. Current risk is estimated at 1:200,000 per unit transfused.
   c. Hepatitis C: Accounts for 98% of all cases of posttransfusion hepatitis. Current risk is estimated at 1 per 3400 units transfused.
7. Metabolic complications
   a. Increased potassium: The potassium levels steadily increase during the period of blood storage. Massive transfusion infrequently produces an increased potassium level. However, transfusions in individuals with impaired renal function may aggravate the chronic hyperkalemia.
   b. Acidosis: The preservatives added to donated blood decrease the pH to approximately 7.2. Continued decreases in pH occur with storage because the red cells continue to be active anaerobically.
   c. Decreased 2,3-diphosphoglycerate (2,3-DPG) levels: The P_{50} of blood decreases from normal of 26 mm Hg to 15 mm Hg after 3 weeks of storage. 2,3-DPG controls the functional capacity of hemoglobin to carry oxygen.
   d. Increased carbon dioxide.
8. Coagulation defects
   a. Dilutional thrombocytopenia: Most common cause of bleeding following transfusion of multiple units of blood. Following 24 hours of storage, banked whole blood does not contain viable platelets. Bleeding diathesis occurs when platelet counts decrease to 50,000.
   b. Decreases in factors V and VIII: Only require 30% activity to maintain normal coagulation; however, these factors are very common in stored blood, decreasing to 40% of normal after 2 weeks of storage.
   c. Disseminated intravascular coagulopathy: A hypercoagulable state caused by the deposition of fibrin within the vasculature, producing fibrinolysis and the consumption of the coagulation factors and platelets.

The administration of coagulation factors and platelets is ill advised, and treatment should be directed at the precipitating cause.

ADDITIONAL READINGS

Fontana, J.L., Welborn, L., Mongan, P.D., et al. (1995). Oxygen consumption and cardiovascular function in children during profound intraoperative normovolemic hemodilution. *Anesthesia and Analgesia, 80,* 219–225.

Holliday, M.A., & Segar, W.E. (1957). The maintenance need for water in parenteral fluid therapy. *Pediatrics, 19,* 823–832.

Sieber, F.E., Smith, D.S., Traystman, R.J., & Wollman, H. (1987). Glucose: A reevaluation of its intraoperative use. *Anesthesiology, 67,* 72–81.

U.S. Department of Health and Human Services. (1988). *Perioperative red cell transfusion. NIH consensus development conference statement* (Vol. 7). Bethesda, MD: The Department.

Weisel, R.D., Charlesworth, D.C., Mickleborough, L.L., et al. (1984). Limitations of blood conservation. *Journal of Thoracic and Cardiovascular Surgery, 188,* 26–38.

Surgical Procedures

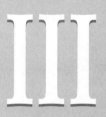

III

8

Anesthesia for Pediatric Ear, Nose, Throat, and Maxillofacial Surgery

Stanley M. Hall, MD, PhD

I. Introduction

A. Otorhinolaryngology is commonly the specialty producing the greatest volume of pediatric surgery cases. Ear, nose, and throat (ENT) procedures are most frequently performed as ambulatory surgery although radical procedures can entail prolonged admission to intensive care.

B. Initially, ambulatory surgery was performed only on healthy patients (American Society of Anesthesiologists [ASA] physical status I or II) for short procedures. Presently, surgeries lasting longer than 6 hours on patients with long-term medical conditions are routinely performed on an outpatient basis.

II. General Considerations

A. Intractable nausea and vomiting is the most common reason for overnight admission for what would otherwise be outpatient surgery. Procedures involving the nose, mouth, and pharynx, which result in the swallowing of blood, have up to a 60% incidence of postoperative nausea and vomiting.

B. Certain ENT and maxillofacial surgeries are performed to correct congenital syndromes or anomalies such as cleft lip and palate.

1. A readily apparent birth defect, such as absent or abnormal external ears, can be associated with less obvious defects, including heart defects (i.e., atrial septal defect [ASD] or ventricular septal defect [VSD]), because the heart and ears develop at about the same time in the fetus.

2. When one birth defect is detected, the presence of others should be suspected until ruled out.

C. At about 6 years of age, children lose their incisors. Preoperative evaluation should include documentation of loose and missing teeth. In addition, the ability to open the mouth and neck mobility are reduced with some facial anomalies.

D. Because of its very low cost, halothane is still commonly used for inhalational inductions of pediatric patients.

　1. ENT surgeons often administer cocaine or epinephrine or both to their patients during surgery to reduce bleeding.

　2. However, the combination of cocaine, epinephrine, and halothane has tremendous dysrhythmogenic potential.

E. Sevoflurane is rapidly gaining popularity as an inhalational agent for pediatric surgery because of its speedy onset and offset of action as well as decreased dysrhythmogenicity.

　1. Compared to halothane, the greater skeletal muscle relaxant effects of sevoflurane mean that less neuromuscular blocker is needed for intubation after inhalational induction.

　2. In addition, sevoflurane's rapid emergence hastens the return of muscle function at the end of surgery.

F. Surgical procedures involving the mouth, pharynx, or larynx frequently use a self-retaining oral retractor (e.g., a Dingman or Jackson retractor). On release of the retractor, especially following prolonged surgery, edema of the tongue can result, obstructing the airway and making reintubation difficult.

G. Many diseases of the head and neck can cause airway obstruction because of their location inside the airway (e.g., laryngeal papillomas, tumors of the tongue or pharynx, aspirated foreign bodies).

　1. Extrinsic airway compression by tumors in this area also can impede ventilation and intubation.

　2. Careful preoperative assessment, preoxygenation, and adherence to the ASA Difficult Airway Algorithm can increase the safety of these risky cases.

　3. Preoperative dyspnea, stridor, and orthopnea are warning signs of potential for catastrophe during anesthesia.

　4. The location of a tumor that compresses the airway can affect the phase of the ventilatory cycle when the greatest obstruction to air flow occurs.

　5. Extrathoracic masses cause their greatest airway obstruction during inspiration, whereas intrathoracic tumors (e.g., mediastinal tumors) restrict air flow more during exhalation. This is because of the tethering effect of the intrathoracic structures, which increase the radius of conducting airways (reducing resistance) during inspiration.

6. Extrathoracic airways retract during inspiration (especially during dyspnea), decreasing their radius and increasing their resistance to air flow.

H. Surgical packs placed during surgery to stop bleeding or decrease the leak of gas from an uncuffed endotracheal tube can be aspirated and obstruct ventilation after extubation if not removed at the end of surgery.

I. Postoperative stridor can have many causes besides retained pharyngeal packs.

J. Mucosal edema resulting from infection or the trauma of intubation or surgery is a common cause.

1. Racemic epinephrine can effectively treat many types of postoperative stridor, but its duration can be limited.

2. Rebound stridor can occur 2 to 3 hours following nebulization.

3. For this reason, discharge from outpatient surgery is routinely delayed for 3 hours following this type of nebulization therapy.

4. This rebound can be reduced by the addition of dexamethasone, 0.1 mg/kg, to the racemic epinephrine nebulization.

III. Ear Surgery

A. Pressure equalization (PE) tubes are inserted usually with the patient under general anesthesia by mask.

1. Although these cases only last 5 to 10 minutes, an intravenous (IV) infusion is routinely started at training institutions to allow rapid administration of drugs if the airway is lost.

2. PE tubes are inserted through an incision (myringotomy) in the tympanic membrane (TM) to treat chronic or recurrent middle ear infection (otitis media) when antibiotics are no longer effective.

3. Myringotomy provides a perforated eardrum, which is desirable in this situation.

4. This allows drainage of the liquid (serous) infected material (pus) when the normal drainage passage of the middle ear, the eustachian tube, is obstructed.

5. In young children, the eustachian tubes can be very narrow or blocked by enlarged or inflamed adenoids.

a. The eustachian tube connects the middle ear to the nasopharynx.

b. The adenoids are in the nasopharynx very near the opening to the eustachian tube.

B. In the absence of chronic serous otitis media (CSOM), a perforated eardrum is undesirable because it decreases the effectiveness of the TM in sound conduction, resulting in hearing loss. Also, the perforation can allow infection to enter the middle ear so water must be prevented from entering the external ear canal following myringotomy.

C. PE tubes are inserted to prevent the rapid sealing of the myringotomy and subsequent recurrence of the otitis media. If the pus does not drain from the middle ear, sepsis, fever, and meningitis can result.

D. Left unattended, CSOM can invade the mastoid air cells in the bone adjacent to the ear canal, requiring opening of the bony mastoid process (mastoidectomy) for drainage.

E. Although mastoidectomy is fairly uncommon presently, it was performed very frequently before antibiotics and PE tubes became routine for treatment of CSOM. Also, cholesteatoma, a growing mass of epithelium and bacteria, can result from chronic infection and can destroy the ear ossicles.

F. Middle ear reconstruction can require revision or replacement of some or all of the ossicles: the hammer (malleolus), anvil (incus), or stirrup (stapes).

G. Middle ear reconstructive surgery can last 4 to 6 hours but still is performed on an outpatient basis.

H. It may be necessary to avoid neuromuscular blocking agents in ear reconstruction cases because of the use of facial nerve monitoring.
   1. The facial nerve passes very near the ear canal (a branch passes through it).
   2. Identifying and monitoring reduce the risk of injury to this structure during surgery.

I. If the eustachian tube is blocked, nitrous oxide can cause rupture of the TM by expanding the air contained in the middle ear.

J. Tympanoplasty entails grafting on a new TM after traumatic rupture, removal of retained PE tubes, or middle ear reconstruction.

K. Usually PE tubes fall out spontaneously within weeks to months following insertion, but they may require surgical removal and restoration of the TM by grafting gelatin film (Gelfilm) or fascia harvested from behind the ear.

L. Nitrous oxide can also interfere with tympanoplasty by dislodging the graft through the creation of negative pressure in the middle ear when the N_2O is turned off.

Discontinuation of the N_2O at least 5 minutes before placement of the graft or avoiding its use altogether will prevent this problem.

M. Nausea and vomiting frequently occur following middle and inner ear surgeries.

1. Effective antiemesis without excessive sedation or expense are factors affecting choice of appropriate anesthetic agent (propofol vs. inhaled agents) and antiemetic drugs.

2. Vomiting or bucking on emergence can result in the TM graft becoming dislodged. Deep extubation or lidocaine administered intravenously or intratracheally can help smooth emergence.

N. Otoplasty is a plastic surgery procedure for absent, deformed, or protruding ears with anesthetic management similar to tympanoplasty.

IV. Rhinoplasty or Septoplasty

A. Although rhinoplasty is much more commonly performed in adults for cosmetic reasons, the occasional pediatric rhinoplasty is more likely to result from trauma or congenital defects such as cleft lip.

B. The endotracheal tube is frequently draped out of sight so the tube must be carefully taped and secured.

C. The placement of an oropharyngeal airway before emergence can facilitate extubation since nose breathing is impossible because of nasal packing.

D. Using the least possible pressure with the face mask can reduce the risk of injuring the nose on emergence but can make airway maintenance difficult.

V. Choanal Atresia

A. Newborns with complete bilateral choanal atresia (obstruction of the air passages between the nasal cavity and the nasopharynx) are at risk of asphyxiation because they breathe only through the nose.

1. The choanae are also called the *posterior nares*.

2. Surgical repair during the neonatal period entails all the attendant problems of neonatal anesthesia, such as heat loss and fluid and electrolyte imbalances.

B. An oropharyngeal airway or oral endotracheal tube is usually present since birth to maintain the airway.

C. For surgery, an oral RAE (Ring, Adair, Ewald) tube, which is shaped to conform to the tongue and jaw and down over the chin, is used to avoid interfering with the surgery.

D. The incidence is about 1:8000 births.

E. Coexisting anomalies must be considered. The CHARGE syndrome includes
   1. C: coloboma (an eye defect)
   2. H: heart anomalies, including tetralogy of Fallot (TOF), patent ductus arteriosus (PDA), double outlet right ventricle (DORV), VSD, ASD, and atrioventricular (A-V) canal
   3. A: atresia of choanae
   4. R: retarded growth (and other central nervous system [CNS] anomalies)
   5. G: genital anomalies (hypogonadism)
   6. E: ear anomalies

VI. Adenoidectomy or Tonsillectomy

A. The adenoids (also called *pharyngeal tonsils*) and the palatine (major) tonsils are both lymphoid tissues that tend to shrink in size after the onset of puberty.

B. Adenoidal hypertrophy can obstruct the eustachian tube resulting in middle ear disease.

C. Recurrent tonsillitis can result in such extreme hypertrophy that the two major tonsils contact each other at the back of the oral cavity (kissing tonsils).

D. Tonsillar hypertrophy can produce airway obstruction resulting in snoring, sleep apnea, and hypoxia. Pulmonary hypertension (caused by hypoxic pulmonary vasoconstriction) can cause right-sided heart failure.

E. The adenoids are near the pharyngeal opening of the eustachian tube. They are also adjacent to the muscles responsible for palate elevation during swallowing (velar muscles).

F. It is important that the patient keeps still during adenoidectomy to avoid injuring this muscle responsible for normal swallowing and speech.

G. Following an inhalational induction, oral intubation with a regular endotracheal tube or an oral RAE tube is secured by taping to the middle of the jaw.
   1. The oral self-retaining retractor inserted by the surgeon holds the endotracheal tube against the tongue but may cause kinking of the tube or endobronchial (one-sided) intubation.
   2. Switching to manual ventilation when this retractor is inserted can speed detection of kinking or dislodging of the endotracheal tube.

H. Blood loss is not as great for adenoidectomy as for tonsillectomy. Preoperative prothrombin time (PT), partial thromboplastin time (PTT), and bleeding times are required by some surgeons.

I. Gentle midline suctioning of the mouth and pharynx with a soft suction catheter (avoiding the lateral tonsillar beds) precedes extubation.

J. Awake extubation is less likely to be associated with laryngospasm than deep extubation.

K. There is no evidence that deep extubation causes less postoperative bleeding (which usually occurs within 4 hours but can be as late as 2 weeks postoperatively).

L. The patient is transported to the postanesthesia care unit (PACU) in the "tonsil" position, which is the lateral position with the head lower than the hips to promote drainage. This position is also called the modified Sims' position.

M. Consideration for postoperative pain control is warranted. Management techniques can include
   1. Administration of a narcotic, such as morphine, 0.1 mg/kg, or fentanyl, 1.0 µg/kg, immediately following the induction
   2. Administration of oral or rectal acetaminophen preoperatively
   3. Local infiltration by the surgeon

N. Patients returning to surgery for bleeding following a tonsillectomy should be treated as having a full stomach and an uncertain intravascular volume.

VII. Endoscopic Sinus Surgery

A. Surgical drainage of chronic sinus infection can be performed endoscopically through the nose.

B. The liberal use of vasoconstrictors (cocaine, phenylephrine, oxymetazoline) to shrink edematous nasal mucosa can produce dramatic systemic side effects, such as hypertension, dysrhythmias, and pulmonary edema.

C. Some surgeons do not like to tape or cover the eyes for these cases so that rupture through the bony wall of the sinuses into the orbit can be more rapidly detected. This appears as periorbital ecchymosis, tenseness, and swelling.

D. Patients with cystic fibrosis make up a large portion of those receiving endoscopic sinus surgery.
   1. Cystic fibrosis is the most common lethal genetic disorder and is characterized by impaired mucus and electrolyte secretion.
   2. Airway obstruction by thick mucus, recurrent lung infections, and hypoxia characterize this disease.

   3. Thus careful pulmonary monitoring and avoidance of respiratory depression are especially important for these patients.

VIII. Epistaxis

A. Recurrent nose bleeds in pediatric patients are most commonly associated with compulsive nose picking, whereas adult epistaxis is usually related to hypertension.

B. Vasoconstrictors, nasal packing, and cauterization are usually adequate treatment for pediatric epistaxis with internal maxillary artery ligation reserved for unresponsive or more severe cases.

C. Nasal intubation frequently causes acute nose bleed, which can be reduced by preintubation (and postextubation) administration of vasoconstrictors.

   1. Selection of a nasotracheal tube one size smaller than would be used orally, copious lubrication, and use of steady, gentle pressure on insertion reduce epistaxis.

   2. Remember that the floor of the nasal cavity (adjacent to the widest airspace) is parallel to the roof of the mouth.

   3. Elevate the apex of the nose to bring the nares in line with the floor of the nasal cavity, and insert the tube straight in (not pointing upward toward the vascular turbinates).

   4. Consider the possibility of coagulopathy.

D. Nausea and vomiting are common when blood is swallowed.

IX. Cleft Lip and Palate Repair

A. These patients commonly have a history that includes aspiration, rhinorrhea, CSOM, growth retardation, or other congenital anomalies.

B. Dental impressions are sometimes obtained following intubation of a patient with a cleft palate in order to make a palatal prosthesis. The material used to make the impression can strongly adhere to the endotracheal tube, resulting in extubation when the impression is removed from the mouth.

C. Oral intubation is performed with a regular or oral RAE endotracheal tube secured in the middle of the mouth against the tongue with tape and the self-retaining oral retractor.

D. Kinking of the endotracheal tube, extubation, and endobronchial intubation are frequent occurrences, especially on insertion of the oral retractor.

E. Nasal intubation should not be performed because it inter- feres with the surgery. Further, patients who have previ- ously had palate surgery should not be nasally intubated for subsequent surgery because of the risk of trauma to the abnormal floor of the nasal cavity.

F. The laryngoscope blade can sometimes become lodged in a large cleft, making intubation difficult.

G. Excessive pressure exerted with the face mask can disrupt cleft lip skin sutures following extubation.

X. Pharyngeal Infections

A. Peritonsillar abscess
1. If the patient has trismus before induction, inadequate opening of the mouth can persist after administration of neuromuscular blocking drugs.
2. Use a smaller endotracheal tube than usual and be careful not to rupture the abscess.

B. Retropharyngeal abscess
1. May cause tracheal deviation.
2. This occurs almost exclusively in children because the lymph nodes atrophy in adults.
3. Surgical drainage is necessary to prevent airway obstruc- tion.
4. Rupture of abscess during intubation attempts can cause aspiration of infected material and fulminant pneu- monia.
5. In some instances, awake intubation or even tracheos- tomy with the patient under IV sedation is performed to reduce this risk.

C. Ludwig's angina (cellulitis of the floor of the mouth)
1. Frequently caused by bacterial infection from poor dental care
2. Progressive trismus, fever, drooling, and voice changes ("hot potato" voice)
3. Swollen tongue with posterior displacement
4. Laryngeal edema with progressive tachypnea, dyspnea, stridor, and cyanosis
5. Airway management includes consideration for an awake or fiberoptic intubation, or tracheostomy

D. Epiglottitis
1. Bacterial infection that can present as acute airway obstruction
   a. Usually caused by *Haemophilus influenzae* type B, although other organisms (streptococcus, staphylococ- cus) may be responsible

b. Symptoms of upper airway obstruction, dysphonia, dysphagia, drooling, and systemic sepsis (dehydration, fever) can be seen.

c. Severity of symptoms depends on the rapidity of the progression of the infection.

2. The incidence has significantly decreased since the development of a vaccine for *H. influenzae* type B

3. Protocols established by most hospitals delineate the management of these life-threatening airway emergencies with the anesthesia department

4. If the child is stable, x-rays are completed before transfer to the operating room

5. Management

a. Inhalation induction with insertion of an oral endotracheal tube

b. Emergency cricothyrotomy or tracheostomy if needed

c. IV hydration and antibiotic therapy

d. Sedatives as needed for postoperative ventilation and care

XI. Bronchoscopy or Laryngoscopy

A. Causes of airway obstruction in the pediatric patient include subglottic stenosis (frequently secondary to prolonged endotracheal intubation), laryngotracheomalacia, foreign bodies in the airway, laryngeal webs, laryngotracheal papillomatosis, tumors, abscesses, croup, and epiglottitis.

B. Bronchoscopy and laryngoscopy are used diagnostically as well as for part of the therapeutic management of many of these problems (i.e., laser laryngoscopy for laryngeal papillomas).

C. Other treatments include tracheostomy, laryngotracheal reconstruction (with cartilage harvested from the rib cage), and nebulization of racemic epinephrine.

D. Sharing the airway with the surgeon greatly adds to the complexity of these cases.

E. However, mandatory pulse oximetry has greatly improved the safety of these cases, reducing the incidence of cyanosis, bradycardia, and cardiac arrest caused by inadequate ventilation while the instruments are in the airway.

F. Oxygenation can be provided via the side arm of the rigid bronchoscope if the viewing end is occluded with a lens or a finger during positive pressure ventilation.

G. Larger patients can be intubated and ventilated with a

flexible bronchoscope passed through the endotracheal tube if the tube is large enough and the scope is small enough.

H. Apneic oxygenation (periods of hyperventilation with 100% oxygen interspersed with brief periods of bronchoscopy or laryngoscopy) can maintain acceptable saturation levels.

I. Adequate oxygenation can also be maintained by jet ventilation (with a Sander's ventilator).
1. Ventilatory rate is kept near normal, while the duration of the breath is guided by chest expansion and pulse oximetry.
2. Allowing adequate time for exhalation is essential for ventilation and perfusion (excessive intrathoracic pressure impedes venous return and cardiac output).

J. Inhaled anesthetics can be administered via a ventilating bronchoscope but not during apneic oxygenation or jet ventilation.
1. Nitrous oxide is avoided, and the depth of inhalational anesthesia can be unreliable.
2. Inadequate anesthesia can produce bronchospasm and dysrhythmias. IV agents, such as propofol, narcotics, and short- to intermediate-duration muscle relaxants, provide adequate depth while matching the duration of anesthesia to the duration of the procedure.

K. A foreign body in the airway can quickly cause death. Attempts to remove an object partially obstructing the airway can dislodge it to a location producing complete airway obstruction.
1. If prompt removal is impossible, pushing the object down into a mainstem bronchus may allow life-saving ventilation (only using 100% oxygen) of the opposite lung.
2. After removal of the foreign body, the airway should be reexamined with the bronchoscope for additional foreign bodies that may not have shown up on x-ray. Two coins side-by-side appear as only one on x-ray.

L. Direct laryngoscopy by the surgeon commonly uses a surgical laryngoscope to observe vocal cord movement (avoiding neuromuscular blockers) or to examine laryngeal anatomy.
1. When paralysis is needed, short- to intermediate-acting muscle relaxants are used with time to reversal minimized by using timing (giving the paralyzing drug immediately before the hypnotic agent) or priming (giv-

ing 5%–10% of the intubating dose 2–3 minutes before induction) techniques.

2. These techniques provide good intubating conditions rapidly while slightly reducing the intubating dosage.

M. Laser laryngoscopy for the removal of polyps or papillomas of the larynx or trachea usually contraindicates the use of nitrous oxide (which supports combustion) as well as oxygen concentrations greater than 30%.

1. The preferred technique for airway and ventilatory management for a specific case depends on factors including the size of the airway, degree of obstruction, location of lesions, and if a tracheostomy is already present.

2. Specially designed, flame-resistant endotracheal tubes with laser reflective wrapping and water-filled cuffs are available.

3. Additional techniques include the use of apneic oxygenation, jet ventilation, or metal tracheostomy tubes.

4. An IV anesthetic technique is helpful to ensure adequate anesthetic depth.

5. Neuromuscular blockade monitoring to ensure patient immobility reduces the risk of laser injury.

6. Avoid hitting or leaning on the operating room bed for any case using a microscope.

XII. Tumors of the Head and Neck

A. These masses can be benign or malignant based on their cell type but can be life threatening by obstructing or compressing the airway

B. Cystic hygroma

1. This congenital mass of the head and neck can extend into the mouth and displace the tongue, causing loss of airway and impeding intubation.

2. These tumors can be quite large and sometimes extend into the pleural cavity.

C. Thyroid and parathyroid tumors

1. Tumors of these endocrine glands are rare in children and are frequently malignant.

2. Softening of the underlying tracheal cartilages (laryngomalacia) can produce postoperative respiratory distress.

D. Hemangiomas

1. These blood-filled tumors can be quite large.

2. Resection can cause massive blood loss.

3. Preoperative type and match as well as blood consents should be in order before starting if indicated.

E. Neurofibromas

1. Multiple tumors are characteristic of von Recklinghausen disease and may reside in the nose, pharynx, or mediastinum.
2. Characterized by brown café au lait spots, this syndrome also has an increased risk of pheochromocytoma.
F. Branchial cleft cysts or fistulas
1. These tumors of embryologic origin are excised mainly for cosmetic reasons unless inflamed.
2. Their lateral location depends on the branchial cleft of origin occurring in preauricular sites or lower in the neck.
G. Thyroglossal duct cyst
1. This cyst is the most common type of midline neck mass in children and frequently involves the hyoid bone.
2. It is excised mainly because of swelling, external drainage, or infection.

XIII. Esophagoscopy or Gastroscopy

A. A common location for foreign bodies to lodge is at the bottom of the pharynx where the conical-shaped cricopharyngeal muscle narrows to begin the esophagus (at the level of the sixth cervical vertebra).
B. Endotracheal intubation is performed to protect the airway from aspiration before attempting to remove the foreign body. Tracheal compression or deviation can make intubation difficult so using a smaller-sized tube can ease insertion.

XIV. Tracheostomy

A. Elective tracheostomy with the patient anesthetized and intubated is much less stressful than when performed as an emergency.
1. After incising the trachea, the endotracheal tube is withdrawn just enough to make room for the tracheostomy tube.
2. Complete removal of the endotracheal tube is not performed until proper placement of the tracheostomy is verified by hearing bilateral breath sounds.
3. If the tracheostomy tube cannot be placed or enters a false passage, the endotracheal tube can be easily advanced to restore ventilation.
B. Emergency tracheostomy on a hypoxic patient with an obstructed airway is riskier and more difficult (because of factors such as patient movement, less time for hemostasis, and inadequate anesthesia).

Develop primary and alternative strategies:

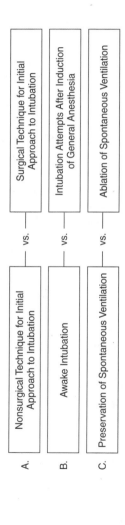

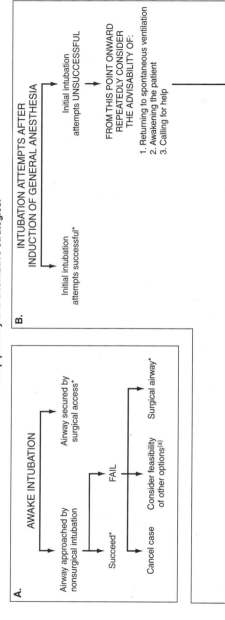

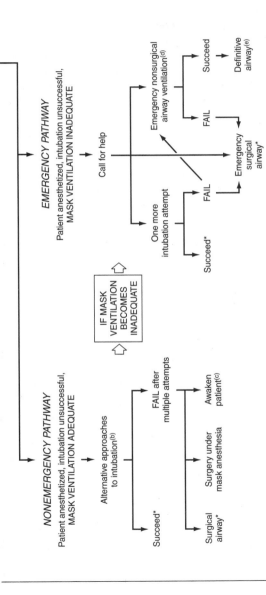

FIGURE 8–1. Difficult airway algorithm. (From American Society of Anesthesiologists Task Force on Management of the Difficult Airway. [1993]. *Anesthesiology, 597–602.*)

*CONFIRM INTUBATION WITH EXHALED CO_2.

(a) Other options include (but are not limited to) surgery under mask anesthesia, surgery under local anesthesia infiltration or regional nerve blockade, or intubation attempts after induction of general anesthesia.

(b) Alternative approaches to difficult intubation include (but are not limited to) use of different laryngoscope blades, awake intubation, blind oral or nasal intubation, fiberoptic intubation, intubating stylet or tube changer, light wand, retrograde intubation, and surgical airway access.

(c) See awake intubation.

(d) Options for emergency nonsurgical airway ventilation include (but are not limited to) transtracheal jet ventilation, laryngeal mask ventilation, or esophageal-tracheal combitube ventilation.

(e) Options for establishing a definitive airway include (but are not limited to) returning to awake state with spontaneous ventilation, tracheotomy, or endotracheal intubation.

NONEMERGENCY PATHWAY
Patient anesthetized, intubation unsuccessful, MASK VENTILATION ADEQUATE

Alternative approaches to intubation(b)

Succeed*

Surgical airway*

FAIL after multiple attempts

Surgery under mask anesthesia

Awaken patient(c)

IF MASK VENTILATION BECOMES INADEQUATE

EMERGENCY PATHWAY
Patient anesthetized, intubation unsuccessful, MASK VENTILATION INADEQUATE

Call for help

One more intubation attempt

Succeed*

FAIL

Emergency surgical airway*

Emergency nonsurgical airway ventilation(d)

Succeed

FAIL

Definitive airway(e)

1. Careful preoperative evaluation can reduce the need for emergency tracheotomy.
2. Anticipate difficult intubation and withhold neuromuscular blockers if there is doubt that the patient can be ventilated after paralysis.
3. The Difficult Airway Algorithm of the ASA contains alternative management techniques (e.g., flexible bronchoscope intubation, retrograde intubation, laryngeal mask airway) and should be reviewed by every anesthesia care provider. See Figure 8–1.

ADDITIONAL READINGS

Bridenbaugh, P.O., Cruz, M.E., & Helton, L.H. (1991). Anesthesia for otolaryngologic procedures. In Paperella, M.M., Shurick, D.A., Bluckman, J.L., & Meyerhoff, W. (Eds.). *Otolaryngology* (vol. 1, 3rd ed.). Philadelphia: W.B. Saunders.

Brown, A.C.D. (1997). Anesthesia. In Cummings, C.W., Fredrickson, J.M., Harker, L.A., et al. (Eds.). *Otolaryngology: Head and neck surgery* (vol. 1, 3rd ed.). St. Louis: Mosby.

Feinstein, R., & Owens, W.D. (1989). Anesthesia for ENT. In Barash, P.G., Cullen, B.F., & Stoelting, R.K. (Eds.). *Clinical anesthesia.* Philadelphia: J.B. Lippincott.

Kirk, G.A. (1993). Anesthesia for ear, nose and throat surgery. In Rogers, M.C., Tinker, J.H., Covino, B.G., & Longnecker, D.E. (Eds.). *Principles and practice of anesthesiology* (vol. 2). St. Louis: Mosby.

Parnass, S.M. (1993). Anesthesia considerations for ambulatory patients undergoing ear, nose and throat surgery. *Anesthesiology Clinics of North America,* 11(3), 525–545.

9

Anesthesia Considerations for Pediatric General Surgery and Gastrointestinal and Hepatobiliary Disease

Tim Palmer, MS, CRNA

I. Introduction

A. Gastrointestinal and hepatobiliary disease in the pediatric patient results from both congenital and acquired conditions.
   1. The most prominent etiologic factors in the neonatal period and infancy are in utero maldevelopment of the gastrointestinal (GI) tract, hypoxia, and other clinical insults secondary to premature birth and low birth weight.
   2. Other causes that may become manifest in later infancy and childhood include infectious disease processes and inflammatory lesions of uncertain etiology.
B. This chapter provides an overview of the most commonly encountered pediatric GI diseases associated with the need for surgical intervention. Basic and pertinent anesthetic considerations will also be elucidated.

II. General Considerations

A. There is a strong likelihood of the presence of concomitant disease processes as a result of prematurity or the presence of congenital anomalies. The special problems of the neonatal period and of the ex-preterm infant must be considered in planning anesthesia care.
B. Optimal preparation of the patient may not be able to be accomplished because of the emergent nature of the lesion. Thus the resuscitative process will need to be continued perioperatively and will likely be further complicated by the stress of anesthesia and surgery.
C. In emergency surgery, full stomach considerations are warranted.

1. Even if there has been no oral intake for a period of time, gastric secretions accumulate and transit times of GI contents will be slowed or halted in the presence of GI obstruction or ileus.
2. Other disease processes (e.g., respiratory failure, cardiac disease) are associated with delayed gastric emptying.
3. For these reasons, awake intubation may be indicated after evacuation of gastric contents and preoxygenation.
4. Rapid sequence induction with cricoid pressure is indicated for older children with acute abdominal disease and prior intravenous (IV) line placement.
    a. This may be accomplished without precurarization (in children less than 10 years of age).
    b. Succinylcholine does not increase intraabdominal pressure in this age-group.

D. Patients requiring relatively minor procedures may have associated pathologic conditions as a result of congenital maldevelopment (e.g., renal, cardiac, or central nervous disorders) necessitating consideration in anesthesia planning.

E. For major procedures (e.g., major abdominal surgery), considerable blood loss is possible. This may have a profound influence on perioperative management, particularly in the presence of preexisting anemia (i.e., in the neonate or premature infant).

F. Placement of IV lines should preferentially be established in the upper extremities because of possible occlusion of the inferior vena cava by retraction of abdominal viscera. Central vascular access may be necessary in the high-risk or severely compromised patient.

G. Optimal communication must be maintained among members of the interdisciplinary care team (i.e., surgeon, anesthetist, neonatologist, postanesthesia recovery staff, intensive care nursing staff).

III. Surgical Disorders of the GI Tract

A. Congenital diaphragmatic hernia
1. Congenital diaphragmatic hernia results from a failure of the pleuroperitoneal canals to separate during embryologic development, allowing herniation of abdominal contents into the pleural cavity (incidence of 1:4000 live births)
2. A variable degree of impaired lung development may be present
3. Pulmonary hypertension may complicate management and may be refractory to therapy

4. Other associated anomalies may include cardiac structural defects (20%) and malrotation of the gut (40%). Additional anomalies may affect the upper airway or the renal or neurologic systems
5. Surgical correction
   a. Congenital diaphragmatic hernia constitutes a surgical emergency.
   b. Closure of the diaphragmatic defect with placement of abdominal viscera back into the abdominal cavity is necessary.
   c. Primary repair is undertaken or a staged procedure is elected if the abdominal cavity is too small.
6. Anesthetic considerations
   a. Prevention of further intrathoracic distention during controlled ventilation performed via passage of a gastric tube and maintenance on low suction
   b. Correction of hypoxemia and acidosis as indicated
   c. Avoid positive pressure mask ventilation to prevent further bowel distention and respiratory distress
   d. Awake intubation with controlled ventilation (100% O_2) preferred
   e. Prevention of pneumothorax by controlled ventilation and reduction of inspiratory pressures
   f. Adequate neuromuscular blockade necessary following intubation
   g. Minimize oxygen demand by maintaining adequate depth of anesthesia and neuromuscular blockade and avoiding hypothermia
7. Anesthetic technique
   a. If the patient is not already intubated, an awake intubation is performed (post-GI decompression) followed by a smooth anesthetic induction (i.e., volatile agent or opioids).
   b. After intubation, use low inspiratory pressures (25–30 cm H_2O) with high ventilatory rates.
   c. If pneumothorax is suspected (hemodynamic and ventilatory deterioration) a contralateral chest tube should be inserted.
   d. Low concentrations of inhalation anesthetics may be employed with high inspired FIO_2. High-dose opioids are also acceptable. Selection of the technique depends on the patient's stability and hemodynamic status.
   e. Avoid N_2O, which can cause further abdominal visceral expansion.

    f. Monitor blood gases, acid-base values, and hematologic parameters; correct as indicated.

8. Postoperative concerns

    a. Extubate when ventilatory parameters are satisfactory and patient is completely awake. Blood gases also must be optimal.

    b. Maintain normothermia (i.e., via incubator).

    c. Maintain gastric suction until distention abates.

    d. Closely monitor fluid intake, urine output, and blood gases (i.e., acid-base $A/a\ DO_2$).

    e. Persistent hypoxemia and acidosis may require continuation of endotracheal intubation and positive end expiratory pressure (PEEP) and high-frequency oscillatory ventilation with 100% O_2 with pulmonary vasodilator therapy (tolazoline, prostaglandin E_1, isoproterenol, glucagon, sodium nitroprusside, calcium channel blockers).

    f. With continued respiratory failure, extracorporeal membrane oxygenation (ECMO) may be employed to support infants who remain refractory to more conventional therapies.

B. Esophageal atresia and tracheoesophageal fistula

1. Esophageal atresia and tracheoesophageal fistula are congenital anomalies that commonly occur together with an incidence of 1:4000 live births

2. Both lesions occur from incomplete separation of the lung bud from the foregut during embryologic development

3. A typical presentation in the infant is variable impairment in respiratory function

4. Associated anomalies (e.g., various cardiac defects) are often seen. The term *VATER* has been used to describe usual associated anomalies: (V) vertebral, (A) anal, (T) tracheoesophageal fistula, (E) esophageal atresia, (R) radial or renal anomalies. Thus anesthetic planning must generally include issues related to prematurity and presence of additional GI and renal abnormalities

5. Surgical correction

    a. Primary repair: ligation of the fistula and esophageal anastomosis

    b. Staged repair: gastrostomy with fistula diversion and latex repair of the esophagus

6. Anesthetic considerations

    a. Prevention of aspiration.

  b. Avoidance of fistula intubation.
  c. Monitoring of ventilatory inspiratory pressures.
  d. Avoidance of high inspiratory pressure.
  e. Correction of fluid and hemodynamic perturbations or continuation of resuscitative efforts (i.e., oxygen-carrying capacity, acid-base, electrolytes).
  f. Optimal fluid balance (i.e., intake and output) is of major importance, keeping in mind that neonatal fluid requirements are low in the first 24-hour period. Electrolyte depletion may not be seen during this time.
  g. Maintain upright position before induction.
  h. Awake suctioning of the proximal pouch is performed before intubation.
  i. For awake intubation, bevel of the endotracheal tube faces posteriorly (to avoid fistula intubation).
  j. Deliberate right mainstem intubation is initially performed. The endotracheal tube is then retracted until equal bilateral breath sounds are ensured, at which point the tube is secured.
  k. After intubation, assessment of inspiratory pressures is mandatory. Excessive pressures may indicate assessment of lip level of the endotracheal tube and possible reintubation.
  l. Anesthesia technique may employ a volatile anesthetic (i.e., isoflurane) combined with IV opioids.
  m. Spontaneous ventilation may be permitted with N_2O, O_2, and isoflurane until the chest is open. The fistula is ligated promptly.
  n. Observe for excessive stomach distention. With stomach distention, discontinue N_2O.
  o. If spontaneous ventilation is inadequate before thoracotomy, institute careful assisted or controlled ventilation.
  p. Administer a muscle relaxant once the chest is open. Control ventilation.
  q. Careful monitoring of inspiratory pressures is warranted.
7. Postoperative concerns
  a. Awake extubation is indicated.
  b. If the infant is lacking vigorous movement and inadequate ventilatory parameters, continue controlled ventilation.
  c. Careful oropharyngeal suctioning is necessary. The

suction catheter must not come close to the anastomosis (to prevent damage).

    d. The catheter distance marking on the oropharyngeal suction catheter must be recorded for future reference.

    e. Usual supportive measures are maintained (i.e., fluid balance, normothermia, nutrient needs, and correction of acid-base and hematologic and electrolyte abnormalities).

8. Later complications
   a. Tracheal diverticulum
   b. Tracheomalacia

9. A staged repair will involve initial placement of a gastrostomy. Otherwise, the same anesthetic considerations apply

C. Necrotizing enterocolitis

1. Necrotizing enterocolitis is a leading cause of neonatal and infantile mortality.

2. The cause is multifactorial; it classically occurs in premature, low–birth weight infants (incidence 4%–7%).

3. The disease represents an ischemia-reperfusion injury subsequent to birth stress. Necrosis of the gut may be localized or involve the entire GI tract.

4. This occurs because of decreased mesenteric blood flow secondary to decreased cardiac output and perinatal asphyxia or hypoxia.

5. Other associated anomalies involving other organ systems must be taken into account in the anesthetic plan. These often include cardiac structural anomalies, bronchopulmonary dysplasia, as well as other organ system derangements from prematurity.

6. Surgical correction.
   a. Resection of the involved intestinal segments with reanastomosis
   b. Possible gastrostomy, ileostomy, or colostomy

7. Anesthetic considerations.
   a. Continuation and modification of hematologic and fluid volume resuscitation may be necessary.
      (1) Fluid requirements may increase to 125 to 150 ml/kg/d in the presence of peritonitis.
      (2) Decreased platelets ($50,000–70,000/mm^3$) and prolonged prothrombin time (PT) and activated partial thromboplastin time (APTT) are common.
   b. Correction of acid-base and electrolyte derangements is essential because infants may be severely compro-

mised as a result of ileus, vomiting, diarrhea (mucoid or bloody), and gastric suctioning.

    c. Gastric decompression may need to be initiated before anesthetic induction.

    d. Optimal respiratory function is established or maintained, with consideration for an awake intubation (if not previously intubated). There is a possible need for high inspiratory pressures and PEEP.

    e. Correction of hypothermia and the maintenance of normothermia are essential.

    f. Induction and maintenance of anesthesia may be achieved with low concentrations of isoflurane, desflurane, or sevoflurane with an air/O_2 mixture.

    g. N_2O is avoided to prevent expansion of intraluminal bowel gas.

    h. Anticipate that some antibiotics may prolong the action of muscle relaxants.

    i. Opioids (e.g., fentanyl) are suitable anesthetic adjuvants.

    j. Perioperative fluid volume resuscitation is monitored and modified by laboratory studies and the clinical picture.

  8. Postoperative concerns.

    a. The infant is returned to the neonatal intensive care unit (ICU) for continued hemodynamic and respiratory support.

D. Omphalocele and gastroschisis

  1. Omphalocele: a herniation of the intestine into the base of the umbilical cord

    a. The defect is variable in size.

    b. An amnion-covered sac contains the exposed viscera.

    c. Incidence is 1:6000 to 1:10,000 live births.

  2. Gastroschisis: a defect of the abdominal wall on the right lateral aspect of the umbilicus through which a variable amount of abdominal viscera protrudes

    a. No sac or membrane covers the defect.

    b. Incidence is 1:30,000 live births.

  3. Omphalocele is associated with a high occurrence of associated anomalies

  4. In contrast, gastroschisis has less incidence of concurrent anomalies, but its presence suggests a likelihood of intrauterine growth retardation and intestinal atresia

  5. Associated conditions

    a. GI malformations

    b. Genitourinary (GU) anomalies

      c. Craniofacial anomalies associated with Beckwith-Wiedemann syndrome (macroglossia, macrosomia, organomegaly)

      d. Cardiac structural maldevelopments

6. Anesthetic considerations

      a. Significant to severe fluid and electrolyte disturbances may be present; possibly hypovolemic shock. Corrective measures are undertaken.

      b. Fluid requirements may be high (up to 150 ml/kg/d) and require the addition of colloid (Plasmanate or albumin).

      c. Blood transfusion may be necessary (100–250 ml of packed red blood cells [PRBCs] should be available).

      d. There is a high incidence of thermoregulatory instability, and therefore warming measures should be instituted. These include increasing ambient room temperature, using heating lamps and forced-air warming blankets, and warming IV fluids.

      e. There is an increased incidence of respiratory instability with aspiration risk.

         (1) The patient is kept semiupright during induction and intubation.

         (2) Gastric decompression is performed before induction.

         (3) Awake intubation is indicated.

      f. High controlled inspiratory ventilatory pressures may be necessary because of impaired diaphragmatic function and increased intraabdominal pressure (bowel distention).

      g. Glucose infusion is initiated in the presence of hypoglycemia (<40 mg/dl).

         (1) Infusion of $D_{10}W$ 2 ml/kg bolus or 8 to 10 mg/kg/min

         (2) Serial glucose measurements monitored perioperatively

      h. Anesthetic technique may include a volatile anesthetic agent (i.e., isoflurane, desflurane, sevoflurane, or halothane) with O_2 and air with an adjunctive opioid.

      i. N_2O is avoided to prevent further bowel distention.

      j. Reduced doses of muscle relaxants are administered.

7. Postoperative concerns

      a. Maintenance of optimal ventilation and oxygenation may require continued controlled ventilation if spontaneous ventilation is inadequate.

      b. Continue supportive measures for fluid and electrolyte resuscitation: hemodynamic stability, restitution of normothermia, and continued gastric decompression.

E. Intestinal obstruction

  1. Duodenal atresia and stenosis are the disease processes responsible for intestinal obstruction

     a. Both diseases occur with equal frequency (1:10,000–1:40,000 live births).

     b. Duodenal atresias result from abnormal canalization of the gut in utero.

     c. The degree of obstruction may be partial to complete.

     d. Polyhydramnios is common in utero.

     e. Associated conditions.

       (1) Cardiac malformations

       (2) Chromosomal abnormalities (e.g., Down syndrome)

       (3) Cystic fibrosis

       (4) GU abnormalities

       (5) Intestinal malrotation, midline defects (e.g., imperforate anus, esophageal atresia), and other GI atretic areas

  2. Jejunoileal atresia

     a. Caused by abnormal canalization of the jejunum or ileum or both in utero

     b. Associated with fewer congenital defects

     c. Polyhydramnios in utero is a common finding, thus contributing to the typical finding of fetal growth retardation seen in infants with this condition

  3. Malrotation and volvulus

     a. Caused by failure of the normal processes of rotation and fixation of the intestinal tract during embryologic development.

     b. Areas of atresia and ischemia develop secondary to twisting of untethered bowel on its mesenteric pedicle with eventual strangulation of the involved segment (volvulus).

     c. Signs and symptoms of intestinal obstruction usually occur 1 or 2 months after birth; however, the possibility for developing this affliction may persist throughout childhood.

     d. Omphalocele and gastroschisis as well as congenital diaphragmatic hernia have been associated with malrotation and volvulus.

4. Intussusception
    a. A length of bowel invaginates into an adjoining segment.
    b. Peristaltic movement contributes to an increasing amount of intestine entering into the intussusception along with its accompanying mesentery.
    c. Eventual luminal closure occurs as well as vascular compromise with ultimate infarction of the involved segment.
    d. The area most at risk is the ileocolic region.
    e. Initial reduction of this condition may be accomplished via sigmoidoscopy with later definitive surgical resection of the involved segment.
5. Anesthetic considerations
    a. Patients may present with symptoms consistent with "acute abdomen" indicated by
        (1) Abdominal distention with or without pain
        (2) Hypovolemia; possible acid-base and electrolyte imbalance
        (3) Lethargy
        (4) Possible fever
        (5) Absent or hyperresonant bowel sounds
    b. Astute preoperative assessment of serum electrolytes, urine output, and volume status is warranted; corrective measures are initiated. Preoperative IV access should be established.
    c. Rapid sequence induction with cricoid pressure is warranted.
    d. Thermal stability is maintained, and resuscitative measures are continued, with modifications based on intraoperative clinical changes.
    e. Anesthesia technique includes a volatile agent, O_2/air, an opioid, and a nondepolarizing muscle relaxant.
    f. Extubation is performed with the patient fully awake and preferably in the lateral position.
6. Postoperative concerns
    a. Provision for postoperative analgesia (e.g., epidural, intrathecal, or parenteral opioids)
    b. Maintenance IV fluids (continue corrective or resuscitative plan as indicated)
F. Meconium syndromes
    1. Meconium ileus
        a. Occurs almost exclusively in patients with cystic fibrosis

b. An obstructive process caused by development of a thick tenacious meconium impaction of usually the distal ileum, which results from a deficiency in pancreatic enzyme secretion

c. Nonsurgical therapy consists of instillation of hyperosmolar contrast enemas. If medical management is ineffective, laparotomy with possible bowel resection is performed

2. Meconium plug syndrome
   a. Unrelated to meconium ileus; diagnosed when the neonate fails to pass meconium within 24 hours of life.
   b. As in meconium ileus, initial management may be employed first (i.e., hyperosmolar contrast enemas) with the goal of passage of meconium and relief of the obstruction.
   c. Of major concern is the possible presence of aganglionic colon (i.e., Hirschsprung disease) that is associated with this condition.

3. Meconium peritonitis
   a. Occurs secondary to obstruction and perforation of the GI tract
   b. Most common cause: presence of meconium ileus
   c. Free meconium in the peritoneal cavity induces fibrous adhesion formation about the perforation, which may form a pseudocyst

4. Anesthetic considerations
   a. Vomiting, diarrhea, fever, and inability to take feedings predispose the infant to fluid, electrolyte, and metabolic derangements warranting corrective IV resuscitation measures.
   b. Gastric decompression is performed before awake intubation and induction of anesthesia.
   c. Severe abdominal distention may impinge on ventilatory mechanics and oxygenation.
   d. Other anesthetic considerations are consistent with those relevant to acute abdomen and bowel obstruction.

5. Postoperative concerns
   a. Ventilatory support and resuscitative measures may need to continue
   b. Controlled or assisted ventilation in the presence of ineffective spontaneous efforts
   c. Restoration of volume and metabolic homeostasis
   d. Provision for analgesic needs

G. Aganglionic megacolon (Hirschsprung disease)
1. Results from a congenital absence of ganglionic cells in the myenteric and submucosal plexuses of the gut (1:5000–1:8000 incidence).
2. The subsequent loss of parasympathetic mediated peristalsis and constriction of the involved segment result in neurogenic intestinal obstruction.
3. Most commonly the rectum and sigmoid are involved, but aganglionosis may extend beyond (15%–25% of cases) and involve the entire colon (10% of cases).
4. Associated conditions.
   a. Cardiac, renal, central nervous system (CNS) anomalies (5%–21% of cases)
   b. Down syndrome (most common; 5% of cases)
5. Definitive surgical correction involves one of a number of laparotomy/pull-through procedures involving resection of the involved segment and reapproximating innervated intestine to the anus.
6. Anesthetic considerations.
   a. Preoperative stabilization or resuscitative efforts are continued, including measures directed toward
      (1) Fluid and electrolyte balance
      (2) Nasogastric decompression
      (3) Antibiotic coverage
   b. A low incidence of prematurity (8%) reflects less possibility of the presence of bronchopulmonary dysplasia. Abdominal distention, however, may be present, warranting appropriate induction and intubation precautions (i.e., gastric decompression before awake intubation).
   c. Other considerations in the intraoperative and postoperative periods are consistent with those employed for acute abdomen and bowel obstruction.
H. Imperforate anus
1. Imperforate anus results from a failure of the intestinal tract to reach the perineum and form a patent anal opening with adequate sphincter control (1:5000 live births).
2. Associated conditions.
   a. GU anomalies (most common)
   b. Vertebral malformation
   c. VACTERL syndrome (vertebral, anal, cardiac, tracheal, esophageal, radial, renal, limb defects)
   d. Chromosomal defects (Down syndrome, trisomy 18)
3. Surgical correction involves construction of the anal

opening with possible bowel resection and temporary colostomy.

4. Anesthetic considerations.
   a. Correction of intravascular volume and electrolyte and metabolic derangements
   b. Particular attention is directed toward possible hypoglycemia (parenteral replacement of glucose, 4–6 mg/kg/min).
   c. Other supportive measures are employed as clinically indicated.
   d. Anesthetic technique and considerations for perioperative care are consistent with those for the patient with bowel obstruction.

I. Pyloric stenosis
   1. Condition in which gross thickening about the circular smooth muscle of the pylorus causes gradual obstruction of the gastric outlet.
   2. The infant is generally 2 to 4 weeks of age and presents with nonbilious projectile vomiting and intolerance of feedings.
   3. Surgical correction involves pyloromyotomy to relieve the stricture.
   4. Anesthetic considerations.
      a. Pyloric stenosis is not a surgical emergency but may be a medical emergency necessitating aggressive IV resuscitation of the hypovolemic or dehydrated patient.
      b. Acid-base disturbances, particularly hypochloremic metabolic acidosis with hypokalemia, may be present because of the loss of electrolyte-rich gastric juices from vomiting.
      c. Preoperative management consists of IV correction of volume and electrolyte deficiencies and continuous gastric decompression.
      d. The airway is secured either by awake endotracheal intubation or rapid-sequence induction.
      e. Pyloromyotomy is a relatively short procedure, and thus short-acting muscle relaxants and newer insoluble volatile anesthetics (i.e., desflurane or sevoflurane) may be useful.
      f. Extubation of the trachea is performed after gastric suctioning and when the infant is fully awake.

J. Gastroesophageal reflux
   1. Common in neurologically impaired infants and children.
   2. The etiology is lower esophageal sphincter incompetence

predisposing to increased risk of regurgitation and aspiration.

3. Besides neurologic impairment (e.g., cerebral palsy) other conditions associated with gastroesophageal reflux include chronic pulmonary disease, esophageal atresia, repair of abdominal wall defects, congenital diaphragmatic hernia repair, and tracheoesophageal fistula repair.

4. Surgical repair consists of an antireflux procedure (e.g., Nissen fundoplication) with gastrostomy.

5. Anesthetic considerations.

   a. Preoperative correction of volume and electrolyte perturbations is undertaken.

   b. Head-up position is maintained until gastric decompression is performed and the airway is definitively sealed.

   c. Postoperative support of ventilation may be necessary in patients with preexisting lung disease or neurologic impairment.

   d. Medical therapy for reflux includes H_2 antagonists, metoclopramide, bethanecol (to increase LES tone), and antisialagogues.

K. Appendicitis

1. One of the most common causes of an acute condition in the abdomen in the child.

2. Generally not associated with congenital anomalies.

3. The pathologic mechanism usually involves obstruction of the base of the appendix by a fecalith, thus causing a closed-loop blockage of the vascular supply with resultant infarction and necrosis.

4. Appendiceal perforation allows for the release of bacterial flora and endotoxin into the peritoneal cavity, resulting in peritonitis.

5. Differential diagnosis should exclude the presence of pyelonephritis, pelvic inflammatory disease, gastroenteritis, or inflammatory bowel disease.

6. Anesthetic considerations.

   a. A major consideration involves the child's fluid and electrolyte status.

   b. Dehydration may be present because of vomiting, diarrhea, anorexia, and fever (fluids should be increased 12% for every 1°C elevation of temperature above normal).

   c. Aggressive fluid and hemodynamic management may be necessary in the presence of peritonitis caused by appendiceal perforation.

      d. In the case of severe illness and peritonitis, anesthetic considerations will be consistent with those for the child with an acute condition in the abdomen.

L. Inguinal hernia, hydrocele, and undescended testis
1. Inguinal hernia repair is the most common elective procedure performed in the pediatric age-group.
    a. Inguinal hernia is caused by a persistence of all or part of the processus vaginalis.
    b. The major risk factor in inguinal hernia is incarceration and strangulation of a loop of bowel within the hernia sac.
2. Hydroceles are collections of peritoneal fluid located anywhere within the course of the processus vaginalis.
    a. The condition is variable in presentation and may mimic an incarcerated inguinal hernia.
3. Cryptorchidism or undescended testis occurs in 1% to 2% of term males, with a higher incidence in preterm infants.
    a. A prominent concern in this condition is not only the potential for infarction of the testis but also a forty-fold higher incidence of testicular carcinoma noted in the undescended testis.
    b. This condition may be accompanied by the presence of an inguinal hernia. The incidence of inguinal hernia and associated abnormalities is increased in preterm infants.
4. Anesthetic considerations.
    a. In the normal, healthy child, surgery may be performed on an outpatient basis.
    b. In the case of bowel incarceration, torsion of entrapped contents with infarction, and other symptomatic evidence of an acute condition in the abdomen, anesthetic care is guided by the concurrent provision for fluid and electrolyte resuscitation, a patent sealed airway, and other supportive measures.

M. Umbilical hernia
1. Occurs because of a defect in the umbilical ring through which a peritoneal sac covered by umbilical skin protrudes.
2. Surgical repair is indicated for a large defect or one that fails to close by 5 years of age.
3. Umbilical herniorraphy is a relatively simple elective procedure that shares essentially the same perioperative considerations and prognosis as inguinal herniorraphy.

N. Inflammatory bowel disease

1. Crohn's disease is a transmural inflammation of the intestine generally affecting the right colon and distal ileum.
   a. It usually affects the small intestine but may affect any part of the GI tract.
   b. Affected areas are usually discontinuous with skip areas.
2. Ulcerative colitis is a diffuse continuous inflammatory disease affecting primarily the mucosal lining of the colon and rectum.
   a. A higher predilection for females is noted in ulcerative colitis.
   b. The causes of both diseases are unknown, although an immunologic defect is suspected in ulcerative colitis.
3. Anesthetic considerations.
   a. Children with Crohn's disease usually have signs and symptoms consisting of growth retardation, abdominal pain, diarrhea, and strictures, which cause intestinal obstruction.
   b. The child with ulcerative colitis usually presents with bloody diarrhea with or without abdominal pain.
   c. Significant metabolic and intravascular volume deficits may be present as well as anemia.
   d. The child with ulcerative colitis may be at risk for the development of toxic megacolon, a surgical emergency.
   e. Toxic megacolon is an acute obstructive process with a high risk of perforation and a high associated mortality (20%–30%).
   f. The potential for malignant transformation of the mucosa also prompts removal of the involved mucosa (proctocolectomy) with construction of a permanent ileostomy. This is usually a curative procedure.
   g. The child with Crohn's disease may require repeated procedures for resection of the involved segment.
   h. Anemia seen in inflammatory bowel disease is usually a result of iron deficiency secondary to inadequate absorption of folate and vitamin B_{12} (i.e., with disease involvement or resection of the terminal ileum).
   i. No specific anesthetic is indicated; however, it is best advised to manage the patient similar to considerations given for acute abdominal disease.

j. Measures for restoration of adequate hemoglobin content and acid-base balance are also indicated.

O. Neoplastic disease

1. Wilm's tumor (nephroblastoma)
   a. Most common abdominal childhood neoplasm
   b. Usually detected as an abdominal mass during pre-school development
   c. The renal mass may be localized or extensive, involving other structures
   d. Usually unilateral but may involve the contralateral kidney
   e. Surgical therapy: radical nephrectomy with lymphadenectomy followed by chemotherapy

2. Anesthetic considerations
   a. Wilm's tumor may be associated with other congenital anomalies.
   b. It may be asymptomatic or be associated with anemia, fever, hypertension, weight loss, and hematuria.
   c. Pulmonary function may be compromised because of metastatic disease or abdominal distention.
   d. An anesthetic plan should be devised to account for possible perturbations in metabolic, hematologic, and intravascular volume status.
   e. Massive blood loss is possible intraoperatively. Have available at least two crossmatched units. Transfuse when warranted (hemoglobin [Hgb] <8.0).
   f. Retraction may compromise cardiac preload with consequent decreased cardiac output.
   g. Hypertension may be severe. Treat with increasing concentration of volatile agent or opioid (IV) and other therapies as indicated (e.g., infused IV vasodilators, angiotensin-converting enzyme [ACE] inhibitors).
   h. Postoperative ventilation with sedation, adequate analgesia, and antihypertensive therapy may be necessary.
   i. Possible intrathecal or epidural analgesia may serve as a useful adjuvant.

P. Polypoid diseases

1. Usually diagnosed later in childhood
2. Polyps arise from the mucosal surface of the colon and may be localized or part of a polyposis syndrome.
3. More common polypoid syndromes
   a. Juvenile polyposis syndrome: associated with a high

likelihood of adenomatous polyp development (considered premalignant)
  b. Familial polyposis syndromes
    (1) Gardner syndrome
    (2) Turcot syndrome
    (3) Preutz-Jegher syndrome
  4. Anesthetic considerations
    a. Long-term rectal bleeding (the primary diagnostic clinical presentation) may dispose the patient to anemia.
    b. Other complications include weight loss (i.e., cachexia) and bowel obstruction or intussusception.
    c. Anesthesia for polypectomy will usually be via general anesthesia.
    d. Provisions in the anesthesia plan must accommodate possible anemia, hypoalbuminemia, and hypovolemia.
    e. Colectomy is usually reserved for refractory disease or complications (disease related or iatrogenic).

IV. Diseases of the Spleen

  A. Numerous syndromes, notably those involving perturbations in metabolic processes (i.e., inborn errors of metabolism) may include splenic dysfunction as part of their clinical appearance.
  B. Examples.
    1. Anderson disease (hepatosplenomegaly)
    2. Cori disease (hepatosplenomegaly)
    3. Hunter syndrome (hepatosplenomegaly)
    4. Hurler syndrome (hepatosplenomegaly)
    5. Ivemark syndrome (splenic agenesis)
  C. Splenic dysfunction may be a morbid secondary manifestation caused by a primary biochemical defect in another related organ (i.e., the liver), or it may be a defining characteristic of a given syndrome.
  D. Syndromes involving defective hematologic or immunologic system function that are noted to present in the presence of splenic disease include
    1. Blackfan-Diamond syndrome (hepatosplenomegaly)
    2. Letterer-Siwe disease (lymphocytic hepatosplenic infiltration)
    3. Moschcowitz disease (thrombotic thrombocytopenic purpura)
  E. Other more familiar disease processes that are definitively managed via splenectomy include idiopathic thrombocyto-

penic purpura, hereditary spherocytosis, and thalassemia (with hypersplenism).

F. As part of the reticuloendothelial system, the spleen assumes a prominent role in the clearance of bacteria and aged or defective erythrocytes and platelets from the blood.

G. Thus a more conservative approach is considered that may involve partial splenectomy and, in the case of blunt trauma to the spleen, primary repair.

H. Anomalies in other organ systems (e.g., cardiac, CNS, pulmonary) are often present; thus the incidence of surgical morbidity and mortality is increased as well as the complexity of anesthetic management.

I. Anesthetic considerations.
  1. Assess the patient's coagulation status, platelet count, and oxygen-carrying capacity (i.e., hematocrit and hemoglobin).
     a. With splenomegaly or hypersplenism, thrombocytopenia and anemia may be present as well as deficits in coagulation factors.
     b. Correction of a low hemoglobin level and platelet count should take place after removal of the spleen.
  2. Other metabolic studies should be assessed (i.e., acid-base status, serum glucose) and correction of deficiencies undertaken.
  3. Many patients are receiving long-term steroid therapy. Thus they should receive supplemental preoperative steroid coverage.
  4. Pneumococcal vaccine should be administered to those requiring elective total splenectomy.
  5. Trauma to the mucosa of the airway should be avoided to prevent upper airway bleeding and edema.

V. Hepatic Tumors

A. Hemangiomas comprise the most common pediatric hepatic tumor. Other types include
  1. Mesenchymal hamartoma
  2. Hemangioendotheliomas

B. Malignant hepatic tumors include
  1. Hepatoblastoma
  2. Hepatocellular carcinoma

C. Hepatocellular carcinoma usually affects older children and adolescents and is associated with a preexisting syndrome of liver dysfunction:
  1. Biliary atresia
  2. Wilson disease

3. Giant cell hepatitis
4. Hypoplastic disease of the intrahepatic bile ducts
5. Von Gierke disease

D. Anesthetic considerations
1. Children presenting with hepatoblastoma infrequently show ascites, jaundice, or anemia.
2. These symptoms are usually present along with fever and lethargy in patients with hepatocellular carcinoma.
3. Basic perioperative considerations include the potential for massive blood loss with concurrent perturbations in coagulation.
4. Disturbances in oncotic intravascular pressure may need to be considered. Modification in the dosages of highly protein bound drugs is warranted to prevent exaggerated responses.
5. Airway considerations are paramount and include aspiration precautions, decreased ventilatory compliance, shunting, and increased inspiratory pressures as a result of ascites. There is a strong likelihood of needing postoperative ventilatory support.
6. Hemodynamic support may require full invasive monitoring (a high cardiac output and low systemic vascular resistance are common in chronic hepatic disease).

VI. Sacrococcygeal Teratoma

A. Usually benign tumors composed of tissues derived from embryologic germ layers
B. May be solid or cystic
C. The size of the tumor along with its position may cause obstruction of the GU and GI tracts
D. Most teratomas are diagnosed late in the second or third trimester.
E. Other anomalies will often be present (18%), including anorectal anomalies, spina bifida, and other musculoskeletal abnormalities
F. Anesthetic considerations
1. The infant may likely be positioned prone for corrective resection.
2. In some cases arteriovenous shunting within the tumor may cause high-output cardiac failure and consumptive coagulopathy.

VII. Neuroblastoma

A. An embryonal tumor arising from neural crest cells.
B. High incidence in the adrenal medulla.

C. Another 25% arise intraabdominally, with the rest arising from the mediastinum, neck, and pelvis.
D. Involvement of the spinal cord is common.
E. Metastases are usually found in the liver, bone marrow, and bone cortex and within the eye orbit.
F. Metabolically active products are often expressed (i.e., catecholamines, catecholamine metabolites, vasoactive intestinal peptide, ferritin).
G. Signs and symptoms may mimic pheochromocytoma or carcinoid syndrome.
H. Anesthetic considerations.
   1. Massive blood loss is possible.
   2. Possible increased catecholamine levels warrant judicious use of vasodilators and antihypertensives.
   3. Have available
      a. Labetalol
      b. Esmolol
      c. Phentolamine
      d. Sodium nitroprusside (for infusion)
      e. Propranolol
      f. Other adjunctive antihypertensives: hydralazine, captopril, fenoldapam, clonidine
   4. Maintenance of an adequate plane of anesthesia via balanced volatile agent–opioid technique is most appropriate.
   5. Prepare for the possible need for invasive hemodynamic monitoring (i.e., arterial line; central venous pressure [CVP] line).
   6. Monitor blood electrolytes and glucose.
   7. Aggressive hydration may be needed to maintain adequate urine output (0.5–1 ml/kg/h) and CVP (9–11 cm H_2O).
   8. Avoid drugs that may induce an increased release of catecholamines (e.g., succinylcholine) or sensitize the myocardium to their activity (e.g., halothane).

VIII. Rhabdomyosarcoma

A. A soft tissue, highly malignant tumor typically found in the lower GI tract, perineal area, bile duct, head and neck
B. In adolescence, it is more commonly found peripherally and in the uterus. No tumor markers are known
C. Anesthesic considerations
   1. The anesthesia plan must consider the extent of the disease and the degree of system decompensation present.
   2. For patients with stage III or IV disease (distant metastases) the prognosis is poor.

3. These patients may present for any number of palliative procedures or those to establish adequate access for pain control and chemotherapy.
4. The anesthetic plan must accommodate the diminished metabolic and hemodynamic reserves of these patients.

D. Early detection with aggressive excision and follow-up therapy (i.e., chemotherapy) has shown encouraging results

IX. Biliary Tract Disease

A. Jaundice in the neonatal period is common and considered physiologic. Its cause is an immaturity in bilirubin conjugation (glucronyl transferase deficiency)
B. Beyond 2 weeks of age it is considered pathologic.
C. The persistence of unconjugated bilirubin is attributed to hemolytic disorders (Rh and ABO incompatibility or hereditary spherocytosis)
D. Causes of biliary obstruction
   1. Biliary atresia or hypoplasia
   2. Bile duct stenosis
   3. Infectious processes (e.g., cytomegalovirus, herpes, hepatitis)
   4. Cholestasis secondary to total parenteral nutrition
E. Other causes of biliary tract disease
   1. Cystic enlargement of the common bile duct
   2. Intrahepatic cystic disease
F. Surgical considerations
   1. A significant presence of developmental anomalies in other systems is found (10%–15%).
   2. The child may have associated cystic fibrosis with compromised respiratory function.
   3. The particular type of biliary atresia will determine the extent of the corrective surgical procedure.
      a. Type I: atresia of the common duct only
      b. Type II: atresia limited to the hepatic duct
      c. Type III: atretic extension to the porta hepatis
      d. Types I and II favor anastomosis of the bile duct to the bowel
      e. Type III will require the more extensive Kasai procedure (the creation of a jejunal conduit to ductal tissue at the porta hepatis)
      f. Liver transplant may in certain circumstances remain definitive therapy
G. Anesthetic considerations
   1. Full assessment of the patient's metabolic, hematologic, electrolyte, and intravascular volume status must be

undertaken with appropriate corrective action initiated or maintained.

2. Other preexisting complications may be present, including diminished pulmonary reserve, renal insufficiency, and derangements in serum glucose.
3. Blood loss may be massive.
4. Adequate IV lines to include possible central access (for volume infusion and hemodynamic monitoring) must be established.
5. Maintenance of normothermia is of utmost importance.
6. Isoflurane/N_2O/O_2 with an adjunctive opioid is appropriate. Muscle relaxation with cis-atracurium may be most appropriate.
7. A strong possibility of the need for postoperative ventilatory support with ongoing restoration of volume, electrolyte, and hematologic deficiencies must be appreciated in postoperative care.

ADDITIONAL READINGS

Adkins, J.C., & Kieswetter, W.B. (1976). Imperforate anus. *Surgical Clinics of North America*, 56, 379–394.

Beasley, S.W., & Myers, N.A. (1988). The diagnosis of congenital tracheoesophageal fistula. *Journal of Pediatric Surgery*, 23, 415–417.

Flake, A.W. (1993). Fetal sacrococcygeal teratoma. *Seminars in Pediatric Surgery*, 2, 113–120.

Grosfeld, J.L. (1997). Pediatric surgery. In *Sabiston textbook of surgery: The biological basis of modern surgical practice* (15th ed.). Philadelphia: W.B. Saunders.

Harberg, F.J., Pokorny, W.J., & Hahn, H. (1979). Congenital duodenal obstruction: A review of 65 cases. *American Journal of Surgery*, 138, 825–828.

Kleinhaus, S., Weinberg, G., & Gregor, M.B. (1992). Necrotizing enterocolitis in infancy. *Surgical Clinics of North America*, 72, 261–276.

Motoyama, E.K., & Davis, P.J. (Eds.). (1990). *Smith's anesthesia for infants and children* (5th ed.). St. Louis: Mosby.

Nakayam, D.K., Bose, C.I., Chescheir, N.C., & Valley, R.D. (1997). *Critical care of the surgical newborn*. Armonk, N.Y.: Futura.

Sermer, M., Benzie, R.J., Pinkston, L., et al. (1987). Prenatal diagnosis and management of congenital defects of the anterior abdominal wall. *American Journal of Obstetrics and Gynecology*, 156, 308–312.

Teitelbaum, D.H., Qualman, S.J., & Caniano, D.A. (1988). Hirschsprung's disease: Identification of risk factors for enterocolitis. *Annals of Surgery*, 207, 240–244.

10

Anesthetic Considerations for Pediatric Orthopedic Procedures

Pamela Friedman, MS, CRNA, and John Aker, MS, CRNA

I. Conditions in Pediatric Orthopedics
  A. Trauma
  B. Congenital abnormalities
  C. Infectious processes
  D. Abnormalities of growth or metabolism
  E. Bone tumors

II. Common Features of Orthopedic Surgery Patients
  A. Children may be chronically ill with prolonged immobilization.
  B. Children with congenital abnormalities return for a series of corrective surgical procedures.
  C. Intraoperative skeletal muscle relaxation is rarely required.
  D. Intraoperative fluoroscopy or series of radiographs require lead shielding of the patient and intraoperative personnel.
  E. Limb tourniquets are used to control hemostasis.
  F. Extremity plaster casts, splints, or skeletal traction may limit patient mobility and positioning.

III. Considerations for Anesthetic Management
  A. Preoperative preparation
    1. Preoperative visit
      a. A preoperative visit allows the anesthetist to review the child's surgical diagnosis and the surgeon's anticipated surgical procedure and to identify factors that may increase the child's operative risk (e.g., family history of malignant hyperthermia).
      b. Preoperative laboratory evaluation should be guided by the patient's medical history, proposed surgical procedure, and anticipated intraoperative fluid and blood loss.
      c. Child and parent or guardian are familiarized with the proposed anesthetic plan and anticipated intraopera-

150

tive monitoring modalities (arterial lines, central lines, regional anesthetic techniques).

d. The incidence of malignant hyperthermia is linked with a number of diseases of skeletal muscle.

e. Latex allergy has been identified as a cause of anaphylaxis in patients with spina bifida, patients who have repeated exposures to latex via self-catheterization, and patients who have undergone diagnostic testing using latex items.

B. Intraoperative considerations

1. Large intraoperative blood loss may occur with extensive surgical procedures (spinal deformity correction). Preoperative determination of hematocrit and body weight facilitates the calculation of allowable blood loss and maintenance of intraoperative fluid requirements.

2. Prolonged tourniquet inflation times may be necessary to complete the surgical procedure.

   a. The maximum time limit for safe tourniquet inflation is not known with certainty; however, 1½ to 2 hours is generally accepted in the clinical setting.

   b. An increasing duration of circulatory arrest in the extremity is associated with progressive decreases in venous pH. Acidosis produces significant biochemical alterations, including muscle fatigue at a pH of 7.0, and a hypercoagulable state.

   c. Decreases in capillary P_{O_2} modify capillary endothelium integrity, increasing capillary permeability to fluid and protein.

3. Techniques.

   a. *General anesthesia* is the most frequently chosen technique for the pediatric patient. Inhalation inductions are generally more acceptable to the child although intravenous (IV) induction may be chosen in special circumstances (full stomach) or when an IV line has been previously placed.

   b. *Regional anesthesia* techniques may be used in conjunction with general anesthesia to provide postoperative analgesia. There are few indications for the use of regional anesthesia as the sole anesthetic technique in children. Regional anesthesia is efficacious for premature infants (<60 weeks' postconceptual age), children with neuromuscular diseases who have decreased pulmonary reserves, children with reactive pulmonary diseases, or children with diagnoses of malignant hyperthermia.

C. Recovery
  1. Recovery is a time of increased risk because the pediatric patient is more likely to experience upper airway obstruction, postintubation croup, or apnea.
  2. Approximately 50% of all pediatric perioperative cardiac arrests are the result of ventilatory dysfunction in the immediate recovery period.
  3. Prompt and effective postoperative analgesia minimizes associated metabolic stresses and allows for timely discharge.
  4. Additional postoperative problems include nausea and vomiting and temperature instability.
  5. Care must be taken to protect the child who awakens in an excited state because the uncontrolled movement of casted limbs may result in self-injury or breach the integrity of the cast or skeletal correction.

IV. Anesthetic Techniques for Trauma

A. Traumatic orthopedic injury is associated with hemorrhage, circulatory shock, and central neurologic injury that requires prompt treatment before orthopedic procedures.
B. Trauma patients have full stomachs and require that the airway be secured with an endotracheal tube of appropriate size.

V. Anesthetic Technique for Surgical Procedures of the Hip

A. Congenital dislocations and developmental dysplasias may require either a closed or an open approach.
  1. Pelvic osteotomy is associated with significant intraoperative blood losses.
  2. Following surgical correction, hip spica casts are applied.
  3. The child should remain asleep and immobile until these cast applications are complete and final radiographs are obtained.
B. Children with slipped capital femoral epiphyses are usually overweight male adolescents.
  1. Increased weight adds stress to the proximal femoral growth plate, causing the femoral head to move in relation to the growth plate.
  2. The increased weight may complicate airway management and positioning.

VI. Anesthetic Technique for Surgical Procedures of the Spine

A. Thoracolumbar deformities have multiple causes and occur in pediatric and adolescent populations

B. Females are affected more often than males (4:1)
C. Preoperative evaluation is conducted the same as any patient being prepared for a major surgical procedure, with emphasis on the cardiovascular and respiratory systems
1. Respiratory system considerations
   a. Abnormalities in pulmonary function depend on the degree of spinal curvature and presence of neuromuscular disease.
   b. Children with curves in excess of 65 degrees have decreased pulmonary function.
   c. Preoperative pulmonary function tests are consistent with a restrictive disease process, with global decreases in lung volumes and decreases in vital capacity and expiratory reserve volume.
   d. Hypoventilation and ventilation-perfusion defects are common with accompanying increases in pulmonary vascular resistance.
   e. Arterial blood gas (ABG) values demonstrate decreased Po_2 with normal $Paco_2$.
   f. Postoperative ventilatory support is required in patients with vital capacity <50% of predicted values and a $Paco_2$ >45 mm Hg.
2. Cardiovascular system considerations
   a. Children with myopathies have degenerative changes in the myocardium that lead to decreases in myocardial contractility.
   b. Tachydysrhythmias are common. Accordingly, these children should have a thorough cardiac evaluation before elective correction of thoracolumbar deformities.
D. Operative approaches for thoracolumbosacral spine deformity
1. Anterior approach
   a. The anterior approach is used in conjunction with a posterior approach to facilitate mobilization of the spine before posterior correction (see below) and generally precedes the posterior surgical approach.
   b. After positioning in the lateral decubitus position, a thoracotomy is performed, with subsequent division of the diaphragm. A chest tube is connected to a Pleurovac drainage system at the time of chest closure.
2. Posterior approach
   a. The posterior approach begins with an incision along the entire length of the dorsal spine.
   b. A hook is fitted in the facet joint of the upper and

lower vertebrae, and a distraction rod is placed between the hooks on the concave aspect of the curve. A compression rod is placed on the convex side of the curve.

   c. The vertebrae are decorticated along their entire length (blood loss may be in excess of blood volume).

   d. Bone graft from the child's iliac crest is placed over the decorticated vertebrae for fusion.

   e. Following distraction of the spine, a "wake-up test" may be conducted.

   f. Intraoperative awakening facilitates the assessment of motor function after spinal distraction.

E. Anesthetic plan

   1. The anesthetic technique must provide profound sedation and analgesia. A continuous opioid infusion (fentanyl) with the simultaneous administration of a low concentration of volatile anesthetic is typically used. This facilitates careful titration and the ability to "turn off" the anesthetic for the wake-up test (see below).

   2. Inhalation anesthetic concentration should be <0.5–1 minimum alveolar concentration (MAC) to minimize interference with somatosensory evoked potential (SSEP) monitoring.

   3. Although muscle relaxation is important, neuromuscular blockade should not exceed two twitches of the train-of-four, facilitating neural stimulation with surgical dissection near important neural structures.

   4. Intraoperative monitoring.

      a. Standard monitoring to meet the standard of care is used (blood pressure, heart rate, pulse oximetry, capnography, electrocardiogram [ECG]).

      b. In addition, selective invasive monitoring modalities (arterial blood pressure, central venous pressure) may be indicated when controlled intraoperative hypotension and large intraoperative blood loss are expected.

   5. Attenuate decreases in core body temperature.

      a. Large incisions and extensive operating times lead to decreases in core body temperature.

      b. The operating room should be warmed before the patient's arrival, the child's head covered to prevent conductive heat loss, lower extremities covered with a forced air warming blanket, and, if possible, administered IV fluids warmed and anesthetic gases humidified.

      c. The surgical team should be encouraged to use warm irrigating solutions.

  6. Controlled hypotension.

      a. Controlled lowering of the mean arterial pressure to a predetermined level will decrease intraoperative blood loss.

      b. It should be conducted with arterial line blood pressure monitoring.

      c. Simultaneous hyperventilation should be avoided to minimize the risk of spinal cord ischemia.

      d. Sodium nitroprusside has a rapid onset and is readily titratable. Simultaneous administration of beta-blockers minimizes reflex tachycardia. Potential exists for cyanide toxicity with large doses and prolonged infusions.

      e. Nitroglycerin decreases preload and cardiac output. Beta-blockers are also used to minimize reflex tachycardia.

      f. Inhalation agents can be used to decrease blood pressure; however, the necessary dose may produce significant cardiovascular depression. Recall that large doses interfere with SSEP monitoring.

  7. Management of intraoperative blood loss and fluid replacement.

      a. Blood loss can be significant. Right lateral decubitus positioning may produce compression of the inferior vena cava, decreasing venous return and producing venous stasis in the operative site.

      b. Two large-bore IV lines (or central venous access) are necessary.

      c. Blood is typed, crossmatched, and readily available. The older child may provide autologous blood before the procedure. Cell saver may be used to harvest shed blood.

      d. Operative sites are locally infiltrated with dilute epinephrine solutions.

      e. Hemodilution may be undertaken using crystalloid or colloid solutions with the simultaneous removal of blood, with a target hematocrit of 25% to 28%.

F. Intraoperative monitoring of spinal cord function

  1. Somatosensory evoked potentials (SSEPs) involve the recording of a brief electrical current that is delivered to a peripheral sensory or motor nerve.

      a. SSEP will determine the integrity of the dorsal spinal column.

    b. Motor deficits that develop are not detected (see discussion of wake-up test).

    c. The posterior tibial nerve is typically selected for spinal cord monitoring.

    d. Inhalation anesthetic agents alter the intraoperative character of SSEPs.

    e. The individual who monitors the SSEP should be made aware of changes in anesthetic technique or the patient's underlying physiologic responses because essentially all anesthetics impact SSEP and influence the baseline recordings.

    f. A steady state of anesthetic depth will aid the interpretation of SSEP.

    g. Increasing concentrations of inhalation agents *decrease* the SSEP amplitude.

    h. Ketamine and etomidate *increase* SSEP amplitudes.

    i. Opioids, benzodiazepines, and muscle relaxants produce less influential changes on SSEPs.

2. Intraoperative wake-up test.

    a. Spinal distraction carries an associated risk of damage to neural structures.

    b. Neural damage may follow arterial occlusion, stretching of neural structures with distraction, or direct pressure on the cord (e.g., hematoma).

    c. The wake-up test is highly specific for motor function.

    d. It requires a cooperative patient to follow commands to move the lower extremities.

    e. Potential risks include damage to the spine from excessive movement, endotracheal extubation in the prone position with attendant hypoxia, and venous air embolism with spontaneous respiratory effort.

    f. The child is instructed before anesthetic induction regarding what verbal phrase will be used (e.g., "move your feet like a windshield wiper") and what accompanying motor response is desired at the time of the test.

    g. The surgeon provides advanced warning of the need to assess motor function (30–45 minutes).

    h. Inhalation agent and opioid infusion is discontinued; skeletal muscle relaxant administration is titrated to allow reversal at the time of the test.

    i. Nitrous oxide is discontinued and 100% oxygen administered. When the end-tidal N_2O approaches 15% to 20%, the child is verbally stimulated and asked to move the feet.

j. With confirmation of bilateral foot movement, sodium pentothal is administered and inhalation agents or opioid infusion is reestablished. If the patient does not move lower extremities following the reinstitution of general anesthesia, the distraction rod will be repositioned with an additional wake-up test to assess motor function.

G. Emergence and recovery
   1. Children who have anteroposterior spinal procedures may require postoperative ventilation.
   2. Children who undergo only posterior procedures may be extubated at the conclusion of the procedure if underlying pulmonary function is acceptable.
   3. IV analgesia is imperative to prevent additional respiratory complications (atelectasis, hypoxia) that can occur secondary to splinting from pain.
   4. The surgeon can administer intrathecal morphine (0.1–0.25 mg) at the time of closure.

VII. Juvenile Rheumatoid Arthritis (JRA; Still's Disease)

A. JRA is a generalized systemic autoimmune disease in which rheumatoid factor is produced and deposited within multiple joints.
B. Rheumatoid factor influences the release of lysosomal enzymes, which leads to joint destruction.
C. Age of onset is between 2 and 4 years; 70% of those affected are females.
D. Preoperative evaluation.
   1. Generalized symptomatology
      a. Fever, rash, joint redness, increased erythrocyte sedimentation rate, and leukocytosis
      b. Microcytic hypochromic anemia that is refractory to exogenous iron therapy
      c. Polyarthritis, lymphadenitis, and splenomegaly with advanced stages of the disease
   2. Respiratory assessment
      a. Altered respiratory function generally follows in those children with severe disease.
      b. Pleuritis, pleural effusions, and recurrent pneumonias may develop.
      c. Respiratory assessment is directed to airway assessment.
         (1) Temporomandibular ankylosis limits mouth opening.

    (2) Mandibular hypoplasia follows long-term steroid use.

    (3) Laryngeal synovial joint involvement produces narrowing of glottis.

    (4) Dysphagia and vocal hoarseness occur from cricoarytenoiditis.

    (5) Atlantoaxial or cervical subluxation is possible.

    (6) Limited cervical mobility follows ankylosis of the apophyseal joints.

    (7) The Sharp and Purser test may be used to assess atlantoaxial instability. In the seated position with the head flexed, pressure is applied to the forehead with simultaneous digital palpation of the spinous process of C2. In 50% of patients with instability a gliding sensation is felt with reduction of the subluxation.

3. Cardiovascular assessment

    a. JRA is a systemic connective tissue disease. As many as 36% of children may have echocardiographic evidence of pericarditis.

    b. Steroids may be prescribed to children with myocardial involvement.

    c. Generalized vasculitis may develop in children with progressive disease.

    d. Preoperative electrocardiograms or two-dimensional echocardiography or both may detail the extent of myocardial involvement.

4. Renal assessment

    a. Renal impairment is common and more prevalent in children with long-standing disease.

    b. Renal impairments result from amyloid deposits and progressive vasculitis.

    c. Preoperative assessments of electrolytes, blood urea nitrogen (BUN), and creatinine are made.

5. Hematologic assessment

    a. Complete blood count (CBC) with differential, platelet count, bleeding time, prothrombin time, and activated partial thromboplastin time

6. Drug therapy

    a. A host of drugs may be prescribed for JRA, including salicylates, nonsteroidal agents, steroids, and gold.

    b. In some cases cytotoxic agents (cyclophosphamide) may be employed.

    c. Salicylates and nonsteroidal antiinflammatory drugs

       precipitate gastritis, peptic ulceration, and gastrointestinal (GI) bleeding. Platelet function is impaired by these agents.

    d. Steroids inhibit normal skeletal growth and suppress the hypothalmic-pituitary-adrenal axis; long-term administration may lead to Cushing's syndrome (excess glucocorticoids).

    e. Gold salts are nephrotoxic (nephrotic syndrome) and produce bone marrow suppression and exfoliative dermatitis.

  E. Anesthetic management.

    1. Supplemental steroid dosing should be considered for children who are prescribed steroids.

    2. Anesthetic agent selection should take into account potential renal involvement (use caution with renally eliminated drugs), myocardial involvement (myocardial depression), and limited reserves.

    3. IV induction may be difficult because of IV access difficulty (fragile veins, low platelet count) and uncertainty of securing the airway.

    4. Strategies for securing the airway include blind nasal intubation (potential for bleeding), careful direct laryngoscopy, or fiberoptic intubation.

    5. Anemic patients may benefit from a higher inspired concentration of oxygen.

    6. Drug therapy may precipitate osteoporosis (steroids) and dermatitis (cytotoxic agents). Careful positioning of the child with adequate padding of joints is imperative to avoid injury.

VIII. Achondroplasia

  A. Achondroplasia, the most common chondrodystrophy, is autosomal dominant and affects 15 per 1 million live births

  B. Approximately 80% of children affected have no previous family history and are new gene mutations

  C. Clinical features

    1. Proximal shortening of the limbs, long trunk, large head with prominent frontal features, depression of the nasal bridge, with a prominent mandible

    2. Tridentate hands with short, broad fingers

  D. Neurologic involvement

    1. These children may come to the operating room for a variety of neurologic problems, including cranial, lumbar, and lower extremity dysfunction.

2. Megacephaly is very common and is associated with mild dilation of the ventricles.
3. Hydrocephalus develops in a small proportion of patients and may be caused by a small foramen magnum. It is associated with spinal cord compression.
4. Spinal cord compression presents as subtle or overt. Failure to make the diagnosis is responsible for a high mortality. Cyanosis after crying, poor head control, or quadriparesis may be the presenting sign. Decompression is via suboccipital craniotomy.
5. Neurologic deficit of lower limbs results from narrow spinal canal and bony abnormality (vertebral tapering from top to bottom instead of normal bottom to top). The characteristic lumbar lordosis does not require surgical intervention.

E. Anesthetic management
   1. Airway management.
      a. Facial abnormalities generally do not inhibit airway management.
      b. Neck extension may be limited by cervical spine abnormalities preventing direct laryngoscopy.
      c. Hyperextension and hyperflexion must be avoided.
      d. Select normal-size endotracheal tube for age of patient.
   2. Controlled ventilation should be provided (musculoskeletal abnormalities).
   3. Regional anesthetic techniques may be problematic (technical difficulties because of spinal abnormalities), and the possibility of additional neurologic impairment exists.
   4. Attentive patient positioning is important to avoid further injury.

ADDITIONAL READINGS

Bernstein, R.L. (1988). Anesthetic management of patients with scoliosis. In *ASA refresher course* (Vol. 16). Philadelphia: American Society of Anesthesiologists and Lippincott-Raven.

Holtby, A., & Kelton, J. (1987). Orthopedic diseases. In Katz, J., & Steward, D.J. *Anesthesia and uncommon pediatric diseases.* Philadelphia: Saunders.

Kabat, K.M. (1991). Anesthetic management of pediatric musculoskeletal disorders. In Bell, C., Hughs, C.W., & Oh, T.H. (Eds.). *The pediatric anesthesia handbook* (revised edition). Department of Anesthesiology, Yale University School of Medicine. St. Louis: Mosby–Year Book.

Rinsky, L., & Lin, Y. (1994). Pediatric orthopedic surgery. In Jaffe, R., & Samuels, S. (Eds.). *Anesthesiologists' manual of surgical procedures.* New York: Raven Press.

Salem, M.R., & Klowden, A.J. (1989). Anesthesia for pediatric orthopedic surgery. In Gregory, G.A. (Ed.). *Pediatric anesthesia* (2nd ed.). New York: Churchill Livingstone.

Zukerman, A.L., & Yaster, M. (1996). Anesthesia for orthopedic surgery. In Smith, R. *Anesthesia for infants and children* (6th ed., pp. 603–632). St. Louis: Mosby.

11

Neuroanesthesia

John Aker, MS, CRNA

I. Cerebral Anatomy and Physiology

A. General considerations

1. The newborn brain weighs 340 g (10%–15% of total body weight), doubles in weight by 6 months, reaching 1000 g by 2 years and adult weight (1200–1400 g) by 12 years of age.

2. The brain receives 15% of the cardiac output and requires 20% of the total body oxygen consumption.

3. Neuronal development and myelination continue from birth into the third year of life. Moro and grasp reflexes allow the continued assessment of neuronal development.

B. Normal physiologic values

1. Cerebral blood flow (CBF) values for pediatric patients

   a. Global CBF in infants and children: 100 ml/100 g/min

   b. CBF in premature infants: 40 ml/100 g/min

   c. Gray matter blood flow: 80 ml/100 g/min

   d. White matter blood flow: 20 ml/100 g/min

   e. Cerebral metabolic rate of oxygen (CMR_{O_2}) utilization: 5 to 6 ml/100 g/min

   f. Brain tissue glucose utilization: 6.8 mg/100 g/min

2. Spinal cord

   a. Ends at intervertebral space of L3, reaching adult level of L1–2 by 8 years of age

   b. Average blood flow: 50 ml/100 g/min

   c. White matter blood flow: 15 to 20 ml/100 g/min

   d. Gray matter blood flow: 60 to 100 ml/100 g/min

3. Cerebral blood volume

   a. Gray matter blood volume: 4 to 6 ml/100 g

   b. White matter blood volume: 1.5 to 2.5 ml/100 g

   c. Changes in cerebral blood volume will parallel changes in cerebral blood flow, except when cerebral perfusion decreases and autoregulation produces vasodilation to maintain a constant flow

4. Autoregulation of CBF

   a. Autoregulation refers to the ability of the central

nervous system to regulate CBF over a wide range of cerebral perfusion pressures:

$$CPP = MAP - ICP$$

where CPP = cerebral perfusion pressure, MAP = mean arterial pressure, and ICP = intracranial pressure.
   b. CBF can be readily altered by the anesthetist to decrease intracranial pressure.
   c. The specific mechanisms of autoregulation are not completely understood but are thought to depend on myogenic (intrinsic response of arterial smooth muscle), metabolic (blood flow regulated via vasodilator metabolites), and neurogenic (vasodilator and vasoconstrictor nerves innervate cerebral vessels) influences.
   d. Complete loss of cerebral autoregulation may occur during hypoxia, severe hypercapnia, blood-brain barrier disruption following head trauma, or administration of high concentrations of inhalation anesthetic agents and vasodilators (nitroprusside).
   e. CBF and spinal cord blood flow are held constant at CPP between 50 and 150 mm Hg.
   f. Autoregulation is rapid (10–120 seconds).
   g. CPP is reduced by increased ICP or a decrease in MAP.
   h. When CPP exceeds the upper limit of 150 mm Hg, cerebral perfusion increases.
   i. Sympathetic stimulation (e.g., hypertension) will shift the lower and upper autoregulation limits to the right, requiring higher CPPs.
   j. CBF is also influenced by $Paco_2$ over the range of 20 to 80 mm Hg. A 1 mm Hg change in $Paco_2$ produces a 4% change in CBF.

II. Pathophysiology of Increased Intracranial Pressure

   A. The supratentorial compartment contains the cerebral hemispheres, which are separated by the falx cerebri into three lobes: frontal, temporal, and parietal-occipital.
   B. The term *increased intracranial pressure (ICP)* represents supratentorial cerebral spinal fluid (CSF) pressure within the lateral ventricles and the overlying cerebral hemispheres.
   C. Increased ICP in the supratentorial compartment produces reductions in cerebral perfusion producing cerebral ischemia (Cerebral perfusion pressure = Mean arterial pressure − ICP).

D. Continuing increases in ICP may produce shifts of intracranial contents resulting in brain tissue compression against the falx, tentorium, or foramen magnum.

E. Determinants of ICP.

1. The cranial vault and spinal canal provide a bony enclosure for the protection of the delicate neural elements.

2. Within the cranium the neural elements compose 70% of the intracranial volume, whereas the extracellular fluid, intracranial CSF, and cerebral blood volume each contribute an additional 10% to intracranial volume.

3. The majority of CSF (80%) is produced by the choroid plexus and the ependymal lining of the ventricular system. The arachnoid villi absorb CSF. The rate of CSF production (0.35 ml/min) is generally balanced by absorption.

4. CSF exits the ventricular system from the fourth ventricle through the foramina of Magendie and Luschka, moving into the cisterna magna, where the cranial and spinal subarachnoid spaces are joined.

5. The pediatric cranial vault is formed by ossified plates that are separated by a fibrous junction (the fontanelles). The posterior fontanelle closes by the second or third month, and the anterior fontanelle closes between 12 and 16 months of age. The fontanelles ossify during the teenage years.

6. Normal ICP in children is approximately 2 to 4 mm Hg compared to the adult values of 5 to 15 mm Hg.

7. Negative ICP may develop following the loss of salt and water (postbirth body weight) within the first days following birth. This negative ICP has been thought to contribute to intraventricular hemorrhage in the low–birth weight premature infant.

8. Any increase in intracranial volume via an increase in cellular content (tumor), intracellular or extracellular water (edema), or CSF volume (hydrocephalus) will increase ICP.

9. Increases in volume of one compartment must be offset by decreases in another.

10. Although cerebral blood volume may be decreased with hyperventilation-induced hypocapnia, CSF plays the greatest role in spatial compensation.

11. As intracranial volume increases, CSF volume will decrease (via translocation, decreased formation, and

perhaps increased absorption) by an approximately equal volume, maintaining near normal ICP.

12. After this compensatory mechanism has been exhausted, small increases in intracranial volume are associated with large increases in ICP.

13. Although the adult cranium is a rigid nonexpandable container, the pediatric cranium has open fontanelles, which may allow for expansion with *slow* increases in intracranial volume. The fibrous fontanelles are unable to accommodate acute increases in intracranial volume.

F. Intracranial hypertension.

1. Intracranial hypertension is defined by sustained increases in ICP that exceed normal physiologic values.

2. Table 11–1 details the signs and symptoms of increased ICP in infants and children.

3. ICP increases more rapidly in the pediatric patient than the adult patient.

4. Exhaustion of compensatory mechanisms (spatial compensation) produces neurologic symptoms of increased ICP.

5. Symptoms of intracranial hypertension: complaints of nausea and headache by older children, vomiting, lethargy, somnolence, and photophobia.

6. Signs of intracranial hypertension: papilledema, Cushing reflex (bradycardia, hypertension), focal neurologic deficits, altered ventilatory function, decreasing consciousness, seizures, and coma.

7. Radiologic findings.

TABLE 11–1. Signs of Intracranial Hypertension in Infants and Children

Infants	Children	Infants and Children
Irritability	Headache	Decreased consciousness
Full fontanelle	Diplopia	Palsies of cranial nerves II and VI
Widely separated cranial sutures	Papilledema	Loss of upward gaze
Cranial enlargement		Vomiting
		Herniation
		Cushing triad, pupillary changes

From Krane, E.J., & Domino, K.B. (1996). Anesthesia for neurosurgery. In Motoyama, E.K., & Davis, P.J. (Eds.). *Smith's anesthesia for infants and children* (6th ed.). St. Louis: Mosby.

    a. Fontanelle suture separation; magnetic resonance imaging (MRI) and computed tomography (CT) scan will identify midline shifts, the presence of cerebral edema, the presence of mass lesions, abnormal ventricular size, and obliteration of the basal cistern.

8. Treatment of intracranial hypertension.

    a. Common etiologies of intracranial hypertension are listed in the box below.

    b. Hyperventilation ($Paco_2$ 25–30 mm Hg): Lowering $Paco_2$ will decrease cerebral blood volume and decrease ICP. Although hyperventilation is of value in decreasing intracranial volume in the intraoperative setting, there is a lack of evidence suggesting a beneficial effect of prolonged hypocapnia.

    c. Administration of diuretics (mannitol, furosemide): These agents remove water from brain tissue and decrease the rate of CSF production. Rapid administration of mannitol may produce a transient increase in ICP that may be attenuated by prior administration of furosemide. Mannitol dose is 0.25 to 1 g/kg. Prolonged mannitol use may produce hyperosmolality and electrolyte imbalance.

    d. Pharmacologic production of cerebral vasoconstriction: Increasing doses of thiopental (1.5–5 mg/kg) decrease

---

Etiologies of Intracranial Hypertension

Increased cerebral blood volume
- Hypertension
- Arterial dilation
- Venodilation
- Hypercarbia
- Hypoxia
- Anatomic abnormalities: arteriovenous malformation

Increased brain volume
- Cerebral edema (global or regional)

Tumor or brain abscess

Posttraumatic
- After anoxia

Increased CSF volume
- Hydrocephalus (obstruction of CSF flow)
- Tumor, abscess, or hematoma

cerebral metabolic rate and cerebral blood volume, with maximal decreases occurring with the onset of an isoelectric electroencephalogram (EEG).

e. Elevation of the head.

f. Control of systemic blood pressure: Maintain CPP.

g. Restrict intravenous (IV) fluids.

h. Corticosteroid administration: Glucocorticoids (dexamethasone) penetrate the blood-brain barrier and decrease ICP and edema associated with mass lesions. In the absence of a mass lesion, glucocorticoid administration may produce pseudotumor cerebri (increased ICP when no mass lesion exists) and papilledema. The majority of clinical trials have failed to demonstrate a beneficial effect, although a recent national study has found improved outcomes in acute spinal cord injury following the administration of large doses of methylprednisolone.

i. CSF drainage: Drainage may only relieve intracranial hypertension.

j. Surgical decompression: removal of hematoma.

III. Preoperative Assessment and Preparation

A. Preoperative history and physical examination

1. The preoperative assessment requires an individualized assessment targeting respiratory, cardiovascular, and neurologic function.

2. Young children are vulnerable to the development of respiratory failure when faced with a major illness. Oxygen consumption is higher per body surface area than in adults, and it increases during illness. The goal of preoperative assessment is the optimization of oxygenation and ventilation.

3. Recall the relationships among preload, heart rate, and afterload that form the basis for cardiac output. Infants and children have fixed stroke volumes and depend on changes in heart rate to maintain cardiac output.

4. Although blood pressure varies with age, hypotension is a late sign of intravascular volume depletion.

5. The adequacy of peripheral perfusion is determined by quality of peripheral pulses, temperature of extremities, and capillary refill.

6. The intrinsic heart rate is higher to meet the high baseline oxygen consumption demands.

B. Assessment of ICP and recognition of intracranial hypertension

1. Serial determinations of the level of consciousness, responses to noxious stimuli, and the presence or absence of brain stem reflexes are crucial for the child with neurologic injury or disease.

2. The Glasgow Coma Scale is a useful and repeatable assessment for scoring altered states of consciousness based on evaluations of eye opening, vocalization, and motor responses (see Chapter 22).

3. Clinical presentation differs according to patient age.
   a. Neonates and infants with increased ICP exhibit increased irritability, lethargy, and poor feeding. Clinical signs of increased ICP include a bulging anterior fontanelle, dilated scalp veins, and a cranial deformity if ICP elevation has been sustained.
   b. Children with increased ICP may exhibit vomiting, disturbances in gait, lower motor deficits, decreasing levels of consciousness, seizures, oculomotor palsies (sunset sign), ptosis (oculomotor nerve [cranial nerve III] palsy), strabismus (abducens [cranial nerve VI] palsy), dysphonia, and dysphagia.
   c. Older children may complain of headache on awakening (sleep-induced hypercapnia) and nausea and vomiting.
   d. Papilledema and absence of retinal venous pulsations may be present in all age-groups.

C. Laboratory evaluation
   1. Suggested tests are guided by the history and physical examination.
   2. Hemoglobin and hematocrit are done to ensure satisfactory oxygen-carrying capacity.
   3. Assessment of electrolytes is important in children with protracted vomiting.
   4. Hypocalcemia, hypophosphatemia, and hypomagnesemia occur in children with shock, sepsis, and multisystem organ failure.
   5. Glucose is a "double-edged sword" because the brain depends on it for an energy source. Hyperglycemia is associated with delayed gastric emptying, osmotic diuresis, increased CO_2 production, and hyperglycemia-associated intracellular lactic acidosis. Animal models suggest worse neurologic outcome when hyperglycemia is present during periods of cerebral ischemia. Accordingly, routine glucose administration is avoided.
   6. Endocrine evaluation may be required for children with supracellar tumors.

D. Radiographic evaluation
   1. Preoperative radiographic evaluation with skull radiographs, ultrasound, CT, or MRI.
   2. "Beaten copper" or "thumb printing" appearance and widening of sagittal sutures on skull radiographs are characteristic of increased ICP.
   3. Brain ultrasound performed through anterior fontanelle at bedside is useful for premature infants and neonates.
   4. CT and MRI are essential neurodiagnostic tools that are invaluable for identification of pathologic conditions, and they assist in tailoring the anesthetic for the specific neurosurgical procedure. These studies generally require anesthetic intervention to ensure a quality study (see Chapter 13).
E. Premedication
   1. Opioids and sedative/hypnotics are avoided to prevent further increases in ICP following hypoventilation-induced hypercapnia and to facilitate continued neurologic assessment before the induction of anesthesia.
   2. The obtunded child should not receive preoperative medications.
   3. However, children with vascular anomalies may benefit from preoperative anxiolysis to minimize hypertension and intracranial bleeding.
   4. Sedation may be accomplished with
      a. Oral midazolam, 0.5 mg/kg.
      b. Oral pentobarbital, 4 mg/kg, will produce sedation and decrease ICP. Barbiturates decrease $CMRo_2$, lowering ICP. Children with increased ICP should not receive preoperative sedation.
   5. Preoperative steroids should be continued in the perioperative period.

IV. Perioperative Monitoring

A. Standard noninvasive monitoring includes auscultation of heart tones and breath sounds (esophageal stethoscope), electrocardiogram (ECG) rate and rhythm, blood pressure, pulse oximetry, capnography, neuromuscular function, and temperature.
B. The application of a radial artery Doppler may be helpful for determining noninvasive blood pressure in neonates.
C. Invasive monitoring (arterial and central venous catheterization) requires an individualized assessment of the risks and benefits for each patient.
D. Arterial catheterization is recommended for intracranial

procedures, providing minute-to-minute assessment of blood pressure and ready access for arterial blood sampling. The system should be electronically zeroed at the level of the circle of Willis, using the tragus of the ear as a reference.

E. A urinary catheter should be considered for all intracranial procedures when osmotic diuretics are employed perioperatively and for neurosurgical procedures of long duration.

F. Neurophysiologic monitoring (e.g., electroencephalography, evoked potentials) may be used for selected procedures.

V. Surgical Positioning

A. Positioning for neurosurgical procedures involves a mixture of physiologic assets and risks

B. General principles of pediatric positioning

1. A patent airway must be ensured before and following alterations of patient position via auscultation of the chest and observance of acceptable capnography tracing.

2. Infants and children have large body surface areas and a limited ability to autoregulate core temperature. The operating room should be warmed before the child's arrival and additional equipment (heating blanket, skull caps when appropriate to prevent evaporative heat loss, overhead heating lamps, forced-air blankets) should be employed to maintain a near normal core body temperature.

3. As previously mentioned, cardiac output in the infant and young child depends on heart rate rather than stroke volume. Accordingly, the pharmacologic manipulation of myocardial contractility (e.g., ephedrine sulfate) has a limited impact on the resultant cardiac output.

4. All the volatile inhalation anesthetics produce dose-dependent myocardial depression by decreasing contractility. Halothane suppresses the baroreceptor response, limiting the increase in heart rate in the older child.

5. The combination of both 2 and 3 may exaggerate the hemodynamic effects that accompany sudden positioning changes in the anesthetized pediatric patient.

C. Considerations specific to neurosurgical procedures

1. Following surgical draping, the pediatric patient cannot be viewed by the anesthetist. Surgical drapes should be suspended to provide direct observation of the child and allow access to the airway and IV and invasive monitoring catheters.

2. The head is elevated to promote venous blood and CSF

drainage. Recall the risk of venous air embolism (VAE) whenever the surgical site is higher than the heart.

3. Excessive neck flexion impedes jugular venous return and increases ICP.

4. The child is positioned either 90 or 180 degrees from the anesthetist following anesthetic induction and endotracheal intubation, necessitating IV and anesthesia circuit extensions.

5. Displacement of the endotracheal tube (ETT) may occur with flexion and extension of the neck. Recall that the position of the ETT "follows the chin": Chin down, ETT moves caudad (bronchial intubation); chin up, ETT moves cephalad (potential for extubation).

6. The ETT must be secured using an adhesive and cloth tape. All breathing circuit connections must be tight to prevent unintended disconnections.

D. Supine position

1. Employed for children undergoing supratentorial neurosurgical procedures (craniotomy, ventriculoperitoneal [VP] shunts, correction of craniosynostosis).

2. The head is placed to the side for posterior access to skull and anterior access to neck. Care must be taken to prevent airway obstruction with flexion or kinking of the ETT.

3. Stability of the anesthesia circuit is important to prevent unintended extubation by the weight of the anesthesia circuit.

4. A roll may be placed under the shoulders augmenting neck extension and is helpful in children with large craniums (hydrocephalus, acromegaly, gigantism).

5. When the head is turned to one side, the external ear may be in direct contact with the bed. The external ear must be protected with foam padding to prevent pressure injury.

6. Foam padding should be placed under the heels, elbows, and the portion of the head that is in contact with the operating table.

7. The arms may be placed at the sides and should be protected from pressure of electrical monitoring cables, IV lines, and leaning surgical assistants. Padding should be placed at the elbows for the protection of the ulnar nerve.

E. Sitting position

1. Infrequently used in young children. Contraindications to the seated position are listed in the box on page 172.

2. CPP decreases 2 mm Hg per vertical inch elevation of the head above the heart. In a normotensive child an MAP

Contraindications for Use of the Seated Position in Neurosurgery

Intracardiac defect (possibility of right-to-left shunt)
Hypovolemia and unstable hemodynamics
Presence of ventriculoatrial shunt
Probe-patent foramen ovale

---

of 55 to 60 mm Hg and Pa_{CO_2} of 25 to 30 mm Hg will maintain acceptable cerebral perfusion.

3. Rapid assumption of seated position may create a large drop in CPP. The seated position should be assumed slowly and hemodynamics aggressively treated to maintain cerebral perfusion.

4. A minimally depressive anesthetic technique (N_2O/O_2 neuromuscular relaxant) produces minimal cardiovascular alterations.

5. Arterial blood pressure monitoring is recommended to evaluate hemodynamic changes and maintain acceptable CPP.

F. Prone positioning

1. Common position for spinal procedures, repair of encephalocele, and suboccipital craniotomy: The child is positioned face down, supported by the ventral body surface.

2. The ventral body surface rarely functions as a weight-bearing structure. Improper positioning produces increased work of breathing from chest compression, and diaphragmatic excursion is limited from abdominal pressure from cranial shift of abdominal contents.

3. Proper positioning (abdomen free from compression, chest supported with bolsters at acromioclavicular joint) increases compliance, decreases required tidal volumes (minimizing barotrauma), and decreases venous congestion.

4. Hemodynamic embarrassment may occur from compression of femoral veins and inferior vena cava, precipitating hypotension consequent to decreasing cardiac output. Proper positioning (bolsters placed under anterior iliac crest) will minimize hemodynamic alterations.

5. ETT must be secured before positioning.
   a. Flexion of the ETT within the oral pharynx may

produce tissue edema and postoperative airway obstruction.

b. Macroglossia may develop during the course of long procedures from inhibited venous drainage from the tongue caused by compression from the ETT, oral airway, and/or bite blocks.

c. Upper airway edema may necessitate continued postoperative ventilation until edema subsides.

6. Adequate personnel must be available to place the child in the surgical position to avoid unnecessary injury.

7. Positioning is begun from the supine position using one smooth motion, with the head supported in the neutral axis, avoiding neck extension. Careful positioning of chest bolsters ensures minimal hemodynamic and respiratory embarrassment.

8. To minimize injury from head positioning, the head should remain in the neutral axis whenever possible.

9. Protective ointment may be placed within the lower eyelid; however, the eyes must be taped closed following anesthetic induction and before positioning.

10. Excessive neck flexion in the final surgical position will increase venous congestion and exacerbate increases in ICP. A foam support, foam "donut," or Mayfield pin holder (in children older than 3 years of age) may be used to support the head following assumption of the position.

G. Lateral position

1. The most unstable of all surgical positions.

2. The head is supported with foam or rolled towel to maintain in neutral position, avoiding strain of neck musculature and avoiding pressure on the external ear or the down-side eye.

3. An axillary roll is placed in older children on the down-side thorax inferior to the axilla to prevent injury to the dependent brachial plexus. A pulse oximetry probe placed to monitor the down-side arm will ensure adequate perfusion following placement of the "axillary roll."

4. The up-side arm is supported by a blanket or pillow and arranged so there is a 90-degree bend in the elbow, with the forearm draped across the chest.

5. The lateral position is maintained by placing a roll both anterior and posterior to the chest and abdomen. Support may also be obtained with the use of a bean bag underneath the child.

6. Excessive flexion or extension of the neck may produce ETT displacement. Auscultation of both lung fields is

important to ensure acceptable ETT position following attaining the lateral position.

7. The anesthesia circuit should be secured with a circuit tree or taping of the circuit to prevent undue weight on the ETT, minimizing unintentional extubation.

8. Hypotension following the assumption of the lateral decubitus position is infrequent. Right lateral decubitus positioning may produce obstruction of the inferior vena cava, reducing venous return and decreasing cardiac output.

9. Recall the redistribution of blood flow and ventilation (dependent lung better perfused, nondependent lung better ventilated).

VI. Venous Air Embolism (VAE)

A. Incidence and etiology.

1. Sitting position is habitually associated with VAE.

2. The risk of VAE during neurosurgery has been variously reported in adult patients between 11% and 60%.

3. VAE occurs in as many as 35% of pediatric neurosurgical cases, whereas clinical symptoms of VAE are exhibited by up to 50%.

4. Peak occurrences are during placement of central venous catheters, skin and muscle incision, exposure of venous sinuses, and opening of dural veins.

B. Signs and symptoms of air embolism depend on volume and rate of air entrainment. Use of nitrous oxide increases the size of embolized air (34 times more soluble than nitrogen).

C. The detection of VAE depends on the sensitivity of the monitor employed. There are a number of monitors with various sensitivities for the detection of air embolism. No single monitor is ideal (see Fig. 11–1); an ultrasonic precordial Doppler should be employed for all sitting cases.

D. Signs and symptoms of VAE.

1. Increased CVP

2. Cardiac dysrhythmias

3. Hypotension

4. Abnormal heart tones (mill wheel murmur)

5. Decreased peripheral resistance

6. Hypotension

E. Treatment.

1. When VAE is suspected, notify surgeon, administer 100% oxygen, apply jugular venous compression (increased venous pressure at surgical site, perhaps decreasing air entrainment).

HIGH SENSITIVITY ──────────────────────── LOW SENSITIVITY

Transesophageal echocardiography

   Doppler

      End-tidal CO_2

         Pulmonary artery catheter

           Cardiac output

              Central venous pressure

                ECG changes

                  Blood pressure

                    Precordial stethoscope

SMALL VAE VOLUME ──────────────────────── LARGE VAE VOLUME

FIGURE 11-1. Sensitivity of VAE detection devices. (From Aker, J. [1995]. Clinical dilemmas in neuroanesthesia. *CRNA: The Clinical Forum for Nurse Anesthetists*, 6, 1, 9–15.)

   2. Jugular compression may produce bradycardia.
   3. Trendelenburg position may be required to stop the air entrainment (surgical site above the level of the heart).
   4. Inotropic agents may be required to increase cardiac output.
   5. If a central venous catheter is in place, attempt to withdraw the entrained air.
  F. Paradoxical air embolism (PAE) occurs with the movement of air from the venous to the arterial side of the circulation.
   1. The embolized air passes through an intracardiac defect (ventricular or atrial septal defect, a probe-patent foramen ovale) or via transpulmonary passage.
   2. Air entering the brain will produce cerebral infarction, whereas air entering the coronary circulation will produce myocardial ischemia and infarction.

VII. Intraoperative Management

  A. Anesthetic induction
   1. Table 11–2 delineates the effects of various anesthetic agents on cerebral dynamics.
   2. The child with increased ICP is ideally induced with IV thiopental (3–6 mg/kg) or propofol (2–4 mg/kg), which produces cerebral vasoconstriction and decreases CMR_{O_2}. IV induction facilitates rapid airway control and subsequent hyperventilation for the control of increased ICP.

TABLE 11-2. Anesthetic Effects on Cerebral Dynamics

Drug	CBF	CMR_{O_2}	ICP	CPP
INHALATION				
Nitrous oxide	↑	↑↓	0	↓
Halothane	↑↑	↓	↑	↓
Enflurane	↑	↓	↑	↓
Isoflurane	↑*	↓	↑	↓
Sevoflurane	↑*	↓	↑	↓
Desflurane	↑*	↓	↑	↓
INTRAVENOUS				
Barbiturates	↓↓	↓↓	↓↓	0/↑
Etomidate	↓↓	↓↓	↓	0
Propofol	↓	↓	↓	↓
Ketamine	↑↑	↑	↑↑	↓
Benzodiazepines	↓	↑	↓	0/↑
Morphine	0/↓	0/↓	↓	↑↓
Fentanyl	0/↓	0/↓	↓	0/↑
Alfentatil	0/↓	0/↓	↓	↓
Sufentanil	0/↓	0	↓	↓
Remifentanil	0/↓	0	↓	↓

CBF, Cerebral blood flow; *CMR_{O_2},* cerebral metabolic rate for oxygen; *ICP,* intrancranial pressure; *CPP,* cerebral perfusion pressure.

Modified from Devane, G. (1997). Neurosurgical anesthesia. In Nagelhout, J., & Zaglaniczny, K.L. (Eds.). *Nurse anesthesia* (p. 796). Philadelphia: W.B. Saunders.

NOTE: Anesthetic drug effects as determined from adult studies.
*Dose-dependent increases in CBF >1 MAC.

3. Multiple attempts to secure IV access may be inadvisable because crying will exacerbate preexisting ICP.

4. IV access may be attempted 15 to 30 minutes following sedation with oral midazolam (0.5 mg/kg in cherry-flavored acetaminophen).* The child must be continuously monitored with pulse oximetry while awaiting the onset of sedation. The administration of 10% rectal methohexital (25–30 mg/kg) will produce sedation in 5 to 10 minutes, facilitating IV catheter placement.

5. When IV access is not attainable, an inhalation induction may be facilitated with halothane or sevoflurane (less coughing or breath holding than isoflurane, which would aggravate the increased ICP).

  a. Recall that cerebral vasodilation is greater with increasing concentrations of volatile anesthetic.

---

*Note that Roche has released an oral preparation of midazolam.

   b. IV access may be attempted once the child is asleep and a patent airway is obtained.
   c. This technique may minimize the needed concentrations of halothane or sevoflurane and allows the induction to be completed with thiopental or propofol.
6. Awake intubations are difficult to perform, are associated with variable decreases in oxygen saturation, and produce increases in ICP via a reduction in venous outflow from the head.
7. Neuromuscular blockade is produced with a selected nondepolarizing agent before laryngoscopy and endotracheal intubation.
8. Children with increased ICP have delayed gastric emptying that may necessitate a rapid sequence induction.
   a. Succinylcholine produces a transient rise in ICP that may be attenuated with IV thiopental and hyperventilation.
   b. Succinylcholine may produce exaggerated increases in serum potassium when administered to children with known myopathies, burn injuries, spinal cord injuries, crushing tissue injuries, or encephalitis.
9. Providing that the preoperative airway examination is acceptable, an IV induction with thiopental or propofol is followed by rocuronium, 1 mg/kg. Mild hyperventilation may be instituted with care to prevent inflation of the stomach while continuous cricoid pressure is maintained by an assistant.
10. Laryngoscopy in a lightly anesthetized child will induce both systemic hypertension and increased ICP. The sympathetic stimulus to laryngoscopy may be blunted with the IV administration of lidocaine, 1.5 mg/kg 2 minutes before laryngoscopy, or small doses of IV opioid (fentanyl, 1–3 µg/kg; alfentanil, 10–20 µg/kg).
B. Anesthetic maintenance
   1. The selection of specific anesthetic agents should be tailored to the individual and the proposed neurosurgical procedure.
   2. The selection of specific agents must take into account their effects on cerebral metabolism, blood flow, and ICP.
   3. Anesthetic maintenance may be accomplished with three separate techniques:
      a. Balanced technique using barbiturate and opioid with N_2O or low inspired concentrations of isoflurane (<1%) in oxygen and a nondepolarizing muscle relaxant. A balanced anesthetic technique facilitates rapid

recovery allowing prompt neurologic evaluation at the conclusion of the procedure.

   b. Isoflurane (up to 1%) in N_2O with hyperventilation is acceptable for anesthetic maintenance. Recall that the volatile anesthetic agents increase CBF, cerebral blood volume, and ICP in a dose-dependent manner.

   c. Nitrous oxide is contraindicated in children with pneumocephalus. In addition, some practitioners eliminate the use of N_2O when the potential exists for VAE.

  4. Skeletal muscle relaxation is important to prevent unexpected patient movement (but should never be used in lieu of anesthetic agent administration). Decreased thoracic pressure following chest wall paralysis increases venous drainage from the cranium and may decrease ICP.

C. Anesthetic emergence

  1. Emergence following neurosurgical procedures should focus on the following considerations:

   a. Elimination of anesthetic agents (volatile and IV) to facilitate awakening and neurologic assessment

   b. Use of a peripheral neuromuscular function monitor to document reversal of residual neuromuscular paralysis

   c. Avoiding sudden increases in ICP

  2. Tracheal extubation is generally completed when the child awakens following the demonstration of protective airway reflexes and adequate respiratory function (avoidance of hypercarbia and accompanying increases in ICP).

  3. Children with neurologic disorders may have altered gastric motility, and this should be considered when making the decision to extubate the child before being awake.

  4. Supplemental oxygen should be administered into the postoperative period and the adequacy of arterial oxygen saturation determined continuously with pulse oximetry.

D. Fluid administration

  1. See Chapter 7 for the calculation of maintenance and deficit fluid requirements and the selection of intravenous fluids.

  2. Specific considerations to the neurosurgical patient.

   a. Fluid homeostasis in the pediatric neurosurgical patient is complicated by the need to replace preoperative fluid deficits to maintain cardiovascular stability with anesthetic administration, the intraoperative administration of osmotic diuretic agents to decrease brain water content, and the difficulty in estimating actual blood loss.

b. Intraoperative fluid or blood administration must be balanced by the need to avoid excessive fluid administration that will contribute to cerebral edema and increased ICP.

c. The goal of fluid therapy should be to maintain circulating blood volume with isoosmolar, isooncotic fluid to maintain cerebral perfusion. Controversy exists as to whether colloid or crystalloid solutions are better for the neurosurgical patient. No clear advantage of either fluid has been demonstrated.

d. Fluid transit from the cerebral vasculature to the brain tissue is prevented by an intact blood-brain barrier. The blood-brain barrier is disrupted following head injury, as in the presence of mass lesions. Electrically charged molecules, such as sodium, and large molecular weight substances, such as albumin and mannitol, are free to cross the disrupted blood-brain barrier.

e. In the child with increased ICP, an osmotic diuretic is administered and followed by a balance of crystalloid or colloid fluid to maintain an isovolemic, isooncotic circulating plasma volume.

f. Perioperative fluids are restricted to minimize the contribution to increases in cerebral edema and ICP. However, limited fluid administration will decrease renal perfusion and may contribute to the development of hypotension following the administration of vasodilating anesthetic agents and the initiation of positive pressure ventilation. A decreased cardiac output decreases pulmonary blood flow, increases pulmonary shunting, and may contribute to the development of hypoxemia (particularly in children placed in the lateral position). Accordingly, Pao_2 may be decreased in the hypovolemic child.

g. Postoperative increases in aldosterone and antidiuretic hormone (ADH) secretion increase fluid retention with parallel decreases in serum sodium concentration. Increases in circulating plasma volume may contribute to rebound hypertension and increased cerebral edema and ICP.

h. Fluid osmolality in large part determines the movement of water across the blood-brain barrier. Hypotonic solutions should be avoided because they contribute to the production of cerebral edema.

i. Routine administration of glucose-containing solutions should be avoided. Cerebral ischemia results in the anaerobic metabolism of glucose, producing lactic acidosis in neuronal tissue. (See additional comments regarding glucose in Chapter 7.)

j. Blood loss is viewed on the surgical drapes and is usually mixed with irrigating solutions when suctioned from the surgical field. Initial blood loss from the scalp can be minimized with the prior injection of a 1:200,000 to 1:400,000 solution of epinephrine. When epinephrine-containing local anesthetics are used, the safe total dose should be determined before injection.

k. Blood loss is replaced to maintain acceptable oxygen-carrying capacity (see additional comments regarding blood replacement in Chapter 7).

VIII. Representative Surgical Procedures

A. Craniosynostosis
   1. Characteristics
      a. Common in infants with craniofacial malformations.
      b. Involves the sagittal suture, the coronal sutures, or both.
      c. Surgical correction is accomplished between 2 and 8 months of age.
      d. Approximately 50% of cases involve the sagittal suture, which produces frontal bossing and increases anteroposterior appearance of the cranium. The anterior fontanelle may be absent.
      e. The coronal suture is involved in 20% of cases.
      f. The forehead may appear flattened on the affected side. The synostosis of multiple sutures occurs in 7% of infants.
      g. Complete cranial reshaping may be required for optimal cosmetic results.
   2. Preoperative considerations
      a. Synostosis may be associated with increased ICP.
      b. Craniectomy includes the turning of large scalp flaps and the opening of thick bone tables along the suture lines, which contributes to the large (greater than 1 blood volume) blood loss and the increased occurrence of VAE.
      c. Ultrasonic precordial Doppler monitoring should be undertaken in infants undergoing craniectomy.
      d. Properly cross-matched blood that has been checked ahead of time must be available in the operating room.

Large blood loss and VAE may occur with the opening of the sagittal suture (underlying sagittal sinus).

3. Intraoperative considerations
   a. Satisfactory IV access must be achieved before surgical incision.
   b. Placement of an indwelling arterial catheter is recommended when multiple craniectomy is anticipated. An indwelling arterial catheter is also needed when induced hypotension is used to decrease intraoperative blood loss.
   c. Airway management may be difficult in infants with craniofacial deformities.
4. Postoperative considerations
   a. Facial edema and upper airway edema may develop at the conclusion of the procedure.
   b. Infants or older children undergoing craniofacial reconstructive procedures should be sedated and remain intubated and ventilated for 24 to 48 hours after the procedure.
   c. There is an increased risk of postoperative subdural and epidural hematoma formation. Occasionally, subarachnoid drains are placed and monitored for 24 to 48 hours postoperatively.
   d. The child should be fully awake with protective airway reflexes before tracheal extubation.

B. Meningomyelocele
   1. Characteristics
      a. Develops from the failure of neural tube closure during gestation.
      b. The neural tissue at the site is exposed to the elements, increasing the risk of neural tissue injury and infection.
      c. Most frequent site of failed neural tube closure is either thoracic or lumbosacral area, producing meningomyelocele at this level.
      d. Meningomyelocele is associated with Arnold-Chiari syndrome and hydrocephalus.
      e. Neural function distal to the defect may be absent or severely limited.
   2. Preoperative considerations
      a. Myelodysplasia is considered a surgical emergency.
      b. Repair is undertaken within the first hours of life to prevent development of meningitis and sepsis, the most common cause of mortality.
      c. Infants with myelodysplasia are at risk for the

development of latex allergy. These children should be treated in a latex-free environment beginning with the first surgical procedure (see Chapter 23).

   d. An open dura will produce CSF leak. Increased IV fluids may be required with CSF leak and increased third-space fluid losses from the defect.

   e. Preoperative antibiotics will be administered and must be continued throughout the perioperative period.

   f. The delicate neural tissue must be protected when placing the child in the supine position before anesthetic induction. A sterile towel should be placed to cover the defect. The infant may be supported with folded sterile towels placed lateral to the defect, allowing the neural tissue to hang freely.

   g. An additional method of positioning involves the use of a foam square cut to allow the neural elements to protrude through the foam. A sterile towel is placed over the foam. The exposed neural elements should remain moistened with sterile normal saline.

3. Intraoperative considerations

   a. Care must be taken to maintain core body temperature. The operating room should be warmed to 80°F before the infant's arrival.

   b. Anesthetic induction and maintenance can be easily accomplished with a volatile agent (halothane or sevoflurane).

   c. Induction may be accomplished in the supine position (see positioning notes above) or in the left lateral decubitus position while maintaining the head in a neutral position.

   d. Following induction and intubation, the infant is placed in the prone position.

   e. Succinylcholine is not associated with hyperkalemic response following administration to infants with myelomeningocele.

   f. Avoid the administration of nondepolarizing muscle relaxants until the surgeon is consulted.

   g. Blood loss rarely exceeds 15 to 30 ml.

4. Postoperative considerations

   a. Infant is positioned to avoid pressure on repair.

   b. Prone positioning may require continued postoperative ventilation until the infant is awake with acceptable respiratory function.

     c. The infant should be placed in a warm Isolette for transport to the recovery area.

C. Tethered spinal cord

  1. Preoperative considerations

    a. The filum terminale (sacral roots) are tethered by fibrous bands originating from the dura.

    b. Without surgical correction, neurologic dysfunction (motor and sensory dysfunction of the bladder and lower extremities) will occur.

    c. Females are affected twice as often as males.

  2. Intraoperative considerations

    a. Succinylcholine is contraindicated because of lower motor neuron involvement.

    b. Nondepolarizing muscle relaxants should not be given until consultation with the surgeon.

  3. Postoperative considerations

    a. Prone positioning may be preferred in the postoperative period.

    b. The child may be extubated in the left lateral decubitus position when awake, followed by prone positioning.

D. Cerebrovascular defects (arteriovenous malformations)

  1. General considerations

    a. Cerebrovascular aneurysm and arteriovenous malformations are uncommon in children.

    b. Fewer than 15% to 18% are diagnosed under the age of 15 years.

    c. These vascular malformation have a large arterial supply that dilates the communicating veins, which produces dilation of both the cerebral and cranial venous systems.

    d. Initial anesthetic intervention consists of general anesthesia for diagnostic cerebral angiography.

  2. Preoperative considerations

    a. Rupture of arteriovenous malformations will produce intracranial hemorrhage, with the compression of adjacent tissue resulting in cerebral infarction.

    b. Congestive heart failure (CHF) and right-sided heart failure may be presenting symptoms in the child with arteriovenous malformation. Left ventricular failure may occur as a result of increased cardiac output and increased pulmonary blood flow.

    c. Physical signs and symptoms may include tachypnea, tachycardia, pulmonary edema, decreased oxygen saturation, and cyanosis.

    d. Accompanying ECG changes may be present.

    e. Low systemic diastolic pressure may compromise coronary blood flow, precipitating myocardial ischemia.

    f. Preoperative sedation before transport to the operating room may decrease anxiety and the risk of intracranial bleeding.

3. Intraoperative considerations

    a. IV access should be secured with one or more large IV catheters before the surgical procedure. Excessive blood loss may occur with intraoperative rupture.

    b. Previously cross-matched blood must be available in the operating room.

    c. Anesthetic induction may be accomplished intravenously (provided a preoperative IV line is in place) or via mask inhalation induction.

    d. The child should be well anesthetized before laryngoscopy and intubation to prevent coughing and a hypertensive response that may elicit intracranial hemorrhage. IV lidocaine (1–1.5 mg/kg) with appropriate end-tidal concentrations of inhalation agent following the administration of a nondepolarizing muscle relaxant is preferred.

    e. Hypocarbia is avoided to prevent the shunting of additional blood to the low-resistance arteriovenous malformation.

    f. Anesthetic maintenance may be accomplished with isoflurane/relaxant or nitrous/oxygen/opioid/relaxant technique.

    g. A hypotensive anesthetic technique (increased inspired concentrations of isoflurane, nitroprusside, or nitroglycerin) is helpful at the time of ligation.

    h. An indwelling arterial catheter is essential following anesthetic induction.

    i. A central venous catheter may also be placed after induction.

    j. Urinary output is best monitored with an indwelling catheter.

4. Postoperative considerations

    a. Postoperative edema following brain retraction may necessitate continued postoperative ventilation and additional remedial therapy.

    b. Children with a preoperative history of CHF require aggressive medical therapy in the intensive care unit.

    c. The goal is to maintain acceptable CPP and avoid intravascular fluid overload.

    d. Antihypertensive agents may be required to prevent hypertension with continued postoperative ventilation and the risk of intracranial bleeding.

    e. Extubation is undertaken with judicious administration of antihypertensive agents or IV lidocaine (1–1.5 mg/kg) to prevent hypertension.

    f. Postoperative analgesics must be carefully administered to prevent excessive sedation, which complicates the postoperative neurologic examination.

E. Ventriculoperitoneal shunt

  1. General considerations (also see discussions of CNS disease, hydrocephalus)

    a. Procedure involves the cannulation of a cerebral ventricle, tunneling the catheter under the scalp subcutaneously through the neck, chest, and abdomen.

    b. The catheter is typically placed within the peritoneal cavity via an abdominal incision, although the distal end of the catheter may be placed into the atria or pleura in selected cases.

    c. Children with VP shunts return frequently for shunt revisions during their childhood years.

  2. Preoperative considerations

    a. Preoperative assessment must include an assessment of the degree of increased ICP.

    b. Increased ICP delays gastric emptying.

    c. A preoperative shunt scan may help delineate the area of shunt dysfunction.

    d. Increased ICP can be controlled with aspiration of the proximal shunt reservoir, removing a small amount of CSF, returning the ICP to near normal levels.

  3. Intraoperative considerations

    a. Anesthetic induction may be accomplished with an inhalation technique or IV technique.

    b. Children with elevated ICP, when possible, should have an IV induction with a barbiturate followed by the application of cricoid pressure.

    c. Hyperventilation is begun with the onset of neuromuscular relaxation. A target end-tidal $Paco_2$ of 25 to 30 mm Hg is sought in individuals with increased ICP.

    d. The child is generally placed in the supine position with the head elevated 20 to 30 degrees.

e. Arterial catheterization is reserved for children with dangerous elevations of ICP.

f. Intravascular fluid replacement may be required for children who exhibit protracted preoperative vomiting secondary to the increase in ICP.

g. Core body temperature is maintained by covering nonsurgical areas with warm blankets and preheating the operating room to 75°F to 80°F.

h. There is minimal blood loss with the procedure. Scalp blood loss can be decreased with the previous injection of a normal saline/epinephrine solution or local anesthetic epinephrine-containing solution.

4. Postoperative considerations

a. Recall the risk of aspiration secondary to delayed gastric emptying.

b. Gastric suctioning before extubation may decrease gastric volume but does not eliminate the risk of vomiting and aspiration.

c. Reversal of skeletal muscle relaxation must be ensured.

d. Supplemental oxygen should be administered and oxygen saturation continuously monitored with pulse oximetry.

e. Postoperative pain is minimal following local anesthetic infiltration of the surgical sites intraoperatively. Judicious use of analgesics is in order to enable continued assessment of children with preoperatively impaired neurologic function.

F. Supratentorial craniotomy

1. The supratentorial compartment contains the cerebral hemispheres, which are separated by the falx cerebri into three lobes: frontal, temporal and parietal-occipital

2. General considerations

a. The supratentorial compartment is the most typical site of solid tumors in children. CNS malignancy is the second most common type of cancer in childhood.

b. Fifty percent of CNS tumors are located in the supratentorial region.

c. Supratentorial tumors are most often responsible for obstructive hydrocephalus.

3. Preoperative considerations

a. Supratentorial tumors are associated with increased ICP.

b. The child should be carefully examined to determine the degree of ICP elevation.

    c. The child with increased ICP has delayed gastric emptying and an increased risk of aspiration and regurgitation.

    d. Fluid and electrolyte imbalance may develop preoperatively secondary to increased ICP and decreases in the level of consciousness (inability to take food and fluid).

    e. The syndrome of inappropriate ADH secretion may also occur secondary to the development of a mass lesion (clinical signs include hyponatremia, increased urine osmolality with decreased urine output).

    f. During transport to the operating room, the head should be elevated at least 10 degrees to promote venous drainage from the head and minimize increases in ICP secondary to obstructed venous outflow from the head.

    g. Marked increases in ICP may necessitate a "preoperative" ventriculostomy before tumor resection.

4. Intraoperative considerations

    a. Anesthetic induction and endotracheal intubation must be smooth to prevent further elevation of ICP.

    b. Preferred induction is accomplished with thiopental/lidocaine/fentanyl and a nondepolarizing muscle relaxant. Cricoid pressure is applied and hyperventilation is initiated following the introduction of low inspired concentration (<1 minimal alveolar concentration [MAC]) of isoflurane.

    c. When using moderate doses of vagotonic opioids (fentanyl, alfentanil, sufentanil) the use of a nondepolarizing skeletal muscle relaxant without cardiovascular side effects (e.g., vecuronium) is associated with marked decreases in heart rate. Pancuronium may be better suited to maintain heart rate, therefore maintaining cardiac output.

    d. Following successful endotracheal intubation, moderate hyperventilation (25–30 mm Hg) is begun to lower Pa_{CO_2}. CPP may be altered with lower levels of Pa_{CO_2}. The induced cerebral vasoconstriction may shunt blood flow away from ischemic areas.

    e. Although positive end-expiratory pressure (PEEP) is helpful, in children with impaired oxygenation, PEEP may reduce jugular venous drainage and contribute to increases in ICP.

    f. Arterial catheterization and/or CVP monitoring is established following induction.

g. A urinary catheter is also placed.

h. Ultrasonic Doppler monitoring is placed before preparation and draping.

i. The child is generally positioned in the supine position with the head elevated to promote venous drainage.

j. Care must be taken to maintain core body temperature. The operating room should be warmed to 80°F. The child can be covered with a forced-air warming blanket or covered with blankets obtained from a heated cabinet. For long surgical procedures, the IV fluids should be warmed with approved devices before infusion.

k. Properly cross-matched blood that has been checked ahead of time must be available in the operating room.

l. For fluid administration, see above discussion of fluid administration.

5. Postoperative considerations

a. See above discussion of anesthetic emergence.

b. Uncontrolled hypertension may precipitate increases in ICP. A combined alpha-beta blockade (labetalol) may be helpful in controlling blood pressure postoperatively.

c. Postoperative pain, hypoventilation with increased $Paco_2$, and a full urinary bladder contribute to postoperative hypertension.

d. Seizures may develop following anesthetic emergence. Intraoperative anticonvulsant administration may be requested by the surgeon.

G. Posterior craniotomy

1. The anatomic boundaries of the posterior fossa are formed by the tentorium cerebelli. The posterior fossa contains the cerebellum, medulla, and pons. The medulla and pons constitute the brain stem

2. General considerations

a. Tumors in the posterior fossa occur more commonly in children.

b. Most common tumors are medulloblastoma, astrocytoma, glioma, and ependymoma.

c. Hydrocephalus is a common preoperative finding in children with posterior fossa tumor.

d. Posterior fossa craniotomy is performed for Arnold-Chiari malformation, a congenital displacement of vermi of the cerebellum.

e. Preoperatively the child with Arnold-Chiari malformation may exhibit gait disturbances, inspiratory stridor, and clinical symptoms of increased ICP. Cardiovascular dysfunction may also accompany this malformation.

3. Preoperative considerations
   a. Children with posterior fossa tumors present with increased ICP and accompanying hydrocephalus. Hydrocephalus may be treated with a ventricular drain or VP shunt before definitive tumor removal.
   b. Gastric emptying is decreased in the presence of a posterior fossa tumor.
   c. A prior history of aspiration and pulmonary dysfunction may be present secondary to chronic aspiration.
   d. Preoperative diuresis for the control of ICP may create fluid and electrolyte disturbances.
   e. Tumors affecting the posterior fossa may produce altered cardiovascular and respiratory function.
   f. Chronic brain stem compression may produce hypertension and altered breathing patterns (sleep apnea).

4. Intraoperative considerations
   a. As outlined above in intraoperative considerations for supratentorial craniotomy.
   b. The child may be positioned in the seated (uncommon), three-quarter lateral, or prone position.
   c. In children at least 3 years of age, the Mayfield pin holder may be used to hold the cranium in the desired surgical position.
   d. Monitoring must include appropriate sensitive monitors for the detection of intraoperative VAE.
   e. Potent inhalation agents produce dose-dependent reductions in amplitude and increase latency of somatosensory evoked potential (SSEP) monitoring. Ketamine and etomidate both increase amplitude. Normothermia is important in maintaining acceptable recordings.
   f. Inspired concentrations of volatile agents should be kept between 0.5 and 1 MAC to minimize alterations in cortical SSEPs.
   g. Bradydysrhythmias and tachydysrhythmias may occur with manipulation of the brain stem. Commonly observed dysrhythmias include bradycardia, ventricular escape beats, sinus arrest, and ventricular tachycardia.
   h. Bipolar cauterization may produce severe hypertension.

i. The anesthetist must be vigilant for these dysrhythmias during the intraoperative manipulation of the posterior fossa contents.

5. Postoperative considerations

   a. See postoperative considerations for supratentorial craniotomy.

   b. Tracheal extubation should only be accomplished when the child is hemodynamically stable and has a regular pattern of respiration.

ADDITIONAL READINGS

Bedford, R.F. (1983). Venous air embolism: A historical perspective. *Seminars in Anesthesia, 2*, 169.

Bissonnette, B., Armstrong, D.C., & Rukta, J.T. (1997). Pediatric neuroanesthesia. In Albin, M. (Ed.). *Textbook of neuroanesthesia with neurosurgical and neuroscience perspectives* (pp. 1177–1246). New York: McGraw-Hill.

Devane, G. (1997). Neurosurgical anesthesia. In Nagelhout, J., & Zaglaniczny, K.L. (Eds.). *Nurse anesthesia* (pp. 795–815). Philadelphia: W.B. Saunders.

Lanier, W.L., Strangland, K.J., Scheithauer, B.W., Milde, J.H., & Michenfelder, J.D. (1987). The effects of dextrose infusion and head position on neurologic outcome after complete cerebral ischemia in primates: Examination of a model. *Anesthesiology, 66*, 39–48.

Newberg, L.A., & Michenfelder, J.D. (1983). Cerebral protection by isoflurane during hypoxemia or ischemia. *Anesthesiology, 59*, 29.

12

Cardiothoracic Surgical Procedures

Claudine N. Hoppen, MSN, CRNA

I. Introduction

A. Pediatric cardiothoracic surgery requires a thorough knowledge of congenital heart defects and their specific anesthetic implications.

B. Refer to Chapter 15 for a review of the anatomy, physiology, and anesthetic implications for each lesion.

II. Repair of Septal and Endocardial Cushion Defects

A. Atrial septal defects (ASDs), ventricular septal defects (VSDs), and atrial-ventricular (AV) canal defects are surgically approached via a midline sternotomy and aortic, caval cannulation for cardiopulmonary bypass.

B. ASDs, VSDs, and AV canal defects are commonly closed via a right atrial incision. Patch closure may be achieved with either synthetic graft or bovine pericardium.

C. Anesthetic implications of septal and AV canal defects.

1. Repair is traditionally performed when the Qp/Qs ratio >3 or the infant has persistent failure to thrive despite medical management.

2. Hyperoxia test results during catheterization are important.

3. Principles of pulmonary overcirculation apply.
   a. Avoid high F_{IO_2}.
   b. Avoid low E_{TCO_2}.
   c. Avoid high systemic vascular resistance (SVR).

4. Strict avoidance of air emboli.

5. Induction techniques are multiple, ranging from an inhalation induction with N_2O + sevoflurane + O_2 to intramuscular injection of ketamine, atropine, and succinylcholine.

6. Surgical repair.
   a. Right ventriculotomy or via the right atrium.
   b. Deep hypothermic circulatory arrest may be used for VSD repair and is commonly used during AV canal repair.

7. After repair: considerations postoperatively for the surgically corrected lesion.

III. Tetralogy of Fallot Repair

A. Occasionally palliative repair is performed before definitive surgical repair (refer to the section regarding surgical shunts).

B. Midline sternotomy and cardiopulmonary bypass with or without circulatory arrest are standard. Closure of the VSD is through either the right atrium or ventricle, and the right ventricular outflow tract obstruction is repaired.

C. Anesthetic management.

1. Preoperative (before surgical repair)
   a. Keep a normal to higher F_{IO_2}.
   b. Maintain a normal pH.
   c. Keep E_{TCO_2} normal to low.
   d. Keep SVR within normal limits; avoid large reductions.
   e. Check hematocrit; if >65%, consider implications of hyperviscosity.
   f. Treatment of hypercyanotic (TET) spells often includes O_2, phenylephrine (Neo-Synephrine), or morphine.
   g. Know preoperatively the location of a Blalock-Taussig shunt if one was placed shortly after birth. The side that the shunt exists on should not be used for invasive lines or blood pressures.

2. Intraoperative management
   a. Induction can be performed with either inhalation (sevoflurane + N_2O + O_2) for pink patients with TET spells or intramuscular ketamine + atropine + succinylcholine for cyanotic patients.
   b. Maintain a higher F_{IO_2} and lower E_{TCO_2}.
   c. Control pulmonary vascular resistance (PVR) with nitroglycerin, prostaglandins, nitric oxide, or tolazoline.
   d. Use extreme care to keep air out of intravenous (IV) lines.
   e. Treatment of TET spell intraoperatively and before bypass.
      (1) Fluids: ensure adequate hydration (10–20 ml/kg)
      (2) Phenylephrine (Neo-Synephrine)
      (3) Oxygen
      (4) Direct aortic compression via surgeon

3. Postrepair implications
   a. Maintain controlled ventilation with a pH of 7.5 and

CO_2 of 30 to 35 mm Hg immediately following repair and after cardiopulmonary bypass.
  b. Avoid right ventricle (RV) failure.
    (1) Keep right atrial pressure (RAP)/left atrial pressure (LAP) ratio less than 8 mm Hg.
    (2) Control PVR with ventilation changes and drugs.
  c. After repair: considerations postoperatively for the surgically corrected lesion.

IV. Surgical Shunts

A. Used when the anatomy involves severe obstruction to pulmonary blood flow
B. Commonly used in patients with tricuspid atresia, pulmonary atresia, severe tetralogy of Fallot, and a single ventricle with severe obstruction to pulmonary blood flow
  1. Blalock-Taussig shunt: a connection placed between the subclavian artery into a branch pulmonary artery on the ipsilateral side
  2. Potts shunt: connects the descending aorta and the left pulmonary artery; rarely used today because pulmonary blood flow can be excessive
  3. Waterston shunt: connects the right pulmonary artery and the ascending aorta; may also result in excess pulmonary flow
  4. Glenn shunt: allows for the systemic venous blood to flow to the lungs; connects the superior vena cava to the right pulmonary artery and can be made bidirectional to both pulmonary arteries
C. Anesthetic implications
  1. Pulmonary flow primarily depends on normal systemic arterial pressures; therefore avoid hypotension.
  2. Balance Qp/Qs ratio with ventilatory changes as indicated.

V. Transposition of the Great Vessels

A. Essentially four surgical repairs exist; however, systemic to pulmonary artery shunts are sometimes placed.
B. Refer to the discussion in Chapter 15 for the anesthetic implications.
C. Corrective repairs.
  1. Arterial switch/Jantene procedure with coronary reanastomosis
    a. Used in infants up to 3 months old
    b. Risks: surgical correction in small neonates; however,

this is no longer as pertinent because of improved capabilities for pediatric cardiopulmonary bypass
  c. Postoperative bleeding via suture lines possible
  d. Use nitroglycerin after bypass because of coronary manipulation
2. Mustard-Senning procedure: atrial switch
  a. Following repair, systemic venous blood is routed to the left ventricle (LV), which is draining into the pulmonary artery. The routing is accomplished via a baffle. Another baffle routes the pulmonary venous blood to the RV and to the aorta.
  b. Risks and problems: The RV is not designed to pump against systemic pressures; hence, RV failure ensues. Baffle obstructions can occur.
3. Rastelli procedure
  a. Used for children 2 to 3 years of age
  b. Primarily for repair of transposition of the great vessels with a VSD and a left ventricular outflow tract obstruction (LVOTO) or pulmonary artery stenosis
  c. VSD is closed with a patch that includes the LV outflow across the aortic valve. Then the proximal pulmonary artery is ligated and a valved conduit is placed from the RV to the main pulmonary artery
  d. Problem: postoperative RV dysfunction
4. Damus-Stansel-Kaye procedure
  a. Right ventriculotomy used to close VSD. Pulmonary artery is transected at the bifurcation, and the proximal portion of the pulmonary artery is anastomosed end to side to the aorta.
  b. A valved conduit is then placed from the RV to the pulmonary artery.

VI. Tricuspid Atresia and the Hemi-Fontan and Fontan Completion

A. This repair is essentially palliative. A midline sternotomy approach is used, as is deep hypothermic circulatory arrest.
B. Hemi-Fontan is the first stage of repair in early infancy. This may include a Blalock-Taussig shunt or a bidirectional cavopulmonary shunt (Glenn shunt connects the superior vena cava to both pulmonary arteries) and later a hemi-Fontan (connects the superior vena cava with the atrial appendage to the main pulmonary artery, obligating half of the systemic venous return to flow passively via the

pulmonary vascular bed). Interatrial communication is also ensured, and a patch or dam is placed to separate the common atrium from the atriopulmonary anastomosis.

C. The Fontan procedure, the second-stage repair at approximately 6 to 12 months old, directs the inferior vena cava blood to the pulmonary arteries via a fenestrated or non-fenestrated tunnel and completes separation of the circuits.

D. Anesthetic implications.
  1. Before hemi-Fontan repair
    a. Strictly avoid preload depletion; NPO time should be kept minimal, possibly 2 to 3 hours preoperatively.
    b. Inhalation induction is acceptable but should avoid depressing myocardial contractility.
    c. Maintain Fio_2 as low as possible, and titrate ventilation to balance Qp/Qs ratio.
    d. Excess pulmonary blood flow will result in higher saturations at the expense of systemic perfusion. This may rapidly result in acidosis and death.
    e. Excess systemic perfusion, at the expense of pulmonary blood flow, will result in increasing cyanosis.
    f. To improve the pulmonary blood flow before repair the following methods can be used.
      (1) Augment intravascular volume.
      (2) Give inotropes: dopamine or dobutamine.
      (3) Reduce PVR by decreasing the $Etco_2$ and increasing Fio_2.
    g. To decrease pulmonary circulation the following methods can be used.
      (1) Avoid increasing Pao_2 >45 mm Hg because this is difficult to reverse and may result in death from insufficient systemic perfusion.
      (2) Decrease respiratory rate and Fio_2; consider adding CO_2 to the circuit.
    h. After hemi-Fontan and Fontan repair.
      (1) Keep CVP high enough to passively drive blood to the pulmonary vascular bed: CVP 15 to 20 mm Hg and LAP <10 mm Hg.
      (2) Minimize PVR by having Fio_2 at 1.0, decreasing $Etco_2$, and increasing tidal volume (VT).
      (3) *No* positive end expiratory pressure (PEEP); minimize peak inspiratory pressures, which will hinder passive pulmonary filling.
      (4) If blood pressure drops, administer volume to maintain an adequate passive pulmonary filling

pressure; then consider dopamine or dobutamine or both.

(5) Avoid agents that may increase PVR.

VII. Hypoplastic Left Heart: The Norwood Procedure

A. Repair is palliative, since the only definitive repair is heart transplantation.

B. Repair is also done via sternotomy, cardiopulmonary bypass, and circulatory arrest.
   1. Stage I repair: Norwood
      a. Creation of a neoaorta with pulmonary homograft
      b. Insertion of a modified Blalock-Taussig shunt
      c. Creation of, or ensuring, a large, nonrestrictive ASD
   2. Stage II: hemi-Fontan
   3. Stage III: Fontan completion

C. Anesthetic implications before Norwood repair.
   1. Maintain patent ductus arteriosus (PDA) with prostaglandin (PGE_1) infusion.
   2. Maintain a balance of Qp/Qs.
   3. Add CO_2 to the fresh gas flow *if* excess pulmonary blood flow is caused by a widely patent ASD (if Qp/Qs ratio >1). This will increase PVR.
   4. Maintain adequate systemic perfusion and cardiac output with dopamine or dobutamine or both (if Qp/Qs ratio <1).

D. Anesthetic implications after Norwood procedure and before hemi-Fontan procedure.
   1. Preserve Qp/Qs = 1.
   2. Keep $Paco_2$ at 40 mm Hg.
   3. Maintain saturations of 75% to 80%.
   4. Manipulate Qp/Qs ratio with ventilation changes and inotropes as needed.
   5. Maintain hematocrit >38%.
   6. Avoid Pao_2 >45 mm Hg because this is difficult to reverse and death may ensue from insufficient systemic perfusion.

E. Refer to the anesthetic implications for before the hemi-Fontan procedure and after the Fontan procedure described under "Tricuspid Atresia."

VIII. Total Anomalous Pulmonary Venous Connection

A. Repair involves dissecting the pulmonary veins from their abnormal position and anastomosing them to the posterior wall of the left atrium.

B. This may require tunneling to the left atrium. Since an

ASD is almost always present this is usually closed during repair.

C. Anesthesic implications.
1. Inhalants are not well tolerated in this population.
2. Narcotic techniques provide the most hemodynamic instability.
3. Considerations for F_{IO_2}
   a. Increasing the F_{IO_2} may not significantly improve oxygenation since this is a fixed mixing lesion.
   b. Consider using higher F_{IO_2} *if* the patient presents with pulmonary hypertension and acute failure.
4. Inotropes such as dopamine and dobutamine are frequently used immediately after repair, because the left ventricle is required to pump a greater volume load.
5. After bypass.
   a. Keep LAP approximately 6 mm Hg to avoid excess stress on suture lines and to prevent fluid overload for the left side of the heart.
   b. Keep the RAP 10 to 12 mm Hg maximum.
   c. If the cardiac output is low, pulmonary edema will ensue and will result in low saturations after bypass. The use of inotropes is recommended.

IX. Patent Ductus Arteriosus
A. Refer to the discussion in Chapter 15.

X. Coarctation Repair
A. Five variations of repair exist. Refer to the anesthetic implications discussed in Chapter 15.
1. Resection and subclavian artery patch angioplasty: left posterolateral thoracotomy. Ductus is ligated, and a clamp is placed between the left carotid artery and the left subclavian artery. A distal clamp is placed distal to the coarctation. The aorta is incised, and a patch from the subclavian artery is used
2. Resection with end-to-end anastomosis
3. Subclavian aortoplasty: uses a Dacron interposition graft, hence similar to the end-to-end anastomosis
4. Patch aortoplasty
5. Bypass grafts occasionally used for long segment coarctations

ADDITIONAL READINGS
Gregory, G. (1994). *Pediatric anesthesia* (3rd ed.). New York: Churchill Livingstone.

Hersley, F.A., & Martin, D.E. (Eds.). (1995). *A practical approach to cardiac anesthesia* (2nd ed.). Boston: Little, Brown.

Katz, J., & Steward, D.J. (Eds.). (1987). *Anesthesia and uncommon pediatric diseases.* Philadelphia: W.B. Saunders.

Lake, C.L. (Ed.). (1993). *Pediatric cardiac anesthesia* (2nd ed.). Norwalk, Ct.: Appelton & Lange.

Motoyama, E.K., & Davis, P.J. (Eds.). (1996). *Smith's anesthesia for infants and children* (6th ed.). St. Louis: Mosby.

13

Pediatric Diagnostic and Therapeutic Procedures

Eva Bowden, MS, CRNA, and John Aker, MS, CRNA

I. Introduction

A. The rapid growth of medical technology has precipitated the development of diagnostic equipment located outside the operating room.

B. Typical pediatric diagnostic procedures are listed in Table 13–1.

C. Not infrequently these pediatric diagnostic procedures require anesthesia provider intervention.

D. Anesthesia care in unfamiliar locations is challenging because of the remote location and the naiveté of health care providers in these diagnostic areas with regard to conscious sedation and general anesthetic procedures.

II. Limitations of Remote Locations

A. Diagnostic and therapeutic suites can be located a great distance from the operating room, requiring the transport of all required anesthesia equipment.

B. Anesthesia care must be to the same standard as the care provided in the operating room.

C. A checklist of equipment needs will aid in organization.

D. Equipment that must be available to ensure safe and effective anesthesia includes:

1. Suction with a selection of suction catheters

2. Full cylinders of oxygen on the anesthesia machine

3. In addition, a cylinder with an oxygen flowmeter should be available to provide oxygen during transport from the diagnostic area to the recovery area

4. Emergency drug cart with defibrillator, pediatric intravenous (IV) access supplies, anesthetic drugs and fluids, pediatric endotracheal tubes, oral airways, laryngoscope and blades

5. Emergency electrical outlets to supply power to the anesthesia machine, and monitoring equipment

TABLE 13–1. Typical Pediatric Diagnostic Procedures

Category	Representative Procedures
Cardiac catheterization	Valvuloplasty, patent ductus arteriosus (PDA) umbrella, electrophysiology studies, percutaneous transluminal angioplasty (renal artery stenosis, arteriovenous grafts, pulmonary valve)
Neuroelectrophysiology studies	Brainstem auditory evoked potential
Angiography	Evaluation and/or embolization of vascular malformations
Nuclear medicine	Diagnostic imaging
Magnetic resonance imaging (MRI), computed tomography (CT)	Diagnostic imaging
Radiation oncology	Radiation therapy
Digestive disease clinic procedures	Gastroscopy or colonsocopy
Clinic procedures	Bone marrow aspiration, percutaneous tissue biopsies

6. Monitoring equipment, including noninvasive blood pressure monitor, temperature, continuous electrocardiogram (ECG), pulse oximetry, and capnography
7. Appropriate sizes of pulse oximetry probes and blood pressure cuffs
8. The ambient temperature of the diagnostic suite is decreased to maintain the electrical equipment
   a. The temperature should be increased to prevent decreases in core body temperature.
   b. Warming blankets, forced air warmers, and diathermy warmers may interfere with diagnostic imaging.
   c. When able, exposed body surfaces should be covered by a warm blanket.
9. Backup light source (flashlight) to view patient and equipment
10. Reliable two-way communication to summon assistance
E. Diagnostic suites have limited space available for anesthesia equipment carts and anesthesia machines.
F. Gas evacuation in compliance with institutional guidelines may require innovative connections from the anesthesia machine to suction devices to facilitate waste gas evacuation.
G. Pipeline source of oxygen and suction are generally available but may be difficult to access.

H. It is unusual to find pipeline sources of air or nitrous oxide unless the diagnostic suite was specifically developed for anesthesia administration.

I. The quality of delivered anesthesia care as mandated by the American Association of Nurse Anesthetists' (AANA's) Standards for Nurse Anesthesia Practice must be followed for anesthesia care delivered in remote locations. These standards are listed in the box below.

Standards for Nurse Anesthesia Practice

Standard I. Perform a thorough and complete preanesthesia assessment.

Standard II. Obtain informed consent for the planned anesthetic intervention from the patient or legal guardian.

Standard III. Formulate a patient-specific plan for anesthetic care.

Standard IV. Implement and adjust the anesthetic care plan based on the patient's physiologic response.

Standard V. Monitor the patient's physiologic condition as appropriate for the type of anesthesia and specific patient needs.

Standard VI. There shall be complete, accurate and timely documentation of pertinent information on the patient's medical record.

Standard VII. Transfer the responsibility for care of the patient to other qualified providers in a manner which assures continuity of care and patient safety.

Standard VIII. Adhere to appropriate safety precautions as established within the institution, to minimize the risks of fire, explosion, electrical shock, and equipment malfunction. Document on the patient's medical record that the anesthesia machine and equipment were checked.

Standard IX. Precautions shall be taken to minimize the risk of infection to the patient, the CRNA, and other health care providers.

Standard X. Anesthesia care shall be assessed to assure its quality and contribution to positive patient outcomes.

Standard XI. The CRNA shall respect and maintain the basic rights of patients.

From American Association of Nurse Anesthetists. (1996). *Scope and standards for nurse anesthesia practice.*

J. Suggested guidelines for the management of conscious sedation for pediatric patients during and after diagnostic and therapeutic procedures are listed in the box below.

Suggested Guidelines for the Management of Conscious Sedation for Pediatric Patients During and After Diagnostic and Therapeutic Procedures

Diagnostic or Procedure Suite: This area must be adequately staffed by individuals trained in the management of conscious sedation who are prepared to attend cardiovascular and respiratory dysfunction that may occur during the diagnostic or therapeutic procedure. Standards for diagnostic and therapeutic suites are generally mandated by state law.

Emergency Care: A policy must be developed that outlines the organization of emergency services for either in-hospital or office-based facilities. Office-based facilities should have a plan for emergency transportation to the nearest hospital emergency department.

Essential Equipment:
- A positive-pressure oxygen delivery system capable of delivering 100% oxygen but never less than 21% oxygen and an essential oxygen supply.
- Equipment designed for the delivery of inhaled anesthetics should contain a fail-safe system and should be calibrated and proper function verified annually.
- A variety of sizes of oxygen masks and airway adjuncts (airways, endotracheal tubes, laryngeal mask airways) must be available to accommodate children of different ages and body weight.
- Essential physiological monitoring should include a continuous electrocardiogram, blood pressure, pulse, respiratory rate, and continuous pulse oximetry (see p. 201, American Association of Nurse Anesthetists Standards for Nurse Anesthesia Practice).
- An emergency cart must be immediately available that contains the necessary drugs and equipment for resuscitation of an unconscious patient and continuous support during

> **Suggested Guidelines for the Management of Conscious Sedation for Pediatric Patients During and After Diagnostic and Therapeutic Procedures** *Continued*
>
> transport to an emergency facility. The emergency cart must be checked and resupplied on a scheduled basis and have accompanying documentation to verify such.
>
> **PREOPERATIVE PREPARATION**
>
> **Preanesthetic Evaluation:** A thorough and complete preanesthetic evaluation must be completed prior to the diagnostic or therapeutic procedure. This evaluation should include a health history, review of systems, a statement as to airway patency, current vital signs, current physical findings, and rationale for sedation.
>
> **Informed Consent:** The anesthetic options (conscious sedation and general anesthesia) must be discussed with the legal guardian. Written consent should be obtained according to the procedure outlines by individual state law.
>
> **Responsible Adult:** The pediatric patient must be accompanied to and from the diagnostic or therapeutic facility by a legal guardian. This individual must remain at the diagnostic or therapeutic facility for the duration of the procedure.
>
> **Documentation:** Documentation must reflect the standards of anesthesia practice and includes all anesthetic interventions and patient responses.

III. Preanesthesia Preparation

    A. All patients receiving anesthesia care in a diagnostic facility require the same, thorough preoperative evaluation as patients receiving anesthesia care in the operating room.

    B. Scheduling of the diagnostic or therapeutic procedure should include the proposed procedure, an approximation of the required duration, required patient position, potential complications, and arrangements for discharge or hospital admission following the procedure.

    C. The child's primary physician should be contacted to obtain a preprocedure history and physical examination.

    D. The anesthetist is responsible for detailing the anesthetic preparation of the child (medications to be continued, duration of NPO period, required diagnostic laboratory testing) and options to the parent or guardian. This may be accomplished by a telephone call to the parent or guardian 1 or 2 days before the procedure.

E. Informed consent is obtained from the responsible parent or guardian through discussions of the risks and benefits of the proposed anesthesia technique.

F. Postanesthesia care.
1. Discussions between the anesthesia provider and physician responsible for the diagnostic examination must resolve where postanesthesia care will be provided before beginning anesthesia.
2. The child may be transported to the postanesthesia care unit (PACU).
3. During transport the child must receive supplemental oxygen administration and have continuous pulse oximetry and electrocardiogram (ECG) monitoring.
4. However, postanesthesia care may be provided in close proximity to the diagnostic suite.
5. All postanesthesia care must be provided by nurses experienced in the immediate postoperative care of children and in an area with suitable monitoring and support services for the care of children.

IV. Conscious Sedation

A. The American Dental Association Council on Dental Education has suitably defined conscious sedation as follows: "a minimally depressed level of consciousness that retains the patient's ability to independently and continuously maintain an airway and respond appropriately to physical stimulation and verbal commands."

B. Pediatric sedation is challenging under the best of circumstances.

C. Successful sedation in the adult population often requires a cooperative patient.

D. Many diagnostic procedures in children require them to be motionless.

E. Repeated doses of IV sedatives and analgesics may promptly produce apnea and unconsciousness with complete loss of protective airway reflexes.

F. Individuals administering sedatives or analgesics must be familiar with the pharmacokinetic and pharmacodynamic differences in the pediatric population (see Chapter 2).

G. Monitoring responsibilities.
1. The individual responsible for the administration of sedatives or analgesics and monitoring of the child must

have no other responsibilities during the diagnostic procedure.

2. This individual should continuously monitor the child during the procedure and establish a record of the child's vital signs throughout the procedure. Areas for monitoring include:

   a. Continuous assessment of the level of consciousness, responsiveness to verbal commands and physical stimulation, and the ability to independently and continuously maintain a patent airway and protective reflexes

   b. Continuous assessment of airway patency (the rate, depth, and character of respirations) and continuous pulse oximetry readings

   c. Assessment of hemodynamic stability with continuous ECG monitoring (heart rate and rhythm) and noninvasive blood pressure determination at least every 5 minutes

   d. The ability to monitor core body temperature by electric thermometry or adhesive skin strips

H. IV access.

1. All pediatric patients undergoing conscious sedation must have a continuous running IV line.

2. IV access may be facilitated with the prior application of EMLA Cream, a eutectic mixture of local anesthetics.

   a. EMLA Cream must be applied 30 to 60 minutes before venipuncture and covered with an occlusive dressing.

   b. For children who arrive from home, EMLA Cream may be provided to the parent during the preanesthesia visit.

3. The anesthesia provider should identify two suitable IV sites by an ink mark directing the parental application of EMLA.

4. Oral midazolam (0.5 mg/kg) may be administered in apple juice or a precalculated dose of acetaminophen 15 to 30 minutes before the procedure. (NOTE: Roche, Nutley, N.J., has released an oral midazolam preparation.)

5. Inhaled nitrous oxide in oxygen may be provided by an anesthesia provider by mask to facilitate IV access. Recall that 50% nitrous oxide may blunt protective airway reflexes, increasing the risk of aspiration and airway obstruction.

V. Administration of IV Radiocontrast Dyes

A. Ionic media are iodinated salts administered intravenously for diagnostic imaging.

   1. Radiocontrast dyes are hyperosmolar ionic or nonionic compounds.
   2. The ionic compounds (Hypaque, Conray, Renografin) have an iodine content of approximately 300 mg/ml and an osmolarity of 2000 to 3000 mOsm/L.
      a. A pediatric dose is approximately 2 ml/kg.
      b. Agents with concentrations of 30% or 60% are used for children.
      c. High iodine and sodium concentrations may produce volume contraction and increased osmolality following administration.
   3. Nonionic radiocontrast compounds (iopamidol, iohexol) have an iodine content of 300 mg/ml and an osmolarity of 700 to 900 mOsm/L.
      a. Like ionic compounds, an appropriate dose is approximately 2 ml/kg.
      b. These agents have a decreased incidence of adverse reactions following administration.
      c. Nonionic compounds are preferred for administration to children.

B. IV administration may release vasoactive substances from mast cells, producing the clinical symptoms of urticaria, hypotension, tachycardia, dysrhythmias, bronchospasm, and nausea and vomiting.

C. Radiocontrast material may produce a true allergic reaction (anaphylaxis) in a small percentage of patients. Patients with a history of food allergy (shellfish), asthma, allergy to iodine, or multiple drug allergies have a greater risk of allergic reaction with radiocontrast dye administration.

D. Hypertonic radiocontrast solutions produce a transient hypertension following administration, which is accompanied by an increase in intravascular volume, central venous pressure, and cardiac output and a decrease in systemic vascular resistance.

E. Children with documented allergy who require radiocontrast administration should receive prophylactic H_2 antagonists, diphenhydramine, 0.5 to 1.0 mg/kg PO or IV 1 hour before the procedure, and methylprednisolone, 0.5 mg/kg PO or IV 12 hours and 1 to 2 hours before the procedure. Prophylaxis *does not prevent an allergic reaction,* since 5% of allergic patients will still experience a reaction, but it does decrease the severity of the reaction.

F. Treatment of an allergic reaction includes the administration of supplemental oxygen, epinephrine boluses in doses of 10 µg/kg (epinephrine infusion of 0.1–1 µg/kg/min IV), and IV crystalloid or colloid to reestablish intravascular volume. Definitive airway management (endotracheal intubation) is required when the airway becomes compromised.

VI. Angiography and Cardiac Diagnostic or Therapeutic Procedures

A. Angiography
1. Angiography procedures involve the intraarterial injection of radiocontrast material to image anatomic structures.
2. Angiography is commonly used for imaging intracranial vascular anomalies or tumors.
3. Anesthesia considerations.
   a. General anesthesia is generally required for the insertion of the arterial catheter and to ensure a motionless child for subsequent imaging.
   b. The airway is generally secured via endotracheal intubation, which secures the airway during imaging of the head and aids the ability to control $Paco_2$.
   c. Hyperventilation produces cerebral vasoconstriction, decreasing the transient nature of intravenously administered radiocontrast dyes.
   d. $Paco_2$ maintained between 30 and 35 mm Hg is sufficient to obtain high-quality images.
   e. The selection of anesthetic agents, whether IV or inhalation, must take into account their effects on cerebral blood flow.
   f. Inhalation agents produce dose-dependent cerebrovasodilation.
   g. Propofol, which reduces cerebral metabolic rate ($CMRo_2$), cerebral blood flow, and intracranial pressure, may produce marked reductions in cerebral perfusion pressure via the accompanying reduction in blood pressure.
4. Hemodynamic instability may occur during cerebral angiography.
5. Tachycardia and bradycardia may occur in up to 20% of patients.
6. In addition, intracranial hemorrhage is accompanied by marked ECG changes, notably T wave inversion.
7. Multiple repeated injections of radiocontrast material may be required.

a. The maximum dose of contrast material that may be safely administered should be determined before the procedure.

8. Neurologic complications, either transient or permanent, are not infrequent following cerebral angiography.

B. Cardiac diagnostic procedures

1. Premature infants, neonates, and older children are scheduled for diagnostic anatomic evaluation of the cardiovascular system.

2. These diagnostic evaluations, using either noninvasive or invasive techniques, require a motionless patient to obtain a qualitative and quantitative evaluation of cardiac function.

3. A steady state cardiovascular function is required for the determination of cardiac chamber pressures and oxygen saturations, the assessment of pressure gradients across stenotic valves, and the calculation of shunt fractions.

4. The chosen anesthetic technique is selected according to the age of the child and the requirements of the diagnostic procedure.

5. It is imperative to be familiar with the cardiovascular effects of various IV and inhalation anesthetic agents.

6. The anesthetist may need to pharmacologically alter preprocedure anxiety associated with transport to the diagnostic suite (to maintain a steady cardiovascular state).

7. Standard monitoring (ECG, pulse oximetry, capnography, noninvasive blood pressure, temperature, neuromuscular function monitor) is afforded for all children during cardiac catheterization.

8. To minimize heat transfer, neonates should have their heads covered and have exposed body portions covered with a warm blanket.

9. Blood sampling for electrolytes (potassium, calcium) and blood glucose may be required for lengthy procedures.

10. The use of fluoroscopy may require positioning of the anesthesia machine and the anesthetist at a distance from the child.

11. IV fluid extensions and circle system circuit extensions may be required.

12. Arterial monitoring will be initiated following femoral or brachial arterial cannulation.

13. The use of fluoroscopy requires the wearing of protective lead shields by all personnel in the diagnostic suite.

These should be available to cover exposed areas of the child.

14. The diagnostic procedure may require IV radiocontrast dye administration. These solutions as well as the flush solutions must be included in the total fluid management calculation.

15. Children generally recover in the pediatric intensive care unit (PICU).

16. Endotracheal extubation is accomplished at the conclusion of the procedure in the PICU.

C. Cardiac catheterization

1. Right-sided heart catheterization is facilitated with cannulation of the brachial or medial cephalic vein (the axillary and femoral veins may also be used).

2. Left-sided heart catheterization is performed via the retrograde insertion of a catheter through the femoral or brachial arteries.

3. Local anesthetic is injected following either sedation or general anesthesia.

4. Following induction, a continuous IV line is established. Endotracheal intubation is generally required for infants and smaller children.

5. For the youngest of children, general anesthesia (either 100% oxygen or oxygen–nitrous oxide with 0.5–1 minimum alveolar concentration [MAC] of inhalation agent) may be administered for catheter insertion and discontinued before hemodynamic assessment.

6. If used, nitrous oxide is discontinued shortly following induction and the selected inhalation agent is administered in 30% oxygen.

7. Nitrous oxide may interfere with reflection oximetry for oxygen saturation determination and should be discontinued at least 10 to 15 minutes before oxygen saturation measurements.

8. Heart catheterization, although not extremely painful, is uncomfortable with the injection of local anesthetic and the pressure of catheter insertion at the selected site. Nausea and vomiting may occur during the procedure.

9. Heart catheterization of the neonate is generally performed on an emergency basis. These neonates can be gravely ill and are usually intubated and ventilated before arrival in the diagnostic suite. Sedation may not be necessary to accomplish the catheterization.

10. Supplemental oxygen administration must be considered for each individual case.

a. An increase in the fraction of inspired oxygen may produce ductus arteriosus constriction in children with aortic stenosis or aortic coarctation.

b. In addition, pulmonary artery pressures and pulmonary vascular resistances are altered with increases in oxygenation.

c. Supplemental oxygen between 20% and 40% may be safely used in these infants.

11. Hypoxemia may be present before or may develop during the course of cardiac catheterization.

a. Hypoxemia is manifest by irritability, depressed consciousness, tachycardia, intercostal and sternal retractions, utilization of accessory muscles of respiration, and an increase in cyanosis (decreasing Spo_2).

b. Occlusion of a stenotic pulmonary outflow tract may precipitate acute decreases in oxygen saturation.

c. Respiratory depression may develop from intravenously administered respiratory depressants.

12. Ventilatory control in the anesthetized infant may affect the cardiac catheterization data via a decrease in mixed venous oxygen content and an increase in left-to-right shunt.

13. Cyanotic children will likely have high hematocrits. Further hemoconcentration may develop following the administration of radiocontrast dyes, which act as osmotic diuretics (see above).

14. Procedure blood loss occurs from the arterial or venous cutdown site and bleeding into the surrounding tissues. IV fluid boluses may be required to maintain acceptable circulating plasma volume.

VII. Radiologic Diagnostic or Therapeutic Procedures

A. Computed tomography (CT) scan

1. CT scan uses ionizing radiation to detect variations in the densities of body tissues.

a. The ionizing radiation source and the accompanying radiation detectors are mounted across from one another.

b. The child is placed on a remote-controlled table into a gantry and positioned between the ionizing radiation source and the radiation detectors.

c. Multiple scans are taken throughout a 180-degree rotation.

d. These individual readings are processed by a computer, which provides images of tissue density.

    e. CT scanning allows the accurate visualization of anatomic structures. CT scanning is used for diagnostic imaging of all body anatomic structures.

2. CT scanning is not painful, but quality images require a motionless patient.

3. Contemporary CT scanners provide rapid imaging (completing scans in 30 minutes).

4. Following the initial scan, IV radiocontrast material may be administered, requiring an additional scan to complete the required diagnostic evaluation.

5. Young children, children who are unable to cooperate with adult instructions, and children with physical disabilities or medical illnesses may require deep sedation or general anesthesia to complete the scan.

6. Positioning of small children can be facilitated by wrapping the child in a warm snug blanket, restraining arm movement.

7. Conscious sedation has been widely used by radiologists in an attempt to avoid general anesthetic techniques.

8. Oral chloral hydrate has been widely used; however, recent concerns regarding the generation of potentially harmful metabolites have decreased its appeal.

9. Ketamine should be avoided because it increases salivation and produces unpredictable spontaneous limb movements.

10. For the aforementioned reason, etomidate should also be avoided.

11. A number of pharmacologic drug combinations have been used for conscious sedation.

    a. The "lytic cocktails," which are composed of an opioid (meperidine or morphine), antihistamine (Benadryl), and phenothiazine (promethazine), have varying degrees of success, producing ineffective sedation in 10% to 20% of patients and extended periods of sedation (up to several hours after the scan).

    b. Rectal methohexital is safe and effective. This technique produces *general anesthesia* and requires anesthesia provider attendance and appropriate monitoring. Deep sedation may be accompanied by airway obstruction and apnea. Rectal methohexital produces minimal alterations in cardiovascular or respiratory function in the healthy child. Recommended dose is 25 to 30 mg/kg of a 5% to 10% solution, which produces sleep in 6 to 10 minutes and lasts 30 to 60 minutes (peak plasma concentrations). Mucosal damage may develop when more concentrated solutions are employed.

    c. A continuous infusion of propofol with oxygen delivery via mask or endotracheal tube is also an acceptable alternative.

12. General anesthesia ensures immobility of the child, increasing the quality of the scanned images.

    a. General anesthesia requires endotracheal intubation or a laryngeal mask airway for airway management since the anesthesia provider will not have access to the face during the scan.

    b. Anesthesia is generally induced with a mask-delivered inhalation agent and maintained with spontaneous ventilation.

    c. A continuous infusion of propofol with oxygen delivery via mask or endotracheal tube is also an acceptable alternative.

B. Magnetic resonance imaging (MRI)

1. MRI has revolutionized the diagnostic assessment of central nervous system pathologic conditions.

    a. MRI produces high-resolution cross-sectional images using the magnetic properties of atomic nuclei.

    b. The child is placed on an adjustable table, which is moved to position the child into a powerful magnet.

    c. An image is computer generated from signals received from the magnetic field.

    d. It is important to note that there is no radiation exposure to the child or personnel in the MRI environment.

    e. However, it is the strength of this magnetic field that produces a number of formidable hazards and challenges for the anesthesia team.

2. The radio frequency pulses create a loud and inconsistent noise. The child should be provided ear protection during general anesthesia or sedation techniques.

3. Ferrous surgical implants may become dislodged, may migrate, and may become dysfunctional in the presence of this strong magnetic field. Children and anesthesia and radiology personnel with ferrous surgical implants (heart valves, aneurysm clips, cochlear or stapedial implants) must be identified to prevent their entry into the MRI suite.

4. Loose ferromagnetic objects may become propelled by the strong magnetic field in the MRI suite.
   a. Ferromagnetic objects (e.g., ink pens, needles, scissors, paperclips, stethoscopes, laryngoscopes, IV poles, ferrous gas cylinders) must be removed before entry into the MRI suite.
   b. Safe nonferrous metals include gold, stainless steel, titanium, tantalum, aluminum, and copper.
5. Radio frequency heating may result from induced currents.
   a. Monitor leads from the ECG and pulse oximeter may heat and produce a patient burn.
   b. The only MRI-compatible temperature monitor available is a wireless skin strip.
   c. Disposable pulse oximeter probes should never be used.
   d. All MRI-compatible wiring must be shielded from direct contact with the child's skin.
6. Physiologic monitoring interference may occur as the static magnetic field distorts and displaces the electric beam images. An MRI-compatible ECG monitor (with artifact suppression) is required for continuous ECG monitoring.
7. There is limited access to the child when positioned into the scanner. A patent IV infusion and properly functioning monitoring equipment (pulse oximetry, noninvasive blood pressure and capnography) is essential before beginning the scan. IV infusion pumps are not compatible within the MRI scanner, and IV regulation is best accomplished with a Buretrol or minidrip infusion set.
8. There are no case reports of tissue injury or oncologic or teratogenic effects from the magnetic field in radiologic personnel. However, the safe use of MRI in the parturient has not been established.
C. Anesthetic considerations
   1. The administration of anesthesia is complicated by the remote location as well as the limitations of the equipment that may be placed within the strong magnetic environment.
   2. To obtain an effective diagnostic image, the child is required to be motionless during imaging.
      a. Imaging may take from 30 minutes to 2 hours depending on the body area to be examined.
      b. Young children will infrequently lie still in the

claustrophobic environment without anesthesia provider intervention.

3. Because of limited access to the child, most anesthesia providers may prefer general anesthesia with either an endotracheal tube or a laryngeal mask airway, which decreases the problems of airway management that may occur during an IV sedation technique.

4. General anesthesia may be induced outside the MRI suite, minimizing the need to eliminate ferrometallic equipment.

5. Following induction, all ferrometallic devices must be removed from the child and anesthesia personnel before transport into the MRI environment.

6. It is acceptable to do a general anesthetic induction inside the MRI suite using appropriate precautions.

7. A continuous IV infusion should be established either before or following mask inhalation induction.

8. A lengthy anesthesia circuit will be required to reach the child when positioned within the scanner.

9. Total intravenous anesthesia (TIVA) is an acceptable method of management. A bolus of propofol (1 mg/kg) followed by an infusion (5 to 10 mg/kg/h) effectively maintains adequate levels of anesthesia and promotes early discharge.

10. Following entry into the MRI suite, MRI-compatible monitoring equipment (noninvasive blood pressure, pulse oximetry, capnography, ECG) is connected to the child.

11. Maintenance of core temperature in small infants and children is difficult because MRI suites are cooled to protect the electrical circuitry.

12. During the MRI scan the magnetic field and radio frequency may actually increase the child's temperature. Temperature monitoring is essential during MRI.

13. MRI-compatible machines are available from both Drager (Telford, Penn) and Datex-Ohmeda (Madison, Wisc).
    a. These machines are composed of nonferrous metallic material.
    b. Gas cylinders are constructed of aluminum.
    c. The MRI suite should have central pipeline connections for oxygen and gas evacuation.

14. Radiocontrast media are frequently administered to enhance image resolution.
    a. Gadopentetate dimeglumine (Magnevist) is a nonionic, renally cleared paramagnetic contrast medium.

     b. This agent will transverse a disrupted blood-brain barrier to image cranial or spinal lesions.

     c. Children with sickle cell disease or trait should not receive Magnevist because sickle cells will align perpendicular to the magnetic field, precipitating a vasoocclusive crisis.

VIII. Nuclear Medicine

A. Nuclear medicine procedures involve the injection of organ-specific radioisotopes with varying degrees of radioactivity that are delivered to the target organ via the bloodstream.

    1. Following a precalculated delivery time (minutes to several hours), the child is returned to the nuclear medicine suite for imaging scanning.

    2. The majority of nuclear imaging uses low radiation isotopes with long uptake and elimination characteristics.

    3. Patient shielding is not required following isotope injection.

B. Positron emission tomography (PET) scans use higher radiation isotopes with shorter uptake and elimination characteristics.

    1. Accordingly the scanning times are shorter.

    2. The treating health care personnel must remain at a distance from the patient following injection and at the time of the scan.

    3. Patients do not require isolation following scan completion.

C. Anesthesia intervention is requested for the period of imaging to ensure a motionless patient.

    1. Anesthetic management may be accomplished with an IV sedation technique or general anesthesia.

    2. Preoperative evaluation is important to assess the child's health, provide parental guidelines for the NPO period, and obtain consent for the proposed anesthetic technique.

D. Abdominal nuclear isotope scans may be hampered by media solution concentration in the bladder. Straight catheterization may be required to empty the bladder.

E. Glucose-based isotope solutions for brain scans depend on cerebral glucose metabolism for isotope uptake. CMR_{O_2} should be maintained near normal for successful study completion.

F. Sedation rather than general anesthesia will minimize the influences on CMR_{O_2}.

G. Movement must be minimized, but this should not be accomplished with increasing depths of anesthesia.

ADDITIONAL READINGS

Forbes, R.B. (1998). Anesthesia for nonsurgical procedures. In Longnecker, D.E., Tinker, J.H., & Morgan, G.E. (Eds). *Principles and practice of anesthesiology* (2nd ed.). St. Louis: Mosby.

Gilles, B.S. (1992). Anesthesia outside the operating room. In Barash, P.G., Cullen, B.F., & Stoelting, R.K. (Eds.). *Clinical anesthesia* (2nd ed.). Philadelphia: J.B. Lippincott.

Patteson, S.K., & Chesney, J.T. Anesthetic management for magnetic resonance imaging: Problems and solutions. *Anesthesia and Analgesia,* 74(1), 121–128.

Wheeler, H.J. (1998). AANA journal course. New technologies in anesthesia: Update for nurse anesthetists. Magnetic resonance imaging. *American Association of Nurse Anesthetists Journal* 57(6), 515–520.

14

Anesthesia for Pediatric Urologic Procedures

Anne Marie Hranchook, MSN, CRNA

I. Introduction

A. Pediatric genitourologic procedures are performed for the correction of congenital or acquired genitourinary defects.

B. Pediatric urologic procedures may account for up to 30% of the total pediatric surgical schedule.

C. The anesthetist must be familiar with the anatomic and physiologic changes that accompany genitourinary congenital defects, the anesthetic requirements for the proposed operative procedure, and the positioning requirements that allow the surgeon anatomic access.

D. Anatomic access to the genitourinary tract for diagnostic or surgical correction of defects may be gained through the urethra via fiberoptic lighted scopes, abdominal laparotomy, or a retroperitoneal approach.

E. Accordingly, the analgesic requirements, muscle relaxation, and required postoperative analgesia will depend on the proposed surgical procedure and the patient's underlying pathophysiology.

F. Table 14–1 lists genitourinary pathologic conditions that may require surgical intervention.

II. Pediatric Renal Development

A. Decreased glomerular filtration rate

1. The newborn has a glomerular filtration rate (GFR) one half to one third of the adult.

2. The premature infant's GFR is only 10% of adult levels.

3. With continuing renal maturity the GFR approaches adult levels by 12 months of age.

4. Although the baseline GFR is acceptable during this time, hypotension, genitourinary infection, systemic viral infections, anemia, or abdominal surgical procedures may further compromise GFR.

TABLE 14-1. Common Pediatric Genitourinary Pathologic Conditions

Category	Pathologic Conditions
Congenital defects	Double renal pelvis and ureters
	Neurogenic bladder
	Exstrophy of bladder
	Undescended testis
	Hypospadias
	Phimosis
Cystic masses	Wilms tumor
	Cystic kidney
	Neuroblastoma
	Pheochromocytoma
Renal dysfunction	Renal biopsy (open, percutaneous)
	Nephrectomy
	Creation of vascular shunts (dialysis)
	Renal transplantation (cadaveric, living related)
Genitourinary infection	Cystitis (cystoscopy)
	Ureteral or renal calculus

   B. Renal tubular function
     1. The newborn has a decreased ability to reabsorb fluid from the renal tubules and a decreased capacity to concentrate urine.
     2. The ability to excrete a solute load is also compromised.
     3. The renal threshold for bicarbonate is decreased, resulting in increased bicarbonate filtration with plasma bicarbonate ranging from 18 to 22 mEq/L.

III. Preanesthetic Assessment

   A. The preoperative assessment must delineate the degree of renal dysfunction.
   B. Repeated urinary tract infections or obstruction may result in progressive renal tubular dysfunction.
   C. The preoperative history should ascertain instances of fever, repeated urinary tract infections, antibiotic therapy, weight loss, and fluid intake.
   D. Urinary output may be ascertained by asking about the number of wet diapers that are changed on a daily basis.
   E. Enuresis, vomiting, fatigue, and pyuria are suggestive of urinary tract infection.
   F. Laboratory evaluation of a urine specimen may include culture and sensitivity and evaluation for protein, hemoglobin, and white blood cells.

G. Serum creatinine (0.4–0.8 mg/dl) and blood urea nitrogen (BUN; 8–20 mg/dl) provide a reliable assessment of renal function.

H. Preoperative radiographic techniques (intravenous pyelogram, ultrasonography, computer tomography) may provide additional information relative to anatomic and physiologic function.

I. Normal pediatric renal function.
   1. Urine output of 0.5 to 1 ml/kg/h
   2. Newborn urine specific gravity of 1.004 to 1.020
   3. Proteinuria: newborn, 240 mg/m^2/d; child, 100 mg/d
   4. Serum creatinine
      a. Age 4 weeks: 0.25 to 0.4 ml/dl
      b. Age 1 to 10 years: 0.4 to 1.0 mg/dl
   5. BUN
      a. Preterm infant: 16 to 22 mg/dl
      b. Newborn: 25 to 31 mg/dl
      c. 12 months to 16 years: 8 to 12 mg/dl

J. Psychologic and emotional preparation.
   1. Congenital urinary problems require repeated physical examinations and surgical procedures.
   2. Urologic surgical procedures are typically performed in children between 6 months and 10 years of age.
   3. Hospitalization and surgical intervention in this age-group generate fear and anxiety associated with
      a. Parental separation
      b. Potential of physical harm
      c. Body injury with accompanying pain
      d. Loss of autonomy and privacy

IV. Urogenital Surgical Procedures

A. Cystoscopy or ureteroscopy
   1. Cystoscopy is generally a brief diagnostic procedure performed with the patient under general anesthesia following an inhalation induction.
   2. Anesthesia is maintained with mask, laryngeal mask airway, and/or endotracheal intubation.
   3. The child should be well anesthetized to prevent laryngospasm with the insertion of the cystoscope or movement during the procedure.
   4. Postoperative regional techniques (caudal or epidural anesthesia) are not necessary because the child experiences little pain following the procedure.
   5. The child is moved to the lower half of the operating table

and placed in the lithotomy position to facilitate access to the external genitalia.

6. Positioning requirements necessitate the movement of monitoring equipment and the anesthesia machine to gain access to the child.

7. The operating room should be warmed and the child covered because exposure of and preparation of the external genitalia with cold solutions will precipitate a decrease in core temperature.

8. Core temperature decreases are also enhanced through the use of room temperature bladder irrigation solution.

9. Rigid ureteroscopy requires an immobile patient.

10. Coughing, bucking on an endotracheal tube, or sudden movement may precipitate ureter rupture.

B. Voiding cystourethrography and urodynamics

1. Urodynamic studies require a depth of anesthesia that is sufficiently light (near the point of awakening) to allow spontaneous voiding to occur.

2. Bladder activity and sphincter tone may be suppressed up to 10 minutes following the administration of thiopental or greater than 1 minimum alveolar concentration (MAC) of an inhalation agent.

3. An anesthetic technique using nitrous oxide in combination with a low concentration of an inhalation agent minimizes the use of intravenous anesthetic agents.

4. Atropine decreases bladder tone, and its prior administration will invalidate a urodynamic study.

5. Lidocaine in a dose of 1 to 1.5 mg/kg will suppress laryngeal reflexes and decrease the risk of laryngospasm during light planes of general anesthesia.

C. Circumcision

1. Circumcision is the most frequent urogenital surgical procedure performed in the newborn period.

2. Newborns undergoing circumcision require anesthesia despite the previously widespread belief that newborns have decreased pain perception.

3. Penile nerve block provides sufficient anesthesia for the procedure as well as postoperative analgesia.

4. Circumcision in older infants and preschool and school-aged children is performed with the patient under general anesthesia.

5. Inhalation induction with nitrous oxide in oxygen is a traditional anesthetic technique.

6. Penile block performed after the induction of anesthesia

but before the surgical procedure will reduce the anesthetic requirement and facilitate a rapid emergence from general anesthesia.

    a. In newborns, 0.8 ml of 1% plain lidocaine produces sufficient anesthesia.

    b. For older children 1 to 3 ml of plain 0.25% bupivacaine provides 4 to 6 hours of analgesia.

    c. Epinephrine-free solutions must be used because the artery supplying the penis is an end-artery. Epinephrine-induced vasoconstriction may precipitate ischemic injury.

7. The caudal instillation of local anesthetic may be accomplished before the surgical procedure and at its conclusion.

    a. Bupivacaine 0.25% with 1:200,000 epinephrine in a dose of 0.5 ml/kg will provide 4 to 6 hours of analgesia.

D. Hypospadias repair

1. Hypospadias occurs in 8 per 1000 male births.

2. Repair is ideally performed when the child is between 6 and 12 months of age.

3. Fibrous chordee tissue is released to straighten the curvature of the penile shaft, followed by the creation of a neourethra from penile skin to advance the urethral meatus to the tip of the glands.

4. The repair may require multiple operative procedures.

5. Associated congenital anomalies are restricted to the lower genitourinary tract and include inguinal hernia, hydrocele, and cryptorchidism.

6. Endotracheal intubation is generally preferred because the surgical procedure may require several hours.

7. For procedures of shorter duration, the laryngeal mask airway may be used in lieu of an endotracheal tube.

8. Anesthesia is generally conducted with an inhalation technique.

9. Skeletal muscle relaxation is not required, and accordingly the child may spontaneously ventilate and receive assisted ventilation.

10. Penile block and/or caudal epidural will reduce intraoperative anesthetic requirements and provide postoperative analgesia.

11. If the duration of the surgery is longer than 2 hours, the caudal anesthesia may be repeated at the conclusion of the procedure using one half to two thirds of the original local anesthetic volume of 0.25% bupivacaine or an equal volume of 0.125% bupivacaine.

12. Penile block is less effective than caudal epidural for postoperative analgesia, especially for repair of proximally located hypospadias.

E. Orchiopexy

1. Cryptorchidism occurs in 0.8% of 1-year-old males.
2. The undescended testis may lie within the abdomen, the inguinal canal, or the external ring just proximal to the scrotum.
3. The chance of complete spontaneous testicular descent after infancy is small.
4. The undescended testis will undergo degenerative changes.
5. Accompanying congenital defects include inguinal hernia and testicular torsion.
6. If the undescended testes are unrepaired, there is an increased chance of testicular malignancy and infertility.
7. Anatomic access for repair is gained through an inguinal incision.
8. A scrotal incision may be required to fixate the testis following its placement in the scrotal sac.
9. When the testis cannot be palpated, inguinal exploration, laparoscopy, or exploratory laparotomy may be necessary to determine the presence of a testis.
10. Abdominal exploration will require endotracheal intubation and skeletal muscle relaxation.
11. Traction of and manipulation of the spermatic cord may elicit bradycardia.
12. For the treatment of bradycardia that does not resolve with cessation of surgical manipulation, atropine (0.02 mg/kg) may be appropriate.
13. Laryngospasm may develop in the lightly anesthetized child.

F. Ureteral reimplantation

1. Ureteral reimplantation is performed to correct vesicoureteral reflux.
2. The duration of the procedure may be as long as 8 to 10 hours.
3. During the procedure the ureter is freed from the bladder and reimplanted in a new, surgically created submucosal ureteral tunnel.
4. This tunnel functions as a valve, preventing the reflux of urine.
5. Ascending bacteria following urine reflux produce renal damage.

6. Bilateral vesicoureteral reflux with accompanying infection may produce atrophic parenchymal scarring followed by developing renal insufficiency and hypertension.
7. Anesthetic considerations.
   a. General anesthesia with endotracheal intubation is required for the lengthy repair.
   b. A caudal or lumbar epidural catheter may be used intraoperatively to decrease the general anesthetic requirement and may be continued postoperatively to facilitate postoperative pain management.
   c. Hypertension may be present in up to 25% of children with reflux who have evidence of renal parenchymal damage.
   d. The continuation of prescribed antihypertensives during the perioperative period should be evaluated on an individual basis.
   e. Invasive monitoring may be required in children with severe renal impairment and hypertension.
   f. Fluid and blood therapy is monitored with serial hematocrit determinations.
   g. Urinary output is unable to be determined, because it will be collected in the surgical field.
G. Prune-belly syndrome
   1. Prune-belly syndrome develops in 1 in every 40,000 births (primarily in males).
   2. Distal urinary tract obstruction leads to multiple organ dysfunction.
   3. Bladder distention leads to the classic pathophysiologic signs, which include bladder wall hypertrophy, abdominal distention, abdominal muscle loss, excess abdominal skin, hydroureter, renal dysplasia, and cryptorchidism. Lower limb abnormalities may also occur.
   4. The severity of organ system involvement allows the classification of these children.
      a. Group I children have severe renal disease and pulmonary hypoplasia and are generally morbid.
      b. Group II children have severe uropathy and urinary tract infection and require multiple corrective procedures.
      c. Group III children have few problems in the newborn period but present later in childhood with urinary tract infection.
      d. Group II and III children develop normally and have normal renal function.

5. Anesthetic considerations.
   a. Decreased abdominal musculature inhibits the ability to cough and clear the pharynx and throat.
   b. Preoperative sedation should be avoided to prevent aspiration and respiratory depression.
   c. The technique of endotracheal intubation should take into account the likelihood of aspiration. Aspiration prophylaxis is warranted.
   d. Controlled ventilation is necessary to prevent hypoventilation and hypoxemia.
   e. Skeletal muscle relaxation should not be required.
   f. Postoperative morbidity originates from pulmonary infection and postoperative aspiration.
   g. Postoperative ventilation may be required in children who undergo lengthy surgical procedures or in children who have significant pulmonary disease.

ADDITIONAL READINGS

Berry, F.A. (1994). Anesthesia for genitourinary surgery. In Gregory, G.A. (Ed.). *Pediatric anesthesia.* New York: Churchill Livingstone.

Cramolini, G.M. (1993). Disease of the renal system. In Katz, J., & Stewart, D.J. (Eds.). *Anesthesia and uncommon pediatric diseases.* Philadelphia: W.B. Saunders.

Davis, P.J., Hall, S., Deshpande, J.K., & Spear, R.M. (1996). Anesthesia for general, urologic and plastic surgery. In Motomoyama, E.K., & Davis, P.J. (Eds.). *Smith's anesthesia for infants and children.* St. Louis: Mosby.

Yaster, M., & Maxwell, L.G. (1989). Pediatric regional anesthesia. *Anesthesiology* 70, 324–338.

Common Diseases

IV

15

Anesthesia for Pediatric Patients with Cardiovascular Diseases

Claudine N. Hoppen, MSN, CRNA

I. Introduction

A. The incidence of congenital heart disease (CHD) remains 8:1000 live births, with 80% to 90% of all lesions falling into 10 general types. Repair may be either corrective or palliative. One-year mortality for severe lesions approaches 25%.

B. Children with CHD may have other congenital lesions or syndromes that will also have anesthetic implications.

C. Chromosome abnormalities or syndromes associated with CHD are listed in Table 15–1.

D. Initial comprehension of congenital heart defects must include a review of both fetal circulation and the balance of pulmonary vascular resistance (PVR) versus systemic vascular resistance (SVR).

E. Fetal circulation is parallel and involves oxygen flowing to the placenta and then to the fetus via the umbilical vein.

1. The flow of blood is then through the ductus venosus → inferior vena cava (IVC) → right atrium (RA) → foramen ovale (FO) → left atrium (LA) → left ventricle (LV) → aorta (Ao) → head vessels.

2. Desaturated blood from the head returns to the heart from the superior vena cava (SVC) → RA → right ventricle (RV) → pulmonary artery (PA) → patent ductus arteriosus (PDA) → descending Ao → lower body. Blood then exits the fetus and placenta via two umbilical arteries.

F. Transitional circulation exists for 2 to 3 days after birth. This is a critical time because of closure of the PDA and FO; in ductal-dependent lesions, closure may result in death.

G. Hypoxemia, hypercarbia, acidosis, sepsis, and persistent pulmonary hypertension can all result in the persistence of the PDA.

H. Factors affecting PVR and the pulmonary:systemic blood flow ratio (Qp:Qs) are listed in Table 15–2. It is vitally important to interpret this information from cardiac cathe-

TABLE 15–1. Chromosome Abnormalities or Syndromes Associated with Congenital Heart Disease (CHD)

Trisomies 13 (Patau syndrome), 18 (Edwards syndrome), 21 (Down syndrome), 9 (mosaic), triploidy, cri-du-chat syndrome, Wolf-Hirschhorn syndrome, 9p, 13q, 18q, 17p (Miller-Dieker syndrome/lissencephaly), 22q (DiGeorge syndrome)
Turner syndrome: sex-linked anomalies
Certain autosomal dominant syndromes (i.e., Apert syndrome)
Brain and neuromuscular anomalies
Skeletal dysplasias
Craniosynostosis syndromes
Major limb defects
VATER: vertebral/anal atresia, tracheoesophageal fistula (TEF), ventricular septal defect (VSD), renal abnormalities
CHARGE: tetralogy of Fallot (TOF), eye anomalies, mental retardation, genital hypoplasia, deafness
Beckwith-Wiedemann syndrome: tetralogy of Fallot (TOF), macroglossia, ear creases, hypoglycemia
Maternal factors: alcohol and drug use, rubella, systemic lupus erythmatosus (SLE), diabetes

terization reports because the anesthetic management of children and infants with heart disease is influenced by Qp:Qs.

I. Determination of the relationship between the pulmonary and systemic blood flow is approximated by the Qp:Qs ratio.

TABLE 15–2. Factors Affecting Pulmonary Vascular Resistance (PVR) and the Role of Pulmonary/Systemic Blood Flow Ratio (Qp/Qs)

INCREASES PVR

Hypoxia	High mean airway pressures
Atelectasis	Light anesthesia
Hypothermia	PEEP
Polycythemia	Acidosis
Cardiopulmonary bypass	Vasoconstrictors
Hypercapnia	Decreased LV output
High peak inspiratory pressures	

DECREASES PVR

High F_{IO_2}	Hypocapnia
Anemia	Vasodilators
Dopamine, 2–10 mg	Alkalosis
Milrinone	Improved LV output

PEEP, Positive end expiratory pressure; *LV,* left ventricular.

1. The Fick method can be used to calculate pulmonary (Qp) and systemic (Qs) blood flow:

   a. $Qp = \dfrac{\text{Oxygen consumption (per m}^2)}{Cp\bar{v}o_2 - Cpao_2}$

   where $Cp\bar{v}o_2$ = pulmonary venous oxygen content and $Cpao_2$ = pulmonary arterial oxygen content

   b. $Qs = \dfrac{\text{Oxygen consumption (per m}^2)}{Cao_2 - C\bar{v}o_2}$

   where Cao_2 = systemic arterial oxygen content and $C\bar{v}o_2$ = mixed venous oxygen content

2. Interpretation
   a. A left-to-right shunt exists when Qp:Qs >1.
   b. A right-to-left shunt exists when Qp:Qs <1.
   c. When Qp:Qs = 1, there is balanced flow, which can indicate a bidirectional shunt of equal magnitude or no shunt.

II. Septal Defects and Endocardial Cushion Defects

A. Atrial septal defects (ASDs)
   1. One of the most common defects; affects females more often than males
   2. Differs from a probe patent foramen ovale (PFO) that may exist in the adult population
   3. Types
      a. Ostium primum: located at or near the PFO
      b. Ostium secundum: located over or near the IVC
      c. Sinus venosus: located at the SVC; may be associated with pulmonary veins draining into the RA
   4. Repair
      a. At 2 to 5 years of age most commonly or if Qp:Qs >2
      b. Problem: left-to-right shunt and pulmonary overflow

B. Ventricular septal defects (VSDs)
   1. Comprise 20% to 30% of all congenital heart lesions
   2. Likely to close spontaneously if size <3 mm
   3. Initial management: medical, with furosemide, digoxin, and/or spironolactone (Aldactone), and high-calorie formula
   4. Repair indicated when failure to thrive exists
   5. Types
      a. Supracristal: close to pulmonary valve

     b. Membranous (75% of VSDs): just below tricuspid valve
     c. Inlet: common in atrioventricular (AV) defects
     d. Muscular: can be multiple
  6. Problems
     a. Left-to-right shunt with chronic pulmonary overload
     b. Left ventricular end-diastolic volume (LVEDV) 2× normal
     c. Normal left ventricular end-diastolic pressure (LVEDP)
     d. Qp:Qs $\geq$3
     e. Pertinent catheterization data
       (1) Existence of a coarctation: very bad prognosis, must repair the coarctation first
       (2) Existence of mitral valve anomalies

C. Atrioventricular canal defect
  1. Most common congenital heart defect in patients with Down syndrome
  2. Types
     a. Partial AV canal: failure of septum primum to fuse with the endocardial cushion; associated with cleft in mitral valve, mitral regurgitation (MR), and left-to-right shunt
     b. Complete AV canal: failure of septum primum to fuse and complete failure of endocardial cushions to fuse with a common interatrial communication, interventricular communication, mitral valve cleft, and abnormal tricuspid valve
  3. Pertinent catheterization data to examine
     a. Systemic pressure in both the right and left ventricles
     b. Large left-to-right shunt
     c. Pulmonary hypertension
     d. Heart failure
  4. Implications of Down syndrome
     a. Airway anomalies or difficulties
     b. Difficult intravenous (IV) and arterial access

D. Anesthetic implications of septal and AV canal defects
  1. Repair traditionally performed when the Qp:Qs >3 or the infant has persistent failure to thrive despite medical management
  2. Hyperoxia test results during catheterization are important.
  3. Principles of pulmonary overcirculation prerepair
     a. Avoid high F_{IO_2}.

   b. Avoid low E_{TCO_2}.
   c. Avoid high SVR.
4. Strict avoidance of air emboli
5. Multiple induction techniques, ranging from an inhalation induction with nitrous oxide (N_2O), sevoflurane, and oxygen (O_2) to intramuscular injection of ketamine, atropine, and succinylcholine
6. Surgical repair
   a. Right atriotomy
   b. Deep hypothermic circulatory arrest: may be used for VSD repair; commonly used during AV canal repair

III. Tetralogy of Fallot

A. Accounts for 15% of all congenital heart defects
B. Includes the following anatomic components: underdeveloped RV infundibulum with a displaced septum, RV outflow tract stenosis, VSD, overriding aorta
C. Right-sided aortic arch in 25% of cases
D. Obstruction to pulmonary blood flow anywhere from the infundibulum to the pulmonary artery, including the pulmonary valve
E. May also have tortuous coronary arteries
F. Associated anomalies: PDA, multiple VSDs, AV canal, dextrocardia
G. Pathophysiologic characteristics
   1. Right-to-left shunt
   2. Decreased pulmonary blood flow
   3. RV and LV sustain the same work load unless the VSD is small or restrictive
   4. Compensatory mechanisms: polycythemia and development of pulmonary collaterals
   5. Hypercyanotic (TET) spells in 20% to 70% of the patients
      a. Present by 2 to 3 months of age (and decrease in severity by 2 to 3 years as a result of adaptive mechanisms)
      b. May be associated with crying, feeding, Valsalva maneuvers, or other responses that increase oxygen demand
      c. Clinical symptoms: hyperventilation, cyanosis, and hypoxemia
      d. A result of the hypoxemia is an increased venous return that increases the right-to-left shunting
      e. Treatment: medications that increase the SVR (phenyl-

ephrine), decrease the venous return (morphine), and reduce the shunt; assuming the "squatting" position also can relieve the symptoms

H. Anesthetic management

1. Preoperative considerations before surgical repair
   a. Maintain a normal to higher F_{IO_2}.
   b. Maintain a normal pH.
   c. Keep E_{TCO_2} normal to low.
   d. Keep SVR within normal limits; avoid large reductions.
   e. Check hematocrit; if >65%, consider implications of hyperviscosity.
   f. Treatment of TET spells often includes O_2, phenylephrine (Neo-Synephrine), and/or morphine.
   g. Know preoperatively the location of a Blalock-Taussig (BT) shunt if one was placed shortly after birth. The side that the BT shunt exists on should not be used for invasive lines or blood pressures.

2. Intraoperative management
   a. Induction can be performed with either inhalation (sevoflurane or halothane) for pink patients or intramuscular ketamine for cyanotic patients.
   b. Maintain a higher F_{IO_2} and lower E_{TCO_2}.
   c. Nitroglycerin, prostaglandins, nitric oxide, and tolazoline can be used to control PVR.
   d. Use extreme care to keep air out of IV lines.
   e. Treatment of TET spell intraoperatively is as follows:
      (1) Fluids: ensure adequate hydration (10–20 ml/kg)
      (2) Neo-Synephrine
      (3) Oxygen
      (4) Direct aortic compression via surgeon

IV. Transposition of the Great Vessels (TGV)

A. TGV includes only 5% to 7% of all congenital heart defects and is not commonly associated with other congenital defects.

B. This defect is essentially parallel circulation where the right ventricle gives rise to the aorta and the left ventricle gives rise to the pulmonary artery.

C. Essentially, this anatomy is incompatible with life unless some form of intercirculatory mixing exists such as a VSD, ASD, or PDA.

D. Five types of lesions may exist, all of which have different forms of intercirculatory mixing (ICM) and variable degrees of pulmonary blood flow (PBF).

E. Diagnosis.
   1. Cardiac catheterization: considered the gold standard
   2. Cyanosis: especially if intercirculatory mixing is small
   3. Congestive heart failure (CHF): especially if there is increased PBF and large ICM
F. Anesthetic implications.
   1. Maintain ductal patency if PDA exists with prostaglandin (PGE_1) infusion.
   2. Maintain heart rate, contractility, preload, and cardiac output.
   3. Avoid agents that decrease contractility.
   4. Preoperative.
      a. Premedication is used only if infant >7 months old; this must be balanced against a tenuous cardiovascular state.
      b. Polycythemia may exist.
G. TGV with both decreased PBF and minimal ICM: anesthetic implications.
   1. Avoid increasing PVR relative to SVR: An increased PVR will decrease PBF and further reduce ICM.
   2. Use ventilatory changes to decrease PVR: increase F_{IO_2} and respiratory rate (RR), decrease E_{TCO_2}, and maintain pH at 7.50 to 7.56.
H. TGV with increased PBF and large ICM: anesthetic implications.
   1. Maintain normal PVR, normal-limit E_{TCO_2}, and low F_{IO_2}.
   2. Do *not* make ventilatory changes to adjust the PVR, because this will only modestly improve saturations at the expense of systemic perfusion.
I. Repairs: For a discussion of both palliative and corrective repairs, refer to Chapter 12.

V. Truncus Arteriosus

A. This is a rare congenital heart defect that occurs as an arrest in embryologic development
B. This defect is almost always associated with the existence of a VSD
C. Following birth, CHF rapidly ensues because of pulmonary overflow
D. Anatomy
   1. Includes four different types, all of which include some form of the main pulmonary artery arising from the truncus
   2. PBF: normal to increased
E. Symptomatology and diagnosis

1. Severe CHF as a result of increased PBF
2. Tachypnea
3. Difficulty feeding
4. Irritability
5. Wide pulse pressure
6. Echocardiogram

F. Prerepair considerations
   1. No premedication is used because repair is in early infancy.
   2. Check for coexisting facial anomalies and difficult airway.
   3. Avoid increasing SVR, which may increase PBF.
   4. Maintain a low F_{IO_2}.
   5. Keep E_{TCO_2} high normal.
   6. Use positive end expiratory pressure (PEEP).
   7. Avoid decreasing SVR too much because this can result in excess systemic flow at the expense of the coronary arteries.

G. Postrepair considerations
   1. Ventricle now has a smaller preload and increased resistance.
   2. Keep pulmonary artery pressure (PAP) low, use high F_{IO_2}, and maintain low normal E_{TCO_2}.
   3. Maintain LV output.

H. Repair is usually during neonatal period: For descriptions of the surgical repair refer to Chapter 12

VI. Single Ventricles

A. Tricuspid atresia
   1. This lesion, along with pulmonary atresia with an intact ventricular septum, results in varying degrees of a hypoplastic right ventricle, an ASD, and PBF dependent on a PDA
   2. Anatomy
      a. Blood flows across the foramen ovale into the left atrium, mixing with the pulmonary venous return. This drains into the left ventricle and is ejected systemically.
      b. The degree of pulmonary blood flow depends on a PDA.
      c. If a large VSD exists, some blood enters the hypoplastic right ventricle and is then ejected. As PVR drops after birth, PBF may become excessive.
      d. Tricuspid atresia may be associated with normally related great vessels or with transposition of the great vessels.

3. Diagnosis
    a. Full-term infant within the first few hours to week of life
    b. Cyanosis and CHF
    c. Tachypnea, feeding difficulties, poor weight gain
    d. Recurrent respiratory infections
4. Repair: For a detailed discussion of palliative repairs please refer to Chapter 12
5. Anesthetic implications
    a. Before hemi-Fontan repair: Strictly avoid preload depletion; NPO time should be kept minimal, possibly 2 to 3 hours preoperatively.
    b. Inhalation induction is acceptable but should avoid depressing myocardial contractility.
    c. Maintain Fio_2 as low as possible and titrate ventilation to balance Qp:Qs. Excess PBF will result in higher saturations at the expense of systemic perfusion. This may rapidly result in acidosis and death. Excess systemic perfusion at the expense of PBF will result in increasing cyanosis.
    d. Methods to improve the PBF before repair.
        (1) Augment intravascular volume.
        (2) Consider inotropes: dopamine and dobutamine.
        (3) Reduce PVR by decreasing the $Etco_2$ and increasing Fio_2.
    e. Methods to decrease pulmonary circulation.
        (1) Avoid increasing Pao_2 >45 mm Hg because this is difficult to reverse and may result in death from insufficient systemic perfusion.
        (2) Decrease respiratory rate and Fio_2. Consider adding CO_2 to the circuit.
    f. After hemi-Fontan and Fontan repair.
        (1) Keep central venous pressure (CVP) high enough to passively drive blood to the pulmonary vascular bed. CVP should be 15 to 20 mm Hg and left atrial pressure (LAP) <10 mm Hg.
        (2) Minimize PVR by Fio_2 1.0, decrease $Etco_2$, and increase tidal volume.
        (3) Do *not* use PEEP, and minimize peak inspiratory pressures, which will hinder passive pulmonary filling.
        (4) If blood pressure drops, administer volume to maintain an adequate passive pulmonary filling pressure; then consider dopamine or dobutamine.
        (5) Avoid agents that may increase PVR.

B. Hypoplastic left heart syndrome (HLHS)
   1. Infants with HLHS are usually full-term infants who do well in utero because of the existence of the ductus arteriosus and foramen ovale
   2. Following birth, as the ductus closes, the infant develops CHF because of excess pulmonary blood flow and a low cardiac output. This is a ductal-dependent lesion before repair
   3. Anatomy
      a. Small left ventricle
      b. Aortic valve atresia
      c. Mitral valve atresia
      d. Hypoplastic ascending aorta
      e. Left ventricle is nonfunctional; therefore the pulmonary venous return is routed to the right atrium via an ASD or stretched foramen ovale
      f. In the right atrium, mixing of systemic and pulmonary circulations occurs
      g. Systemic blood flow is via the ductus arteriosus to the aorta with retrograde filling of the ascending and transverse aortic arch
      h. Before repair if PVR decreases too much, the ductus arteriosus will close and thus systemic flow ceases despite improving saturations
   4. Repair
      a. Palliative repair
         (1) Norwood: stage I
         (2) Hemi-Fontan: stage II
         (3) Fontan: stage III
      b. Heart transplantation: definitive repair
   5. Anesthetic implications
      a. Before Norwood repair
         (1) Maintain patent PDA with PGE_1 infusion.
         (2) Maintain a balance of Qp and Qs.
         (3) Add CO_2 to the fresh gas flow *if* excess pulmonary blood flow from a widely patent ASD is the situation (if Qp:Qs >1). This will increase PVR.
         (4) Maintain adequate systemic perfusion and cardiac output with dopamine or dobutamine (if Qp:Qs <1).
      b. After Norwood repair; before Hemi-Fontan repair
         (1) Preserve Qp:Qs = 1.
         (2) Keep Pa_{CO_2} 40 mm Hg.
         (3) Maintain saturation at 75% to 80%.

(4) Manipulate Qp:Qs with ventilation changes and inotropes as needed.

(5) Maintain hematocrit >38%.

(6) Avoid Pao_2 >45 mm Hg because this is difficult to reverse and death may ensue from insufficient systemic perfusion.

c. Refer to the anesthetic implications for before Hemi-Fontan repair and after Fontan repair described under "Tricuspid Atresia"

VII. Total Anomalous Pulmonary Venous Connection (TAPVC)

A. TAPVC may present early in the neonatal period as a result of pulmonary hypertension, cyanosis, tachypnea, and hypoxemia

B. Some infants present a few weeks after birth with poor feeding, cyanosis, and poor weight gain. TAPVC is a mixing lesion resulting in variable degrees of cyanosis

C. Anatomy: types of TAPVC

1. Supracardiac (type I): pulmonary venous return into the right, or possibly left, subclavian vein or into the innominate

2. Intracardiac (type II): pulmonary venous return to the coronary sinus

3. Infracardiac (type III): pulmonary venous return to either the inferior vena cava, portal vein, or hepatic vein; often constitutes a true neonatal cardiothoracic emergency because of the development of critical pulmonary hypertension and CHF

D. Symptoms

1. Patients often develop early right-sided heart failure.

2. A cyanotic mixing lesion occurs.

3. Saturations usually are in the range of 80% to 90%.

E. Anesthesia implications

1. Inhalants are not well tolerated in this population.

2. Narcotic techniques provide the most hemodynamic instability.

3. Fio_2

a. Increasing the Fio_2 may not significantly improve oxygenation since this is a fixed mixing lesion.

b. Consider using higher Fio_2 *if* the patient presents with pulmonary hypertension and acute failure.

4. Inotropes such as dopamine and dobutamine are frequently used immediately after repair, because the left ventricle is required to pump a greater volume load.

F. After bypass
  1. Keep LAP approximately 6 mm Hg to avoid excess stress on suture lines and to prevent fluid overload for the left side of the heart.
  2. Keep the right atrial pressure (RAP) 10 to 12 mm Hg maximum.
  3. If the cardiac output is low, pulmonary edema will ensue and will result in low saturations after bypass. The use of inotropes is recommended.

VIII. Patent Ductus Arteriosus (PDA)

A. One of the most common congenital heart defects, especially among premature infants; includes failure of the fetal ductus arteriosus to close after birth
B. Results in a shunt between the descending aorta and the pulmonary artery
C. Diagnosed by an echocardiogram
D. Symptoms
  1. Pulmonary congestion because of left-to-right shunt
  2. Widened pulse pressure because of diastolic runoff
  3. Machinery murmur
  4. Feeding difficulties
E. Repaired by surgical ligation of the ductus, most commonly via a left thoracotomy approach; results in an increased diastolic pressure
F. Anesthetic implications
  1. A secure IV line is essential; however, an arterial line is not mandatory.
  2. Use of pulse oximeters and blood pressure cuffs on both upper and lower extremities is prudent, especially during test occlusion.
  3. Adequate anesthesia and analgesia are vital, especially in preterm neonates who are unable to tolerate surgical stress.
  4. Anesthetic techniques are variable; good hemodynamic control can be achieved with fentanyl 5 to 10 µg/kg, pancuronium (Pavulon) 0.1 mg/kg; and low-concentration isoflurane.
  5. Older children may be able to have cardiac catheterization occlusion of the PDA while they are under sedation.
  6. Maintain adequate volume status and be prepared to give packed red blood cells or whole blood if needed. All the implications of neonatal anesthesia apply here.

IX. Coarctation of the Aorta

A. This is a congenital malformation with >20% of all cases diagnosed in adolescence or adulthood.

B. Severe coarctation may result in CHF as early as the neonatal period.

C. Occasionally a patient is asymptomatic until the onset of a cerebrovascular accident, ruptured aorta, or endocarditis.

D. Anatomy: two types.

1. Preductal (neonatal or infantile)

a. Local narrowing proximal to the ductus or diffuse narrowing of the aortic arch

b. May be associated with other congenital defects, such as VSD, PDA, or TGV

c. Infants often critically ill

2. Postductal (child or adult)

a. This primarily involves the aorta immediately distal to the left subclavian artery.

b. Complications may include cerebral hemorrhage or thrombosis, ruptured aorta, or necrotizing arteritis.

c. Obstructions may also be near or by the left carotid or subclavian arteries.

E. Symptoms.

1. Upper limb hypertension with diminished femoral pulses

2. Chest pain

3. Bounding carotid pulsations

4. CHF

F. Repair: Refer to Chapter 12 for a description of the types of repair.

G. Anesthetic implications.

1. Right thoracotomy approach is common.

2. Pulse oximeters are used on the right hand and lower extremity.

3. Insert a right radial arterial line and place blood pressure cuffs on both upper and lower extremities.

4. Cool the room and use a cooling blanket prn to protect against spinal cord ischemia.

5. The principles of complete and partial aortic cross clamping apply. Be aware that cardiopulmonary bypass, either full or partial, is occasionally used.

6. Postoperative problems include paradoxical hypertension, which is responsive to sodium nitroprusside (Nipride) or esmolol, and spinal cord ischemia.

7. In older children or adults, one-lung ventilation may be required.

ADDITIONAL READINGS

Gregory, G. (1994). *Pediatric anesthesia* (3rd ed.). New York: Churchill Livingstone.

Hersley, F.A., & Martin, D.E. (Eds.). (1995). *A practical approach to cardiac anesthesia* (2nd ed.). Boston: Little, Brown.

Katz, J., & Steward, D.J. (Eds.). (1987). *Anesthesia and uncommon pediatric diseases*. Philadelphia: W.B. Saunders.

Lake, C.L. (Ed.). (1998). *Pediatric cardiac anesthesia* (3rd ed.). Stamford, CT: Appleton & Lange.

Motoyama, E.K., & Davis, P.J. (Eds.). (1996). *Smith's anesthesia for infants and children* (6th ed.). St. Louis: Mosby.

16

Anesthesia for Pediatric Patients with Respiratory Diseases

John Aker, MS, CRNA, Rex A. Marley, MS, CRNA, RRT, and
Ronald J. Manningham, MS, CRNA

I. Introduction

A. Respiration is essential for normal growth, maturation, and survival of the human organism. Because of its importance, a number of redundant voluntary and involuntary controls ensure the availability of oxygen for delivery to the tissues. The act of breathing must be closely coordinated with swallowing, speech, coughing, metabolism, thermal control, defecation, and micturition.

B. The anesthetist must remember that respiration is inextricably tied to cardiovascular function. Accordingly, respiratory disease often has a significant impact on cardiovascular function.

II. Pediatric Airway

A. Airway anatomy

1. Table 16–1 lists mean values for anatomic pulmonary volumes and respiratory parameters compared with adults.

2. Newborn pulmonary function is dramatically different in the extrauterine environment. Extrauterine respiration depends on a functioning central nervous system and sufficient skeletal-muscular strength to allow lung expansion.

3. Although covered extensively in Chapter 6, the following is a brief review of the differences between the pediatric and adult airway:

   a. The infant has a large tongue that may predispose to upper airway obstruction.

   b. The infant larynx is located in a more cephalad position (C3–4 interspace) compared to the adult (C5–6 interspace).

TABLE 16–1. Comparative Mean Values for Normal Infant and Adult Airway Parameters

Parameter	Infant	Adult
ANATOMIC DIFFERENCES		
Narrowest portion of airway	Cricoid ring	Epiglottis
Epiglottis	Narrow, short, U-shaped	Broad
Tongue	Large	—
Glottis location	C3–4	C5–6
Tracheal length (mm)	57	120
Tracheal diameter (mm)	4	16
LUNG VOLUMES		
Tidal volume (V_T; ml/kg)	7	7
Anatomic dead space (V_D; ml/kg)	2–2.5	2.2
V_T/V_D ratio	0.3	0.3
Residual volume (ml/kg)	19	16
Closing volume (ml/kg)	12	7
Closing capacity (ml/kg)	35	23
Functional residual capacity (ml/kg)	27–30	34
Vital capacity (ml/kg)	35	70
Total lung capacity (ml/kg)	70	80
RESPIRATION		
Frequency (breaths/min)	30–50	12–16
Alveolar ventilation (ml/kg/min)	100–150	60
Airway resistance (cm H_2O/L/sec)	18–29	2–3
Oxygen consumption (ml/kg/min)	7–9	3

    c. The infant epiglottis is narrow, U-shaped, short, and stiff.

    d. The cricoid cartilage is the narrowest portion of the infant airway.

    e. The infant head is larger (particularly the occiput).

III. Regulation of Respiration

    A. Pulmonary maturity is not complete until after the first year of life. Although airway development is completed early during gestation, alveolar formation does not begin until the final month of gestation. At birth there are 30 to 40 million terminal alveoli. Alveolar development continues, reaching the adult level of 300 million by 18 months of age.

    B. The traditional view of the beginning of respiration at the time of birth (stimulation from fetal hypoxia and hypercarbia) has been challenged. The establishment of ventilation at birth is complex and is likely the result of a combination of increasing Pa_{O_2} with chemical and hormonal mediation.

Neonatal breathing begins in utero; however, the purpose of these respiratory efforts is unknown.

C. Rhythmic extrauterine breathing is initiated by several events, including umbilical cord clamping and the increase in Pao_2 when compared to the Pao_2 of the fetal environment. Although increasing $Paco_2$ does not interrupt this breathing pattern, subsequent hypoxia will depress breathing or produce apnea. Peripheral chemoreceptor regulation of breathing at birth is minimal, since continuous rhythmic breathing is not affected by carotid denervation.

D. Respiratory control depends on input from both peripheral and central chemoreceptors and sensors (see Fig. 16–1). The central pattern generator (CPG), a collection of respiratory neurons located within the brain stem, receives input from central and peripheral chemoreceptors, stretch receptors within the airway and pulmonary parenchyma, and pharyngeal and laryngeal chemoreceptors. The CPG produces an efferent impulse through the phrenic nerve, regulating respiratory rate and tidal volume.

E. The pharyngeal and laryngeal chemoreceptors and sensors can inhibit the CPG producing apnea. In utero, these receptors may be stimulated by amniotic fluid to inhibit respiratory efforts.

F. Upper airway receptors are particularly sensitive in the newborn. The Hering-Breuer reflex originates from receptors located within the airway smooth muscle and the

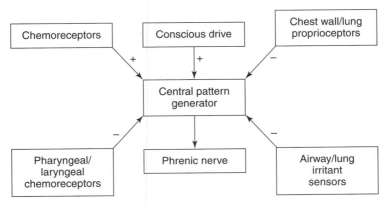

FIGURE 16–1. Respiratory control and interaction of peripheral chemoreceptors and sensors. (From Galinkin, J.L., & Kurth, D. [1998]. Neonatal and pediatric apnea syndromes. In Yaster, M. (Ed.). *Problems in pediatric anesthesia* [p. 445]. Philadelphia: Lippincott.)

bronchial endothelium. With inspiration these receptors produce inhibitory afferent stimuli to the CPG, stopping lung inflation. This reflex is very active in the premature infant and may be a holdover of the fetal inhibition of ventilation. In addition, stimulation of the superior laryngeal nerve may produce respiratory depression and subsequent apnea. This suggests that newborn neural inputs are immature.

G. Irritating volatile anesthetic agents (e.g., enflurane, isoflurane) may stimulate the upper airway receptors resulting in reflex responses, such as coughing, breath holding, and laryngospasm.

H. Hypoxia in premature and newborn infants will initially stimulate an increase in ventilation followed by respiratory depression and perhaps apnea. Hypothermia will abolish this brief increase in ventilatory drive. Hypoxemia will produce a reflex hyperventilation after 4 weeks of extrauterine life. Recall that the period of apnea to cardiovascular collapse is shorter in the child than the adult.

I. The newborn will increase ventilation in the presence of hypercapnia, but the response is less vigorous than that of the adult. The slope of the CO_2 response curve increases with age, suggesting an increase in chemoreceptor sensitivity.

J. Central apnea and periodic breathing are common in preterm infants suggesting an immature central nervous system. Periodic breathing (quiet breathing with 10–15 second periods of apnea) may occur in up to 80% of full-term infants and 95% of preterm infants. These episodes may be accompanied by bradycardia (heart rate less than 100 beats/min).

IV. Pediatric Pulmonary Function

A. General principles
   1. The newborn is an obligate nasal breather.
   2. Respiratory muscular function (chest, abdomen, diaphragm) is controlled by respiratory centers within the brain stem (see Fig. 16–1).
   3. The respiratory musculature (diaphragm and internal intercostal muscles) is active with inspiration and passive with expiration during quiet breathing. Forceful inspiration is inefficient because the accessory muscles of respiration (sternocleidomastoid, anterior serratus, external intercostals) are not developed and the newborn chest

is very compliant. The compliant chest wall will retract with forceful inspiratory efforts. The chest wall becomes less compliant within 6 to 12 months, and the ventilation musculature becomes more developed.

4. The diaphragm is composed of a smaller number of type I sustained-twitch fibers. This increases the potential for diaphragmatic fatigue.

5. The neonatal oxyhemoglobin dissociation curve is shifted to the left because of the presence of fetal hemoglobin (P_{50} of 19 mm Hg compared to 27 mm Hg for the adult). Accordingly, the neonate requires greater hemoglobin levels to ensure oxygen transport.

6. Infants are prone to develop postoperative hypoxemia (see box, p. 246).

B. Anesthetic effects on pulmonary function

1. Anesthetic agents, surgical site (thoracic and abdominal surgical procedures), patient disease, and position will alter lung volumes.

2. As the lung volume is decreased toward residual volume, dependent airways begin to close. This volume (closing volume and residual volume) is referred to as the closing capacity. Although closing capacity is independent of body position, decreases in functional residual capacity (FRC) will result in tidal volumes within closing capacity range.

3. FRC, composed of residual volume and expiratory reserve volume, is equal to the volume of gas that remains within the lung at the end of a normal tidal volume. The FRC serves as a buffer to minimize marked changes in Pao_2 and $Paco_2$. FRC decreases approximately 25% in the supine position and following the induction of general anesthesia. This decrease in FRC results in small airway closure, ventilation-perfusion mismatch, and the development of hypoxemia. With the decrease in FRC following general anesthesia, the infant will breath within the closing capacity during spontaneous ventilation. Assisted ventilation or the application of continuous positive airway pressure will prevent small airway closure and resulting hypoxemia.

4. Vital capacity is minimally reduced with peripheral surgical procedures but may be decreased as much as 70% with intrathoracic procedures.

5. Tidal volume decreases up to 25% with concurrent administration of potent inhalation anesthetics.

Etiology of Infant Postoperative Hypoxemia

1. Infants have immature respiratory control and irregular breathing pattern.
2. Infants have small functional residual capacity (FRC) and high oxygen demands.
3. FRC is reduced following anesthetic induction resulting in atelectasis and airway closure.
4. Infants are prone to upper airway obstruction.
5. Fetal hemoglobin has a high oxygen affinity and low ability to unload oxygen (left shift of oxyhemoglobin dissociation curve).
6. The neonate and infant have twice the oxygen requirements of the adult.
7. Hypoxia is a ventilatory depressant.
8. Trace anesthetic agents will abolish hypoxic ventilatory response.

Modified from Motoyama, E.K. (1996). Respiratory physiology in infants and children. In Motoyama, E.K., & Davis, P.J. (Eds.). *Smith's anesthesia for infants and children* (p. 59). St. Louis: Mosby.

CHILDHOOD RESPIRATORY DISORDERS

V. Apnea of Prematurity and Upper Respiratory Infection
   A. See Chapter 3.

VI. Asthma
   A. Epidemiology
      1. Asthma is the predominant chronic pulmonary disease in children. The past 2 decades have witnessed an increase in the incidence of asthma (doubled) and the deaths attributable to asthma (tripled) in the United States. It is important to note that pediatric death from asthma is infrequent. Asthma contributes to activity restrictions and is the leading cause of school absences and childhood hospitalizations.
      2. Approximately 4.3 million children (7% of children under the age of 18 years) have asthma. More than 5000 individuals died as a result of the disease in 1995. Children whose parents have asthma are three to six times more likely to develop asthma than children whose parents are free of the disease.

B. Pathology
   1. The mechanism of bronchial hyperreactivity is unknown.
   2. The development of asthma is multifactorial with clinical (rhinitis/sinusitis), immunologic (increased incidence in children with atopy), physiologic (air flow limitations caused by bronchoconstriction), and pathologic (cellular inflammatory changes of airway) foundations.
   3. Immunologic components include the release of cytokines, interleukins, and lipid mediators from mast cells following immunoglobulin E (IgE) destabilization of the mast cell membrane.
C. Clinical presentation
   1. Table 16–2 lists the categories of asthma with accompanying clinical history and pulmonary function.
   2. Clinical diagnosis includes persistent cough and wheezing (reversible bronchial hyperreactivity) precipitated by allergy, dust (animal dander), cigarette smoke, exercise, temperature changes (particularly inspired cold air), anx-

TABLE 16–2. Clinical Categories of Asthma

Category	Clinical History	Pulmonary Function
Infrequent episodic asthma	75% of pediatric population; wheezing interval once every 4–6 wk; wheezing occurs with heavy exercise	Normal pulmonary function; no prophylactic medications
Frequent episodic asthma	20% of pediatric population; more frequent attacks of wheezing; wheezing apparent with moderate exercise	Near normal pulmonary function; beta$_2$-agonists administered before exercise
Persistent asthma	5% of pediatric population; frequent acute episodes; wheezing with minor exertion; sleep disturbance, coughing, chest tightness require daily medication	Increased pulmonary resistance; severe air flow limitations; requires beta$_2$-agonists more than three times per week

Modified from Warner, J.O., & Naspitz, C.K. (1998). Third International Consensus Statement on the Management of Childhood Asthma. *Pediatric Pulmonology,* 25, 1–17. Reprinted by permission of Wiley-Liss, Inc., a division of John Wiley & Sons, Inc.

iety, or acute upper respiratory infection (respiratory syncytial virus [RSV], influenza).

3. Aspirin and nonsteroidal antiinflammatory drug–induced asthma is becoming more prevalent and has an increased incidence with a concurrent history of rhinitis or sinusitis.

4. The clinical history is significant for a pattern of sleep disruption as a result of coughing and wheezing.

5. Asthma may also be provoked following aspirin administration and in children with esophageal reflux.

6. These triggering factors provoke spasm of bronchial smooth muscle, increase mucous production and create airway edema and mucous plugging that results in airway obstruction, an increased work of breathing, and a mismatch of ventilation and perfusion.

7. The clinical consequences include respiratory muscle fatigue, with the subsequent development of hypoxemia, hypercapnia, and eventual respiratory failure.

D. Diagnostic testing

1. Chest radiograph demonstrates lung hyperinflation with flattened diaphragms.

2. Pulmonary function tests in older cooperative children will demonstrate reversible airway obstruction. Peak inspiratory flow measurements are encouraged to judge the effectiveness of inhaled pharmacologic agents.

E. Pharmacologic therapy

1. Goals of medical management for asthmatic patients

a. Treatment and resolution of acute symptoms

b. Control of environmental factors (i.e., cigarette smoke, dust) to minimize acute exacerbations

c. Use of prophylactic medications (inhaled beta-adrenergics, corticosteroids, anticholinergics) to optimize pulmonary function, prevent sleep disturbances, and prevent exercise-induced exacerbations

d. Figure 16–2 provides a therapeutic algorithm for the treatment of infrequent, frequent, and persistent asthma

2. Beta$_2$-agonists

a. Table 16–3 presents the comparative pharmacology of selective beta$_2$-adrenergic agonist bronchodilators. These drugs are widely employed for relief of acute bronchospasm in mild acute asthma episodes.

b. Beta$_2$-agonists may be delivered using a metered dose inhaler (MDI), nebulization, or enteral or parenteral routes.

c. Inhaled medication should be administered with a

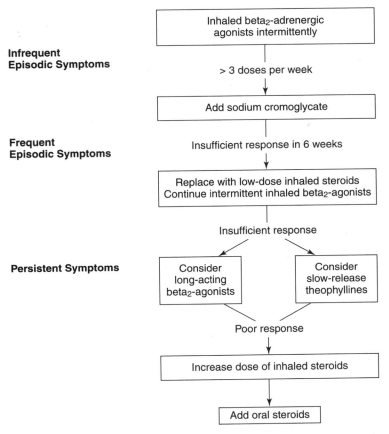

FIGURE 16–2. Asthma treatment algorithm. (From Warner, J.O., & Naspitz, C.K. [1998]. Third International Consensus Statement on the Management of Childhood Asthma. *Pediatric Pulmonology, 25,* 1–17.)

      spacer, which allows the delivery of larger doses of the selected drug to the lung rather than being deposited within the pharynx.

    d. Inhaled beta$_2$-agonists provide a more rapid bronchodilation with fewer systemic side effects.

  3. Cromolyn sodium

    a. Prophylactically administered via inhalation, MDI, or nebulization in an attempt to prevent bronchospasm

    b. Thought to stabilize the mast cell membrane, preventing the release of mediators

    c. Cough is the predominant but minor side effect

TABLE 16-3. Comparative Pharmacology of Selective Beta$_2$-Adrenergic Agonist Bronchodilators

	Beta$_2$ Selectivity	Peak Effect (min)	Duration of Action (h)	Dose (μg/puff)	Method of Administration
INTERMEDIATE-ACTING (3–6 h)					
Albuterol	++++	30–60	4	90	MDI, oral
Metaproterenol	+++	30–60	3–4	200	Oral, subcutaneous
Terbutaline	++++	60	4	200	MDI, oral, subcutaneous
Isoetharine	++	15–60	2–3	340	MDI, solution
Bitolterol	++++	30–60	5	370	MDI
LONG-ACTING (>12 h)					
Salmeterol	++++		>12	21	MDI

++, Minimal stimulation; +++, moderate stimulation; ++++, marked stimulation; *MDI*, metered dose inhaler.

From Stoelting, R.K. (1999). Sympathomimetics. In *Pharmacology and physiology in anesthetic practice* (3rd ed., p. 275). Philadelphia: Lippincott.

4. Corticosteroids
   a. Decrease airway inflammation.
   b. Beclomethasone or budesonide are effective in low doses (200–400 µg/day).
   c. Large doses (>800 µg/day) may be associated with subcapsular cataracts, delayed growth, decreased bone density, and suppression of the hypothalamic-adrenal-pituitary axis.
   d. Systemic effects may be reduced with the use of a spacer device for inhalation.
   e. Oral corticosteroids may be prescribed for acute attacks, whereas intravenous administration is reserved for persistent acute asthma. Inhaled or oral corticosteroids are a mainstay of asthma management.
5. Anticholinergics
   a. Anticholinergic administration (ipratropium bromide [Atrovent]) produces cholinergic bronchodilation and does not affect mucociliary function, sputum viscosity, or sputum removal.
   b. Administration is via an MDI.
6. Methylxanthines
   a. Theophylline, a bronchodilator and perhaps an immunomodulator, is the traditional methylxanthine with a narrow therapeutic margin of safety and significant systemic side effects (nausea and vomiting, headache, seizures, cardiac dysrhythmias, particularly in the presence of halothane).
   b. However, theophylline has been found to have antiinflammatory characteristics when prescribed in low dosages.
F. Anesthetic management
   1. Preoperative considerations
      a. Preoperative preparation should ensure the child is in an optimal state of health before elective surgery.
      b. Elective surgical procedures should be postponed for children with acute exacerbations.
      c. A detailed history is essential. In addition to the standard medical history (allergies, medications and dosages, etc.) the clinical assessment should include a detailed discussion with the parent or caretaker regarding
         (1) Sleep disturbance from cough and wheezing
         (2) Morning chest tightness and cough requiring beta$_2$-agonist administration

(3) Number of acute asthmatic episodes during the past month

(4) Last hospitalization or emergency visit for an acute attack

(5) Daily medication and rescue medication for acute exacerbation

(6) Prophylactic medication dosage and times of administration

d. The child should remain on the prescribed pharmacologic therapy through the perioperative period.

e. The prophylactic administration of inhaled beta$_2$-agonists before anesthetic induction may decrease the risk of bronchospasm.

f. Children who have been taking long-term corticosteroid therapy may require supplemental corticosteroid coverage if there is evidence of hypothalamic-pituitary-adrenal axis suppression.

g. Laboratory evaluation may include chest radiography, arterial blood gas, serum theophylline levels, and complete blood count to determine eosinophil count.

2. Intraoperative considerations

a. The etiology of intraoperative wheezing may not be simply from bronchospasm.

b. Additional causes of wheezing should be ruled out (endotracheal tube obstruction, endobronchial intubation, aspiration, pulmonary embolism, pneumothorax).

c. Airway instrumentation is a potent stimulus provoking bronchospasm.

d. Anesthetic depth should be increased with increased concentration of volatile agent, intravenous lidocaine, and/or opioids before endotracheal intubation.

e. Likewise, tracheal suctioning should not be attempted in light levels of anesthesia.

f. Endotracheal intubation may be avoided with the use of face mask anesthesia or a laryngeal mask airway when appropriate.

g. Regional or local anesthesia avoids airway instrumentation and may be a suitable anesthetic alternative.

h. Inspired gases should be actively humidified to prevent drying of airway secretions.

i. When instituting intraoperative mechanical ventilation, consideration should be given to minimizing lung inflation pressure, utilizing slow inspiratory rates, and increasing expiratory time to avoid air trapping.

j. Potent inhalation agents produce bronchodilation. Halothane may produce cardiac dysrhythmia in patients taking concurrent $beta_2$-agonists or theophylline. Desflurane may produce breath holding and laryngospasm. Sevoflurane with its attendant bronchodilation and minimal airway irritation is acceptable for mask induction.

k. Intraoperative bronchospasm should be initially treated with hand ventilation, increasing the depth of anesthesia with inhalation agents, followed by $beta_2$-agonist administration via a metered dose technique (albuterol, metaproterenol). Intravenous epinephrine in boluses of 0.1 to 1 μg/kg may be required.

l. Timely intubation may better be accomplished with intravenous propofol, which decreases the incidence of postintubation wheezing when compared to thiopental. Ketamine produces bronchial smooth muscle relaxation via catecholamine release and is a suitable intravenous induction agent. Intravenous lidocaine in a dose of 1.5 mg/kg prevents reflex bronchospasm. Intratracheal administration of lidocaine should not be attempted in light planes of anesthesia because it may provoke bronchospasm.

m. Histamine-releasing pharmacologic agents (D-tubocurare, atracurium, morphine, thiopental) should be administered cautiously.

n. Deep extubation places the child at risk for regurgitation and aspiration. The wheezing child should be extubated following the attenuation of airway reflexes with opioid (fentanyl) or intravenous lidocaine, 1.5 mg/kg.

3. Postoperative considerations
   a. Humidified supplemental oxygen should be administered in the immediate postoperative period.
   b. The prescribed bronchodilators should be reinstituted according to the preoperative prescribed schedule.

VII. Bronchopulmonary Dysplasia

A. Epidemiology
   1. Bronchopulmonary dysplasia (BPD) is a chronic pulmonary disease that develops following the development of respiratory distress syndrome and resultant lung injury.

    2. The underlying lung injury occurs most often in the premature infant who requires
       a. Mechanical ventilation for the first three or more days of life, and
       b. High inspired oxygen concentrations of supplemental oxygen for 28 days or longer
    3. The development of BPD is greater in low–birth weight infants (<1500 g) and the more immature (gestational age and birth weight are closely linked).
    4. Infants with BPD are at risk for sudden death. Contributing factors to sudden death include chronic hypoxia and hypercarbia, immaturity of ventilatory control, and recurrent airway obstruction from bronchospasm.
    5. Risk factors for the development of BPD are listed in the box on page 255.
  B. Pathophysiology
    1. Prematurity is associated with pulmonary immaturity and surfactant-deficient alveoli, the ingredients for the development of respiratory distress syndrome.
       a. The very treatment required to maintain satisfactory oxygenation and ventilation produces pulmonary injury. Initial high inspired oxygen concentrations and continued supplemental oxygen lead to the production of oxygen free radicals and subsequent oxygen toxicity.
       b. Airway inflammation follows. The premature lung lacks the necessary antioxidant system to cope with oxygen free radical formation.
    2. Positive pressure mechanical ventilation of the surfactant-deficient alveoli leads to overdistention and the transudation of fluid into the alveoli, with the subsequent development of hyaline membrane disease. Barotrauma is also an inevitable consequence of continued positive pressure ventilation of the noncompliant lung.
    3. Bronchoconstriction and increased airway reactivity (manifest clinically as wheezing) develop in up to 80% of those with BPD.
    4. Bronchoconstriction develops in response to respiratory infection or following inhalation of airway irritants.
  C. Clinical presentation
    1. The general presentation of the disease includes tachypnea with retractions, inspiratory crackles, and wheezing (suggestive of pulmonary edema) accompanied by an abnormal chest radiograph.

Risk Factors for the Development of Bronchopulmonary Dysplasia

PRINCIPAL RISK FACTORS
Birth weight and gestational age
Development of respiratory distress syndrome
Severity of initial pulmonary dysfunction

CONSEQUENTIAL RISK FACTORS
Aggressive mechanical ventilation
Exposure to high concentrations of supplemental oxygen
Development of pneumothorax or interstitial emphysema
Iatrogenic fluid overload
Presence of patent ductus arteriosus with hemodynamic or
  respiratory instability

ADDITIONAL RISK FACTORS
White race
Male gender
Multiple births
Low Apgar scores

Modified from Farrell, P.A., & Fiascone, J.M. (1997). Bronchopulmonary dysplasia in the 1990's: a review for the pediatrician. *Current Problems in Pediatrics*, 27(4), 135.

2. Pulmonary dysfunction
    a. Destruction of the pulmonary vascular bed results in increased pulmonary vascular resistance and increases pulmonary artery pressures (increased right ventricular afterload precipitating right ventricular hypertrophy).
    b. Cor pulmonale may develop subsequent to these changes. Cor pulmonale is associated with recurrent pulmonary edema, hypoxia, and sudden death.
    c. Immaturity may also be associated with decreased ventilatory control. Infants with BPD may have an abnormal hypoxic ventilatory response.
    d. Children with BPD have a decreased pulmonary reserve and are at risk from viral respiratory infections (influenza A and B and parainfluenza, although RSV predominates in this population).
3. Cardiovascular dysfunction
    a. Systemic hypertension, whose etiology is unknown, develops in as many as 40% of BPD patients.

b. Left and right ventricular hypertrophy may develop. Left ventricular hypertrophy may increase the incidence of sudden death in children with BPD. Diastolic dysfunction develops secondary to the stiff left ventricle as a result of hypertrophy. The stiff ventricle requires higher filling pressures. This may contribute to pulmonary edema formation.

4. Impaired growth and development
   a. Generally caused by inadequate nutrition or inadequate oxygenation

5. Neurobehavioral development
   a. Developmental delay is common in premature infants.
   b. The premature infant is at an increased risk for the development of retinopathy of prematurity, hearing loss, and cerebral palsy. These complications are inextricably tied to low birth weight rather than BPD itself.

D. Medical management of BPD
   1. Supplemental oxygen is provided to maintain Pao_2 greater than 55 to 60 mm Hg (corresponding Spo_2 of 90% at sea level). Minimizing hypoxemia will decrease pulmonary injury and growth retardation.
   2. Mechanical ventilatory pressures should be minimized to decrease the development of barotrauma.
   3. Beta$_2$-agonists are employed for bronchodilation, minimizing the restrictions of air flow and decreasing bronchial reactivity.
   4. Additional pharmacologic agents include the methylxanthines and anticholinergics (see discussion of treatment of asthma above).
   5. Pulmonary edema is treated with spironolactone, furosemide, and/or thiazide diuretics.
   6. Corticosteroids may be administered to combat airway edema.

E. Anesthetic management
   1. Preoperative considerations
      a. A thorough history includes examination of the medical records, reviewing the initial treatment (ventilation, oxygenation, pharmacologic therapy).
      b. It is important to note any additional problems attendant with prematurity (apnea, bradycardia, intraventricular hemorrhage, congenital heart disease).
      c. Pulmonary function should be optimal before elective surgical procedures.

d. The prescribed bronchodilators, corticosteroids, and diuretics should be continued until the time of surgery.

e. Laboratory evaluation may include a hemoglobin and hematocrit, selected pulmonary function tests, and arterial blood gas analysis.

f. Cardiovascular evaluation should include the determination of ventricular hypertrophy (previous echocardiogram) and the presence of systemic hypertension and cor pulmonale.

2. Intraoperative considerations

a. The prevalence of bronchospasm and airway reactivity should be considered when planning the anesthetic technique and selecting specific anesthetic agents (see discussion of asthma management above).

b. Hand ventilation allows the determination of pulmonary compliance and may decrease the risk of barotrauma and pneumothorax.

c. Underlying pulmonary hypertension is aggravated by systemic acidosis, hypoxia, hypercarbia, and hypothermia. These conditions are avoided through the monitoring of ventilation via capnography, the administration of oxygen to maintain acceptable oxygen saturation (Pao_2 greater than 55–60 mm Hg), and the use of forced-air warming.

d. The operating suite should be warmed to 78°F to 80°F before the child's arrival.

e. Nitrous oxide administration is safe since it has not been demonstrated to aggravate pulmonary hypertension in the child.

f. Intravenous fluids should be judiciously administered to prevent aggravation of or the development of pulmonary edema. Congestive heart failure is a risk in those with underlying right ventricular dysfunction.

3. Postoperative considerations

a. Postoperative ventilation is generally required following intracavitary procedures. Mechanical ventilation may reduce the incidence of atelectasis but increases the risk of pneumothorax.

b. Prolonged ventilation may necessitate a planned tracheostomy.

c. Pulmonary bronchodilators should be resumed.

VIII. Cystic Fibrosis

A. Pathophysiology

1. Cystic fibrosis (CF) is an inherited autosomal recessive

disorder brought on by mutations of a single gene on the long arm of chromosome 7.

2. Progressive sinopulmonary disease, exocrine pancreatic insufficiency, gastrointestinal obstruction, and excess sodium and chloride in sweat are hallmark manifestations.

3. Impaired lung secretion clearance secondary to increased mucous viscosity and defective transport, and acute respiratory infection lead to chronic lung disease as exhibited by obstructive ventilatory pattern, dyspnea, and productive cough.

B. Epidemiology
  1. CF is the leading fatal disorder affecting the white population (1 in 29 persons are carriers).
  2. In most cases the family history is negative for known disease.
  3. The incidence of CF in the United States varies among races:
    a. Whites: 1 in 3200 births
    b. Blacks: 1 in 15,000 births
    c. Asian Americans: 1 in 31,000 births
  4. Survival has increased dramatically over the past 2 decades. The median age of survival is 31 years.

C. Clinical presentation
  1. Clinical manifestations
    a. The common physical and physiologic features are listed in the box on page 259.
    b. Acute or persistent respiratory symptoms develop in only 50% of affected individuals.
    c. Chronic endobronchial infection (*Pseudomonas aeruginosa*) and inflammation with subsequent cor pulmonale are the leading cause of morbidity and mortality.
  2. Diagnostic tests
    a. The quantitative pilocarpine iontophoresis sweat test is the current gold standard for the definitive diagnosis of CF.
    b. The test quantifies the salt sweat concentration (concentrations greater than 60 mmol/L indicative of CF).

D. Basic therapies
  1. The treatment strategies depend on the extent of the disease and the specific organs affected
  2. Pulmonary management is directed to minimize the occurrence of infection and maintain pulmonary function
  3. Infection control
    a. Prophylactic antibiotics are administered to prevent pulmonary infection.

Common Physical and Physiologic Features of Cystic Fibrosis

1. Chronic sinopulmonary disease
   a. Persistent colonization and infection with typical CF pathogens including *Staphylococcus aureus,* nontypable *Haemophilus influenzae,* mucoid and nonmucoid *Pseudomonas aeruginosa,* and *Burkholderia cepacia*
   b. Chronic cough and sputum production
   c. Persistent chest radiographic abnormalities (e.g., bronchiectasis, atelectasis, infiltrates, hyperinflation)
   d. Airway obstruction as evidenced by wheezing and air trapping
   e. Nasal polyps; radiographic or CT abnormalities of the parasinuses
   f. Digital clubbing
2. Gastrointestinal and nutritional abnormalities
   a. *Intestinal:* meconium ileus; distal intestinal obstruction syndrome; rectal prolapse
   b. *Pancreatic:* pancreatic insufficiency; recurrent pancreatitis
   c. *Hepatic:* chronic hepatic disease as evidenced by clinical or histologic evidence of focal biliary cirrhosis or multilobular cirrhosis
   d. *Nutritional:* failure to thrive (protein-calorie malnutrition); hypoproteinemia and edema; complications secondary to fat-soluble vitamin deficiency
3. Salt-loss syndromes: acute salt depletion; chronic metabolic alkalosis
4. Male urogenital abnormalities: obstructive azospermia

From Fosentein, B.J., & Cutting, G.R. (1998). The diagnosis of cystic fibrosis: a consensus statement. Cystic Fibrosis Foundation Consensus Panel. *Journal of Pediatrics,* 132(4), 589–595.

   b. Recently approved, aerosolized preservative-free antibiotic therapy (e.g., TBOI [tobramycin solution for inhalation]) facilitates the delivery of a concentrated dose of antibiotic for deposition within the lung.
4. Airway clearance
   a. Clearance of secretions is managed with chest physiotherapy three times or more per day, with postural drainage to promote secretion clearance.

b. The administration of mucus-thinning pharmacologic agents (e.g., acetylcysteine [Mucomyst], dornase alfa [Pulmozyme]) lowers mucous viscosity.

c. In addition, exercise is beneficial because it also aids the loosening, mobilization, and expectoration of mucus.

5. Bronchodilator therapy
   a. Beta$_2$-adrenergic bronchodilators are the standard therapy for CF patients who exhibit bronchial hyperreactivity.

6. Antiinflammatory agents
   a. Ibuprofen is administered twice daily and has been shown to reduce pulmonary inflammation and may decrease the progression of the lung disease without noticeable toxicity.
   b. Aerosolized corticosteroids are under investigation.

7. Nutritional support
   a. Gastrointestinal dysfunction in the CF patient results in malnutrition and possible fluid and electrolyte imbalance.
   b. Supplemental nutrition is prescribed to provide 150% of the individual's normal caloric requirements.
   c. The adequacy of the diet is monitored by history of the stool pattern, presence of abdominal distention, and the gain or loss of weight.
   d. Pancreatic enzymes are prescribed to assist in nutrient absorption.
   e. Supplemental vitamins are also generally prescribed.

E. Anesthetic management
   1. Preanesthetic considerations
      a. During the preoperative history and examination, the severity of the disease should be established, including the constellation of symptoms (mild to severe).
      b. Baseline pulmonary function and current pulmonary disease involvement should be determined. Chest physiotherapy should be continued throughout the perioperative period.
      c. Acute infectious processes must be treated with appropriate antibiotics.
      d. Current pulmonary medications (e.g., mucolytics, corticosteroids, beta$_2$-adrenergic bronchodilators) should be continued until the surgical procedure.
      e. Elective surgical procedures should be delayed until optimal respiratory function is established.

    f. The current nutritional condition should be reviewed. A nutritional consultation may be required for supplemental nutritional support (i.e., parenteral or enteral) preoperatively and postoperatively.

    g. Adequate preoperative hydration through a minimization of the perioperative fasting interval is important to reduce airway desiccation and facilitate secretion mobilization. Preoperative intravenous fluid therapy should be instituted early in the preoperative period if possible.

2. Intraoperative considerations

    a. If possible, establish intravenous access and replace deficit fluids before anesthetic induction.

    b. Consider regional or local anesthetic techniques where appropriate, avoiding airway instrumentation and respiratory impairment postoperatively following general anesthesia.

    c. The current nutritional status may impact baseline coagulation (vitamin K deficiency secondary to malnutrition), contraindicating the administration of central axial regional anesthetic techniques.

    d. No specific general anesthetic agent or technique is more beneficial than another.

    e. Because of the concurrent pulmonary disease, inhalation anesthetic uptake may be prolonged.

    f. Nitrous oxide should be avoided if cystic lesions have been identified by chest radiography.

    g. A higher than normal F_{IO_2} may be required to maintain satisfactory oxygen saturation.

    h. Endotracheal intubation is recommended to provide controlled ventilation (higher than normal peak inspiratory pressures may be required because of pulmonary disease).

    i. Short-acting anesthetic agents (e.g., desflurane, propofol, alfentanil) are employed to afford rapid recovery.

3. Postoperative considerations

    a. Supplemental humidified oxygen should be administered in the immediate postoperative period to maintain acceptable oxygen saturation and facilitate secretion mobilization.

    b. Deep breathing, coughing, pharyngeal suctioning, and chest physiotherapy (postural drainage) should be reinstituted.

    c. Early ambulation will also aid the removal of pulmonary secretions.

   d. Postoperative opioids will depress the cough reflex and inhibit pulmonary secretion expectoration.
   e. The administration of long-acting local anesthetics for operative regional anesthetic techniques or via local infiltration by the surgeon decreases postoperative opioid requirements.

IX. Postobstructive Pulmonary Edema (Negative Pressure Pulmonary Edema)

A. Etiology
   1. Postobstructive pulmonary edema (incorrectly referred to as negative pressure pulmonary edema) is a complication of upper airway obstruction in both pediatric and adult patients.
   2. The development of postobstructive pulmonary edema is frequently unrecognized or not diagnosed until after airway patency is reestablished.
   3. Airway obstruction as brief as 30 seconds may precipitate pulmonary edema.
   4. The onset of pulmonary edema following airway obstruction generally ranges from 3 to 5 minutes to as long as 2½ hours.
   5. Croup, supraglottitis, and laryngotracheobronchitis are etiologic in more than 50% of the pediatric cases.
   6. Pediatric patients at risk include those with obstructive sleep apnea, tonsil and adenoid hypertrophy, and nasopharyngeal or pharyngeal masses.

B. Pathologic findings
   1. In the spontaneously breathing patient, subambient intrapleural pressure is generated with inspiratory efforts against a closed glottis (Müeller maneuver, the opposite of Valsalva maneuver).
   2. Intrapleural pressure decreases to -5 cm H_2O during normal respiration, but with the Müeller maneuver it may decrease to -50 to -100 cm H_2O.
   3. Subambient intrapleural pressure increases venous return to the heart, increasing pulmonary microvascular pressure, left ventricular afterload, left ventricular end-diastolic volume, and left ventricular end-diastolic pressure.
   4. Increased pulmonary venous pressure and pulmonary capillary permeability produce subsequent leakage of fluid and blood into the alveoli.
   5. The clinical signs and symptoms of postobstructive

pulmonary edema may be mild or severe and include dyspnea, cyanosis, tachycardia, progressive hypoxemia with attendant hypercarbia (and the accompanying sympathetic stimulation), and the presence of pink frothy pulmonary secretions. Metabolic acidosis may develop, increasing pulmonary vasoconstriction.

6. The translocation of plasma volume into the pulmonary alveoli may create hypovolemia. Fluid resuscitation is required for patients with severe cases of postobstructive pulmonary edema.

7. Pulmonary edema may develop as a result of fluid overload, anaphylaxis, or anaphylactoid reactions as well as cardiac failure. These causes of pulmonary edema must be ruled out.

C. Treatment
1. Postobstructive pulmonary edema is generally self-limiting, requiring only supportive therapy (patent airway, supplemental oxygen to maintain satisfactory oxygen saturation as determined by pulse oximetry).

2. Children who develop postobstructive pulmonary edema may require overnight hospitalization for continued monitoring and observation.

3. Children identified at risk for postobstructive pulmonary edema (see above) or those who have experienced intraoperative airway obstruction may need to be observed for a longer period of time before dismissal from an outpatient facility.

4. For mild cases, supplemental oxygen via mask (with or without continuous positive airway pressure) may be all that is required to maintain acceptable oxygen saturation.

5. For severe cases the majority of pediatric patients will require endotracheal intubation and mechanical ventilation with positive end expiratory pressure.

6. In severe cases the anesthetist must resist the temptation to administer diuretics and restrict fluid administration.

ADDITIONAL READINGS

Farrell, P.A., & Fiascone, J.M. (1997). Bronchopulmonary dysplasia in the 1990's: a review for the pediatrician. *Current Problems in Pediatrics*, 27(4), 133–163.

Fosentein, B.J., & Cutting, G.R. (1998). The diagnosis of cystic fibrosis: a consensus statement. Cystic Fibrosis Foundation Consensus Panel. *Journal of Pediatrics*, 132(4), 589–595.

Sulek, C.A. (1996). Negative pressure pulmonary edema. In Gravenstein, N., & Kirby, R.R. (Eds.). *Complications in anesthesiology* (pp. 191–198). Philadelphia: Lippincott-Raven.

Warner, J.O., & Naspitz, C.K. (1998). Third International Consensus Statement on the Management of Childhood Asthma. *Pediatric Pulmonology,* 25, 1–17.

Zetlin, P.L. (1998). An update on asthma in the 90's. In Lake, C.L., Rice, L.J., & Sperry, R.J. (Eds). *Advances in anesthesia* (vol. 16, pp. 193–224). St. Louis: Mosby.

17

Anesthesia for Pediatric Patients with Musculoskeletal System Diseases

Mary Karlet, PhD, CRNA

I. Introduction

A. Musculoskeletal disorders have a wide range of causes, from autoimmune destruction of tissue to genetically determined defects in muscle membrane protein.

B. Management of cases involving musculoskeletal pathologic conditions must consider preoperative drug therapy, anatomic and physiologic changes, and the variable effects of anesthetic agents and muscle relaxants.

C. In many patients with musculoskeletal disease, associated congenital anomalies decrease cardiac or respiratory reserve, reducing the margin of safety with anesthesia and surgery.

D. Patients undergoing upper abdominal or thoracic surgery are at particular risk for postoperative respiratory morbidity.

II. Duchenne Muscular Dystrophy

A. Etiology

1. Muscular dystrophy is a heterogeneous set of inherited myopathies that includes Duchenne muscular dystrophy, Becker muscular dystrophy, and others (see Table 17–1).

2. Duchenne muscular dystrophy, also known as pseudohypertrophic muscular dystrophy, is the most common and most severe form.

3. It is inherited as an X-linked recessive disease that presents in early childhood between 2 and 6 years of age.

4. Duchenne muscular dystrophy is clinically evident in males and has an incidence of 30 in 100,000 live male births.

5. Patients with Duchenne muscular dystrophy have a mutation in the gene that produces the muscle membrane protein dystrophin.

6. Muscle membranes of patients with Duchenne muscular dystrophy have an absence or a severe deficiency of

TABLE 17–1. Types of Muscular Dystrophies

Muscular Dystrophy	Pathophysiology and Genetics	Clinical Features and Anesthetic Implications
Duchenne	X-linked recessive inheritance; absence or severe deficiency of dystrophin; onset in early childhood	Progressive muscle weakness, especially of proximal muscle groups; kyphoscoliosis; respiratory failure; cardiomyopathy
Becker	X-linked recessive inheritance; deficiency or defect of dystrophin; onset in early to late childhood	Progressive muscle weakness, especially of proximal muscle groups; more benign course than Duchenne dystrophy; cardiomyopathy; respiratory failure after the fourth decade
Facioscapulohumeral	Autosomal dominant inheritance; onset in childhood or adolescence	Slowly progressive weakness of the face, shoulder girdle, and respiratory muscles; later involvement of the hips and back may cause kyphoscoliosis
Limb-girdle	Autosomal recessive or autosomal dominant transmission; affects males and females; onset between the first and third decades	Represents several dystrophic disorders; slowly progressive weakness of the shoulder and hip girdle muscles; variable cardiac involvement; respiratory insufficiency
Emery-Dreifuss	X-linked recessive inheritance	Involves distal muscles of upper and lower extremities; neck contractures may limit movement; predominant risk is cardiac (dysrhythmias, cardiomyopathy) rather than skeletal muscle weakness

dystrophin, which alters sarcolemma permeability and stability.

7. Becker muscular dystrophy results from allelic defects of the same gene as Duchenne, but it is 10 times less common and follows a milder course.

B. Clinical manifestations

1. Infiltration of fibrous and fatty tissue into the muscle creates pseudohypertrophy, especially apparent in calf muscles.

2. A progressive degeneration and necrosis of muscle groups and an unremitting weakness, especially of the pelvis and shoulders, characterize Duchenne muscular dystrophy. The deterioration of muscle strength forces most affected boys to be wheelchair bound by the early teens.

3. Degeneration of respiratory muscles and the development of kyphoscoliosis lead to an ineffective cough and a restrictive type of ventilatory impairment. Forced vital capacity decreases 4% for each year the patient is wheelchair bound and another 4% for each 10 degrees of scoliosis.

4. Cardiac abnormalities (cardiomyopathy, conduction abnormalities, dysrhythmias) occur in 50% to 70% of patients with Duchenne muscular dystrophy but are clinically significant in only 10% of patients—usually during the terminal stages. Mitral valve prolapse is demonstrated by echocardiography in 10% to 25% of patients.

5. The patient's compromised cardiac and respiratory conditions may be masked by the limited activity imposed by skeletal myopathy.

6. Death often occurs in late adolescence or early adulthood and is usually caused by congestive heart failure or respiratory infection. Corticosteroid therapy may slow the disease progression in some patients.

C. Preoperative evaluation

1. A restrictive pattern of respiratory dysfunction may result in chronic hypoxemia and pulmonary hypertension.

2. Pulmonary function tests and arterial blood gases help define the severity of the respiratory involvement. Preoperative vital capacity measurement less than 30% to 35% of predicted value suggests an increased risk for serious postoperative complications and ventilatory dependence.

3. A preoperative chest radiograph is necessary to rule out infiltrates.

4. Tachypnea, use of accessory muscles, and frequent alterations in the respiratory pattern indicate weakness. Room air pulse oximetry readings provide a simple but valuable assessment of lung function, especially in patients who are capable of fairly normal activities.

5. A preoperative electrocardiogram (ECG) will help identify dysrhythmias and conduction abnormalities. ECG changes characteristic of preclinical cardiomyopathy include a large or polyphasic R wave in lead V_1, deep Q waves in the lateral precordial leads (V_4 through V_6), and premature beats. Resting tachycardia is common.

6. Consider supplemental perioperative corticosteroids in patients receiving long-term steroid treatment.

7. When possible, local or regional anesthesia should be considered.

8. Preoperative sedation should be omitted or minimal.

9. Serum creatinine phosphokinase (CK) levels are markedly elevated but decrease as muscle atrophies.

D. Intraoperative management

1. Smooth muscle involvement results in intestinal tract hypomotility and acute gastric dilation.

   a. The potential for delayed gastric emptying plus the presence of weak laryngeal reflexes dictate that the anesthesia plan of care include measures to guard against aspiration of stomach contents.

   b. Prophylactic use of a nasogastric tube helps prevent acute gastric dilatation.

2. Generalized muscle weakness, especially in the advanced stages of muscular dystrophy, makes these patients exquisitely sensitive to the respiratory depressant properties of opioids, sedatives, and general anesthetic agents. The smallest possible amount of anesthetic agents should be used.

3. The sensitivity to nondepolarizing muscle relaxants is marked, and the effects of nondepolarizing muscle relaxants must be scrupulously monitored. Peripheral nerve stimulator monitoring must be interpreted cautiously because patients with proximal muscle weakness (e.g., accessory muscles of respiration, bulbar muscles) may show a relatively normal response to distal muscle stimulation.

4. Decreased cardiac reserve makes these patients sensitive to the myocardial depressant effects of potent inhalation anesthetics.

5. Judicious administration of intravenous fluids is war-

ranted. The sudden occurrence of tachycardia during anesthesia may herald heart failure.

6. Succinylcholine should not be used in patients with muscular dystrophies. The altered sarcolemma can lead to massive breakdown of muscle fibers (rhabdomyolysis), exaggerated potassium release, and cardiac arrest after succinylcholine administration.

7. Duchenne muscular dystrophy is included among the myopathies that are associated with malignant hyperthermia (MH). Although a genetic linkage has not been established, precautions against MH should be taken and a high degree of suspicion maintained for this disorder.

8. Case reports of delayed postoperative respiratory deterioration mandate continued close observation in the postanesthesia care unit and make outpatient surgery inadvisable.

III. Myotonic Dystrophy

A. Etiology
1. The myotonias are a set of disorders characterized by the persistent contracture of skeletal muscle after stimulation (see Table 17–2).
2. Myotonic dystrophy (Steinert disease) is the most common (13 per 100,000 live births) and most severe form of the myotonias.

B. Clinical manifestations
1. A slow, progressive deterioration of skeletal (especially limb, sternocleidomastoid, and facial), cardiac, and smooth muscle occurs over the course of the disease.
2. Myotonia generally antedates the muscle atrophy and weakness, often appearing by age 5 years. The myotonia may be induced by mechanical, chemical, or electrical stimulation of the muscle.
3. Extramuscular manifestations of myotonic dystrophy include cataracts, gonadal atrophy, mental retardation, and endocrine abnormalities.
4. Fifty to ninety percent of patients with advanced myotonia have myocardial conduction defects. Bradycardia and first-degree atrioventricular block are common.

C. Preoperative evaluation
1. A preoperative ECG is indicated for all patients.
2. Preoperative evaluation should strive to identify the degree of muscle wasting. Arterial blood gases and spirometry testing provide useful baseline values for defining the patient's respiratory reserve.

TABLE 17–2. Types of Myotonic Muscle Disease

Type of Myotonia	Pathophysiology and Genetics	Clinical Features and Anesthetic Implications
Myotonic dystrophy (Steinert disease)	Autosomal-dominant mode of inheritance; most common age of onset between second and fourth decades; genetic defect: myotonin-kinase gene	Slowly progressive muscle atrophy and weakness, especially of the facial, sterno-cleidomastoid, and distal muscles; myotonia precipitated by mechanical or electrical stimulation, succinylcholine, propofol, anticholinesterase medications, cold; cardiac dysfunction
Congenital myotonic dystrophy	Affects 25% of children born to mothers with myotonic dystrophy	Feeding difficulties; mental retardation; poor respiratory function
Myotonia congenita (Thomsen disease)	Autosomal dominant inheritance; rare occurrence; genetic defect: chloride channel gene; childhood onset	Widespread myotonia
Myotonia fluctuans	Genetic defect: sodium channel gene	Prolonged myotonia, induced particularly by activity and potassium; correlation of masseter muscle rigidity with positive in vitro halothane caffeine contracture test for malignant hyperthermia

3. Quinidine, procainamide, mexiletine, and tocainide are used to decrease the myotonia in some patients; their use may compound cardiac conduction abnormalities.
4. Pharyngeal, palatal, and tongue weakness produces an impaired swallowing mechanism. Poor gastric motility compounds the danger of aspiration. Preoperative aspiration prophylaxis is advised.

D. Intraoperative management
1. Avoid succinylcholine because it may induce intense,

generalized myotonic contraction. Reversal of muscle relaxation with anticholinesterase drugs may precipitate or enhance myotonia. Descriptions of propofol-induced myotonia have been reported.

2. The patient should be kept warm, since cold and shivering worsen myotonia.
3. Myotonic contractions may impede the ability to maintain a patent airway and ventilate the lungs. Contractions are not abated by regional anesthesia, muscle relaxants, or dantrolene; warm temperature and injection of local anesthesia may attenuate the contraction.
4. Patients are sensitive to nondepolarizing muscle relaxants and respiratory depressants. Prolonged and profound effects have been reported—especially in advanced cases with muscle wasting.
5. Close ECG monitoring is mandatory in the perioperative period.
6. Inconstant associations between the myotonias (especially myotonia fluctuans) and MH have been described. The conservative approach is to avoid MH-triggering agents in patients with myotonia.

IV. Myasthenia Gravis
A. Etiology
   1. In the United States, approximately 3 individuals in 100,000 have myasthenia gravis (MG).
   2. Most patients with MG develop symptoms in adulthood, but patients younger than 16 years account for 10% of all cases.
   3. Microscopic examination of the neuromuscular junctions of patients with MG shows a decrease in the number of functional postsynaptic acetylcholine (ACh) receptors.
      a. The ACh receptor lesion appears to be caused by immune-mediated destruction or inactivation.
      b. Approximately 85% of patients have antibodies to skeletal muscle ACh receptors.
B. Clinical manifestations
   1. The hallmark of MG is generalized skeletal muscle weakness that is exacerbated by exercise and improved by rest.
   2. Thymic hyperplasia is common, especially in young patients.
   3. Pediatric cases are described as one of three types:
      a. *Neonatal transient myasthenia* affects the infant of a mother with the disease. Approximately 20% of new-

born infants born to myasthenic mothers will be affected. The myasthenic neonate typically displays weakness and difficulty in feeding. Symptoms persist for 1 to 8 weeks and may require anticholinesterase therapy.

b. *Congenital (neonatal persistent) myasthenia gravis* is a rare form of the disease that affects the infant in the first few months of life. Symptoms, usually mild, persist for life.

c. *Juvenile myasthenia gravis* affects young people 2 to 20 years of age, with a female predominance. The pathophysiology and presentation are similar to that in adults. The onset may be abrupt or insidious, and the course is often fluctuating, marked by periods of exacerbations and remissions.

C. Preoperative evaluation
1. Patients demonstrate a wide range of symptoms from mild (ptosis) to severe generalized muscle weakness (respiratory failure). Careful preoperative evaluation is necessary to define the severity of the disease. Patients in remission may appear well compensated until stressed by sedatives, secretions, surgery, or infection.
2. Muscles of the mouth, eyes, pharynx, and shoulder girdle are most often affected. Oropharyngeal weakness produces dysarthria, dysphagia, and nasal speech.
3. Patients are treated with anticholinesterase medications, immunosuppressive agents, and surgical thymectomy.
    a. A delicate balance must be reached with dosages of anticholinesterases, because too little (myasthenic crisis) or too much (cholinergic crisis) produces muscle weakness.
    b. Anticholinesterase therapy inhibits pseudocholinesterases and may prolong the effects of succinylcholine, mivacurium, and ester local anesthetics.
    c. Continuation of anticholinesterase therapy into the preoperative period is controversial and should be individualized.
4. Consider perioperative supplementation for patients taking corticosteroids.
5. Avoid preoperative sedative medication.

D. Intraoperative management
1. Regional or local anesthesia should be considered in the cooperative pediatric patient if the surgical procedure warrants it.
2. Weakness of the pharyngeal musculature impairs the

ability to clear secretions and increases the risk of perioperative aspiration. Prophylactic measures to decrease aspiration risk should be implemented.

3. Avoid all muscle relaxants if possible. Intubation is often easily performed with an inhalation agent only.

4. Succinylcholine's muscle-relaxing effect may be unpredictable, and phase II block occurs frequently even at low doses.

5. Patients are exquisitely sensitive to the effects of nondepolarizing muscle relaxants. Pretreatment with even a defasciculating dose may be hazardous. If necessary, nondepolarizing muscle relaxants should be administered at 5% of the usual dose and titrated to effect. Aminoglycoside antibiotics exacerbate the muscle weakness.

6. Reverse muscle relaxants cautiously to avoid cholinergic crisis.

7. Peripheral nerve stimulator monitoring must be interpreted cautiously because patients with proximal muscle weakness (e.g., accessory muscles of respiration, bulbar muscles) may show a relatively normal response to ulnar nerve stimulation.

8. Close monitoring of respiratory function should be continued postoperatively. The ventilation and airway must be supported until the patient demonstrates adequate recovery. Postoperative management in an intensive care unit may be the prudent choice.

V. Juvenile Rheumatoid Arthritis (Still Disease)

A. Etiology
1. Juvenile rheumatoid arthritis (JRA) is a chronic systemic disease characterized by synovitis and extraarticular manifestations in children younger than 16 years of age.
2. The pathophysiology is similar to adult-onset disease, involving an autoimmune assault against cartilage, ligaments, and tendons, creating dislocation and dissolution of contiguous skeletal structures.
3. The disease typically follows a course of remissions and exacerbations.
4. The incidence of JRA is 9 to 15 cases per 100,000, and it accounts for 5% of all patients with rheumatoid arthritis.

B. Clinical manifestations
1. Symptoms usually begin between 2 and 4 years of age.
2. Multiple joint involvement is common; the jaw and neck are often affected. Joint inflammation may result in

temporomandibular ankylosis and limitation of mouth opening.

3. Involvement of the cervical spine may be extensive, limiting movement of the neck or predisposing to cervical instability and atlantoaxial (C1–C2) subluxation.
4. Cricoarytenoid joints of the larynx may be swollen, inflamed, and fixed in a position that obstructs air flow, but this is less common in JRA than in the adult-onset form of the disease.
5. Systemic features include pleuritis, myocarditis, pleural effusion, an erythematous macular rash, fever, and cardiac valvular changes. Echocardiographic evidence of pericarditis has been found in 36% of children with JRA.

C. Preoperative evaluation
1. Mandibular hypoplasia, temporomandibular ankylosis, deviation of the trachea, fusion of the arytenoids, and cervical spine instability create airway and intubation problems and mandate careful airway assessment preoperatively. Preoperative indirect laryngoscopy is indicated in the JRA patient demonstrating dysphagia, stridor, hoarseness, or dyspnea.
2. Radiographic examination of the cervical spine is necessary to establish the extent of cervical spine involvement and to evaluate atlantoaxial joint stability.
3. Hypochromic, microcytic anemia is common.
4. An ECG, pulmonary function tests, and echocardiogram allow preoperative definition of any cardiorespiratory involvement.
5. The patient's preoperative medication regimen may have side effects that affect anesthesia care (see Table 17–3).

D. Intraoperative management
1. Limited joint mobility, contractures, and deformities

TABLE 17–3. Drugs Used to Treat Juvenile Rheumatoid Arthritis

Medications	Anesthetic Implications
Aspirin and nonsteroidal antiinflammatory drugs (NSAIDs)	Platelet dysfunction; exaggerated surgical bleeding
Cytotoxic drugs	Hepatic and pulmonary toxicity; bone marrow suppression
Gold salts	Bone marrow suppression, stomatitis, dermatitis, renal dysfunction
Glucocorticoids	Adrenal suppression; peptic ulcer disease; diabetes; osteoporosis

necessitate generous padding and careful positioning intraoperatively.

2. Anesthetic maneuvers such as laryngoscopy or head rotation may place the spinal cord at risk if cervical spine instability is present. Care must be taken to avoid neck flexion or extension during laryngoscopy, if possible, and to maintain the neck in a neutral position.

3. An awake fiberoptic-guided intubation may be necessary for the patient with cervical spine instability or an anticipated difficult airway. Children with an anticipated difficult airway should have an intravenous infusion started before induction.

4. A smaller than normal endotracheal tube may be required because of an inflamed and narrowed glottic opening.

5. Myocardial depressant drugs will be tolerated poorly in patients with myocarditis and valvular disease.

6. Observe closely for postextubation airway obstruction.

7. Regional blocks have obvious advantages and should be considered if the surgery and patient history warrant their use.

VI. Central Core Disease

A. Etiology

1. Central core disease is a rare congenital myopathy involving an aberration of the central areas (cores) of type I muscle fibers.

2. Defects in the ryanodine receptor gene have been identified in patients with the disease.

B. Clinical manifestations

1. Hypotonia and abnormal or delayed motor function (walking, running, stair climbing), especially involving the lower extremities, are characteristic findings. Muscle weakness is nonprogressive or slowly progressive.

2. Skeletal abnormalities include congenital hip dislocation, scoliosis, and pes cavus.

3. Serum CK levels are usually normal.

C. Preoperative evaluation

1. Evaluate the degree of motor dysfunction.

2. A restrictive pattern of respiratory impairment may develop with resulting chronic hypoxemia and pulmonary hypertension.

D. Intraoperative management

1. Patients with central core disease have a known predisposition to MH. Maintain assiduous monitoring for

signs and symptoms of MH, and deliver a trigger-free anesthetic.

2. Patients are exquisitely sensitive to nondepolarizing muscle relaxants. Avoid if possible.

VII. Osteogenesis Imperfecta

A. Etiology

1. Osteogenesis imperfecta (OI) is a congenital connective tissue disorder that causes a generalized decrease in bone mass (osteopenia) and results in fragility of bone with recurring fractures.

2. The underlying biochemical abnormality appears to involve defective collagen synthesis.

3. The disease is inherited as an autosomal dominant or recessive trait with an incidence ranging from 1 in 20,000 to 1 in 60,000 live births.

4. Progression of OI usually arrests in puberty.

B. Clinical manifestations

1. Patients have clinical features of blue sclera (thinness of the collagen layers of the sclera allows the choroid layers to be seen), dental abnormalities, and brittle bones.

2. Associated problems include deafness (10%), abnormal platelet function, increased serum thyroxine levels, increased basal metabolic rate and O_2 consumption, cleft palate, vascular fragility, hydrocephalus, spina bifida, and aortic and mitral regurgitation.

3. Scoliosis occurs in about 50% of patients with the severe form of the disease.

C. Preoperative evaluation

1. Patients have short necks, large tongues, and fragile teeth, jaws, and cervical vertebrae. Careful evaluation of the airway is indicated.

2. Spinal curvature and thoracic cage involvement are associated with decreased vital capacity and a restrictive pattern of ventilation. Pulmonary function tests should be obtained in patients with respiratory involvement. Arterial blood gases define the patient's ability to oxygenate.

3. Pulmonary hypertension may occur secondary to chronic hypoxia.

4. Old and current fractures should be documented.

5. Seek and investigate signs and a history of bleeding abnormalities.

6. Patients have a tendency to become hypermetabolic and hyperthermic with anesthesia. Explore the patient's history and chart, and question family members regarding

any abnormal temperature increases, especially intra-operatively.

7. A preoperative echocardiogram can diagnose valvular lesions; antibiotic prophylaxis may be required.

8. Ascertain whether the patient has normal hearing.

D. Intraoperative management

    1. Patients are prone to fractures with even minor physical stress (e.g., application of a blood pressure cuff or tourniquet). Careful patient positioning and padding are critical.

    2. Fragility of the teeth, mandible, and cervical spine mandates caution during intubation and airway management. Succinylcholine is not advised because of the possibility of fasciculation-induced fractures.

    3. Intraoperative hyperthermia usually responds to surface cooling and is not believed to be related to MH. Many authorities, however, advise against the administration of MH-triggering agents in OI patients. Maintain a high degree of suspicion for MH-like signs and symptoms.

VIII. Miscellaneous Disorders with Associated Musculoskeletal Abnormalities

A. Several disorders or syndromes have associated musculo-skeletal abnormalities that may impact anesthetic management (see Table 17–4).

IX. Down Syndrome

A. Etiology

    1. Down syndrome (trisomy 21) is a congenital syndrome associated with a varied set of anomalies including those involving the musculoskeletal system.

    2. It occurs in approximately 1 of every 660 live births.

B. Clinical manifestations

    1. Approximately 20% of patients with Down syndrome have ligamentous laxity of the atlantoaxial joint that may allow C1–C2 subluxation and may predispose to spinal cord injury.

    2. Joint laxity may also predispose to temporomandibular subluxation with jaw thrust.

    3. Most Down syndrome patients with atlantoaxial joint instability are asymptomatic. Patients with peripheral ligamentous laxity seem most at risk for atlantoaxial subluxation.

    4. Associated disorders include mental retardation, large tongue, small mouth, and intestinal obstruction.

TABLE 17–4. Syndromes and Inherited Conditions with Associated Musculoskeletal Abnormalities

Syndrome Name	Clinical Features and Anesthetic Implications
Arthrogryposis multiplex	Airway problems caused by temporomandibular joint ankylosis and cervical spine immobility; severe contracture and generalized joint immobility; gastroesophageal reflux disease; congenital heart disease
Ellis–van Creveld syndrome	Airway and intubation problems from mandibular hypoplasia and other skeletal defects; congenital heart disease; chest wall anomalies produce restrictive ventilatory impairment; cleft lip and palate
Goldenhar syndrome	Vertebral instability and hemifacial microsomia result in difficult airway and intubation; congenital heart disease
Pierre Robin syndrome	Micrognathia, cleft palate, glossoptosis produce very difficult intubation; tracheostomy may be required; congenital heart disease
Prader-Willi syndrome	Difficult airway management and intubation from craniofacial and cervical abnormalities; frequent kyphoscoliosis; obesity; aspiration pneumonitis, pulmonary hypertension; hypo- or hyperglycemia
Rett syndrome	Multiple orthopedic and motor movement disorders; gastroesophageal reflux; abnormal control of ventilation; thoracic deformities; diffuse muscle wasting; autism; dementia
Treacher Collins syndrome	Mandibulofacial dysostosis; difficult mask fit and intubation; obstructive apnea; congenital heart defects

    5. Fifty percent of patients have associated congenital heart disease; 8% of patients have cyanotic heart disease, usually tetralogy of Fallot.

  C. Preoperative evaluation

    1. Echocardiography is a useful tool to obtain a noninvasive preoperative assessment of cardiac involvement.

    2. Routine radiologic examination of the cervical spine before anesthesia and surgery is recommended by some authorities but is controversial.

3. A small oral cavity, mandibular hypoplasia, congenital subglottic stenosis (20%–25%), and a large tongue make airway management challenging and warrant careful preoperative evaluation and planning.

4. Preoperative referral to an orthopedic surgeon or neurosurgeon should be sought for those patients with neurologic symptoms (neck pain, arm pain, upper extremity weakness, torticollis) or for those patients whose physical or radiographic examination suggests cervical spine instability. Stabilization of the cervical spine may be indicated before other surgery is undertaken.

D. Intraoperative management

1. Anesthetic maneuvers such as laryngoscopy or head rotation may place the spinal cord at risk if cervical spine instability is present. Care must be taken to avoid neck flexion and extension during laryngoscopy.

2. Placement of a soft collar after induction helps stabilize the spine in a neutral position and serves to remind perioperative providers to avoid extreme flexion, extension, or rotation of the neck.

3. Patients are predisposed to upper airway obstruction.

4. A smaller than normal endotracheal tube may be necessary because of subglottic narrowing.

5. Meticulously avoid inadvertent intravenous injection of air, because systemic embolization may occur with right-to-left shunt.

X. Klippel-Feil Syndrome

A. Etiology

1. Klippel-Feil is a congenital syndrome with an estimated incidence of 1 in 40,000 live births.

B. Clinical manifestations

1. The syndrome consists of (a) a short neck with fusion of two or more cervical vertebrae, (b) cervical spine immobility, and (c) a low posterior hairline.

2. Associated disorders include scoliosis (60%), spina bifida (45%), central alveolar hypoventilation, renal anomalies (35%), and cardiac defects (ventricular septal defect [VSD], atrioventricular [AV] conduction pathway abnormalities). Facial asymmetry, cleft palate, and vocal cord dysfunction may also be present.

C. Preoperative evaluation

1. A thorough assessment of the cervical spine anatomy and evaluation for instability and immobility are warranted.

Radiographs of the cervical spine should be available preoperatively.
2. In addition to involvement of the cervical spine, abnormalities predisposing to difficult airway include micrognathia, mandibular malformations, and cleft palate.
3. An ECG and echocardiogram allow preoperative definition of cardiac function.

D. Intraoperative management
   1. A difficult intubation should be anticipated. The laryngeal mask airway has been used successfully for management of the difficult airway in children with Klippel-Feil syndrome. Awake fiberoptic-guided intubation may be indicated.
   2. Maintain the cervical spine in a neutral and stabilized position during intubation and positioning.
   3. Patients are prone to bradydysrhythmias.
   4. Meticulously avoid inadvertent intravenous injection of air, since systemic embolization may occur with right-to-left shunt.
   5. Extubation should be performed with the child fully awake, after adequate return of laryngeal reflexes.

ADDITIONAL READINGS

Bourke, D.L., Yates, A.J., & Yates, H.M. (1998). Evaluation of the patient with musculoskeletal disease. In Longnecker, D.E., Tinker, J.H., & Morgan, G.E. (Eds.). *Principles and practice of anesthesiology.* St. Louis: Mosby.

Maxwell, L.G., Zuckerberg, A.L., Motoyama, E.K., et al. (1996). Systemic disorders in pediatric anesthesia. In Motoyama, E.K., & Davis, P.J. (Eds.). *Smith's anesthesia for infants and children.* St. Louis: Mosby.

Mendell, J.R., Griggs, R.C., & Ptacek, L.J. (1998). Diseases of muscle. In Fauci, A.S., Braunwald, E., Isselbacker, K.J., et al. (Eds.). *Harrison's principles of internal medicine.* New York: McGraw-Hill.

Miller, J.D., & Rosenbaum, H. (1998). Muscle diseases. In Benumof, J.L. (Ed.). *Anesthesia and uncommon diseases.* Philadelphia: W.B. Saunders.

Vetter, T.R. (1994). Acute airway obstruction due to arytenoiditis in a child with juvenile rheumatoid arthritis. *Anesthesia and Analgesia, 79,* 1198–1200.

Vollers, J.M. (1991). Preoperative evaluation of the pediatric patient. In McGough, E.K., & Monroe, M.C. (Eds.). *Problems in anesthesia.* Philadelphia: Lippincott.

18

Anesthesia for Pediatric Patients with Endocrine System Diseases

Mary Karlet, PhD, CRNA

DIABETES INSIPIDUS

Diabetes insipidus (DI) is a syndrome characterized by elevated plasma osmolality and hypotonic polyuria. It results from insufficient antidiuretic hormone (ADH) release from the posterior pituitary (neurogenic DI) or insensitivity of the renal tubules to ADH (nephrogenic DI). Common causes include pituitary or hypothalamic injury or ischemia from neoplastic, surgical, infectious, vascular, or traumatic origins. DI commonly occurs in the immediate postoperative period after pituitary surgery.

I. Clinical Manifestations

A. Hypotonic urine of high volume results in dehydration with associated polydipsia, hypernatremia, hypotension, and electrolyte loss (see Table 18–1).

B. In some surgical patients DI is transient, with resumption of normal ADH activity occurring 24 to 36 hours postoperatively.

II. Preoperative Evaluation

A. Goals of perioperative management are to preserve normal fluid and electrolyte balance, maintain urine output, and support hemodynamic stability.

B. The urine volume may be prodigious with DI, reaching as high as 10 to 20 ml/kg/h, and urine osmolality is hypotonic (usually <200 mOsm/L) relative to the plasma.

C. Evaluate the child's hydration status. The patient with DI may require gradual hydration with hypotonic or isotonic solution preoperatively.

D. Evaluate serum electrolytes, directing particular attention to sodium and potassium concentrations. Ensure normal levels before elective surgery.

III. Intraoperative Management

A. Monitor urine output, urine osmolality, serum electrolytes, and serum osmolality frequently in the perioperative period.

TABLE 18-1. Comparison of Diabetes Insipidus (DI) and Syndrome of Inappropriate Antidiuretic Hormone (SIADH)

Laboratory Test	DI	SIADH
Urine osmolality	<200 mOsm/L	>200 mOsm/L
Serum osmolality	>280 mOsm/L	<280 mOsm/L
Serum sodium	Usually >148 mEq/L	Usually <132 mEq/L
Urine sodium	<20 mmol/L	>20 mmol/L

Adapted from Maxwell, L.G., Zuckerberg, A.L., Motoyama, E.K., et al. (1996). Systemic disorders in pediatric anesthesia. In Motoyama, E.K., & Davis, P.J. (Eds.). *Smith's anesthesia for infants and children* (p. 831). St. Louis: Mosby.

B. Intraoperative fluid management must consider preoperative volume status, intraoperative blood loss, and urine output. Replace urine losses with a hypotonic solution.

C. If the urine output is greater than 3 ml/kg/h and plasma osmolality exceeds 290 mOsm/L, administration of aqueous vasopressin (continuous infusion starting at 0.5 mU/kg/h) or desmopressin (DDAVP) (starting dose 2.5 µg by nasal insufflation or 0.5 to 4 µg by intravenous [IV] injection) may be used to control the symptoms.

D. Generalized vasoconstriction can occur with large doses of vasopressin; however, side effects are minimal at doses used for antidiuresis.

SYNDROME OF INAPPROPRIATE ANTIDIURETIC HORMONE SECRETION

The syndrome of inappropriate antidiuretic hormone secretion (SIADH) occurs when excessive quantities of ADH are produced in the absence of a physiologic stimulus. This condition exists most commonly in association with central nervous system (CNS) diseases of traumatic, inflammatory, neoplastic, or vascular origin.

I. Clinical Manifestations

A. Hyponatremia, decreased serum osmolality, reduced urine output, and high urine osmolality are the hallmarks of inappropriate ADH secretion.

B. Peripheral edema and hypertension are usually not present.

II. Preoperative Evaluation

A. Serum electrolytes and fluid volume should be normalized before elective surgery.

B. Initial treatment for SIADH includes restriction of fluid intake, which may be sufficient for mild cases and asymptomatic patients. Demeclocycline, lithium, furosemide, and hypertonic saline (3%) may be necessary in more severe cases unresponsive to fluid restriction.

C. Signs of increased intracranial pressure (headache, vomiting, papilledema, tense fontanelles in infants, alterations of consciousness) must be sought in children with SIADH secondary to brain tumors.

III. Intraoperative Management

A. Monitor urine output, urine osmolality, serum electrolytes, and serum osmolality frequently in the perioperative period.

B. Intraoperative fluid management must consider preoperative volume status, intraoperative blood loss, and urine output.

DIABETES MELLITUS

Diabetes mellitus (virtually all type 1, insulin-dependent) is the most common endocrine disease in childhood, affecting approximately 1 in every 500 school-age children. It is now generally believed that type 1 diabetes evolves over a period of months to years, manifesting as weight loss, polyphagia, polyuria, and dehydration. Stresses such as surgery, trauma, and infection may markedly exacerbate elevations in plasma glucose.

I. Complications Associated with Diabetes in the Perioperative Period

A. Hyperglycemia is associated with osmotic diuresis, electrolyte loss, and dehydration. Hyperglycemia has also been associated with poorer outcomes in patients who experience CNS ischemia.

B. Diabetic end-stage complications of renal, cardiac, and eye disease seldom occur before adulthood.

C. Hypoglycemia is the most serious perioperative complication. Common signs of low blood sugar include anxiety, trembling, tachycardia, diaphoresis, and hypertension. These signs may be blunted or masked with the patient under anesthesia or mistaken for "light anesthesia."

D. Infection and decreased wound healing are more prevalent in the diabetic population.

II. Preoperative Evaluation

A. Document the insulin regimen of the child and the degree of blood sugar control. Knowledge of the kinetics of the patient's insulin regimen is necessary (see Table 18–2). Patients with poorly controlled diabetes mellitus may need hospitalization before surgery for optimal preparation.

B. Determine blood sugar (BS) and electrolyte levels on the morning of surgery. Marked hyperglycemia (>250 mg/dl) should be treated with insulin before surgery.

C. Elective surgery should be scheduled as early in the morning as possible.

D. Maintain standard preoperative fasting protocols.

E. Emergency surgery should be delayed, if possible, until ketoacidosis (BS >300 mg/dl, ketonemia, dehydration, acidosis) is treated.

III. Intraoperative Management

A. Regional or general anesthesia is acceptable for the child with diabetes, and the selection of specific anesthetic agents is not affected by the diagnosis.

B. Intraoperative BS control in the diabetic child is challenging, and various perioperative management options have been proposed. All regimens aim to minimize metabolic derangements and avoid hypoglycemia and severe hyperglycemia.

C. Mild hyperglycemia usually does not present serious problems in the pediatric surgical patient, but hypoglycemia can have serious consequences, including permanent neurologic derangements. Important in all diabetic regimens is the frequent determination of plasma glucose in the perioperative period. Three glucose management regimens are highlighted:

  1. Glucose-free, insulin-free technique: This regimen is frequently implemented for operative procedures of short duration after which prompt resumption of oral intake is expected.

    a. Determine morning BS. Withhold morning insulin dose.

    b. If indicated for the procedure, administer glucose-free IV fluids (e.g., lactated Ringer's solution).

TABLE 18–2. Commonly Used Insulins

Insulin	Route	Onset (h)	Peak (h)	Duration (h)
Regular	Intravenous	0.5–1	2–3	5–8
Regular	Subcutaneous	0.5–1	2–4	6–8
NPH	Subcutaneous	1–2	6–12	6–24
Lente	Subcutaneous	1–2.5	7–15	10–20
Ultralente	Subcutaneous	4–8	10–30	24–36

  c. Administer 40% to 60% of the usual daily dose of insulin in the postoperative period after oral fluids are taken and tolerated.

2. Nontight (classic) regimen.

  a. On the morning of surgery, start an IV infusion of 5% dextrose in 0.45% saline solution at 1500 ml/m^2/d (63 ml/m^2/h).

  b. After the IV infusion is started, administer one fourth to one half of the usual morning dose of insulin.

  c. Check the BS at the start of surgery and at least every hour intraoperatively. Finger stick glucose estimations performed with reflectant glucometers provide results that are within 10% of laboratory glucose determinations. Visual estimation of BS using chemical strips is less accurate.

  d. Plasma glucose concentrations are maintained between 100 and 250 mg/dl. Supplemental IV doses of regular insulin can be given on a sliding scale to maintain the desired plasma glucose level.

  e. Continue the IV infusion and frequent BS determinations in the postanesthesia care unit (PACU) until the patient is taking and tolerating oral fluids.

  f. The usual insulin regimen can generally be resumed the next day.

3. Continuous insulin infusion or tight control regimen: This alternative technique is implemented for procedures lasting longer than 1 hour or for diabetics with labile BS.

  a. On the morning of surgery, start an IV infusion of 5% dextrose in 0.45% saline solution at 1500 ml/m^2/d (63 ml/m^2/h). Add 1 to 2 units of regular insulin for each 100 ml of 5% dextrose. Flush the IV tubing with 60 ml before starting to saturate insulin binding sites.

  b. Determine blood glucose on the morning of surgery and at least every hour intraoperatively. Maintain the BS between 100 and 250 mg/dl by adjusting the insulin infusion as needed.

  c. Crystalloid solutions are administered separately to replace blood or fluid losses.

  d. Hypoglycemia can be treated with a 50% dextrose solution (0.1 g/kg will raise the BS level by approximately 30 mg/dl).

  e. Continue the insulin and dextrose infusions until the patient is awake and tolerating oral fluid.

PHEOCHROMOCYTOMA

Pheochromocytoma is a catecholamine-producing tumor derived from chromaffin tissue (usually the adrenal medulla). Children account for 5% of all reported cases. Most pheochromocytomas produce norepinephrine and epinephrine, and clinical manifestations are the result of increased plasma concentrations of these hormones. Elevated levels of catecholamines or their metabolites (vanillylmandelic acid [VMA], normetanephrine) in blood or urine confirm the diagnosis. Neuroblastomas may also increase catecholamine production but less so than pheochromocytomas.

I. Clinical Manifestations

A. The hyperdynamic cardiovascular system associated with catecholamine elevation produces paroxysmal hypertension and tachycardia. There may also be a history of palpitations, headaches, diaphoresis, and vomiting.

B. Tumor manipulation, activation of the sympathetic nervous system, and histamine favor hormone release. Between episodes of catecholamine release, the tumor may be quiescent and the patient totally asymptomatic.

C. Abdominal pain may be present.

D. Sustained hypertension contracts the intravascular volume and increases the hematocrit.

E. Pheochromocytomas may occur as part of the multiple endocrine adenomatosis syndromes, types II or III, and the patient should be evaluated for associated endocrinopathy (see Table 18–3).

II. Preoperative Evaluation

A. Anesthesia is dangerous in the undiagnosed or unprepared patient. The patient should be admitted before surgery

TABLE 18–3. Multiple Endocrine Adenomatosis Syndromes

	System	Disorder
Type I, Werner's syndrome	Pituitary	Hypoglycemia
	Parathyroid	Hypercalcemia
	Pancreas	
Type II, Sipple's syndrome	Thyroid	Thyroid carcinoma
	Parathyroid	Parathyroid hyperplasia
	Adrenal medulla	Pheochromocytoma
Type III	Nervous system	Neuromas
	Thyroid	Medullary carcinoma
	Adrenal medulla	Pheochromocytoma

for evaluation and to ensure adequate control of hypertension.

1. Phenoxybenzamine may be used to produce preoperative alpha-adrenergic blockade. Usually 10 to 14 days are required for adequate alpha-receptor blockade as evidenced by a consistently normal blood pressure and a decrease in hematocrit as the blood volume expands. Beta-adrenergic blockade is usually unnecessary in children, and it should be instituted only after the onset of adequate alpha-blockade.

B. An electrocardiogram (ECG) and echocardiogram are helpful for evaluating cardiac size and myocardial function.

C. These children benefit from preoperative anxiolytics to reduce stress-related catecholamine release.

III. Intraoperative Management

A. An overall goal is to control sympathetic outflow.
   1. Avoid medications that induce histamine release: morphine, atracurium, curare.
   2. Avoid vagolytics and sympathomimetics: atropine, pancuronium, succinylcholine.
   3. Avoid medications that may sensitize the myocardium: halothane.
   4. Avoid indirect catecholamine stimulators: droperidol, ephedrine, metoclopramide, ketamine.

B. Do not initiate anesthesia without an IV line in place.

C. Tailor the anesthetic to decrease sympathetic stimulation. An inhalational agent-O_2-N_2O technique effectively blunts sympathetic outflow activity.

D. Adjunctive use of epidural anesthesia further reduces the stress response and catecholamine release.

E. Anticipate major blood loss with pheochromocytoma tumor resection. A central venous pressure monitor helps guide fluid management.

F. An intraarterial catheter allows for assiduous blood pressure monitoring and serial measurements of arterial blood gases, electrolytes, and blood glucose concentrations.

G. Temperature, urine output, and ECG should be monitored closely.

H. Ensure availability of medications to control intraoperative hypertension and dysrhythmias. Infusion of a short-acting vasodilator (e.g., nitroprusside) or an alpha-adrenergic antagonist (e.g., phentolamine) allows rapid blood pressure control. Esmolol, as an infusion, provides titratable beta-adrenergic blockade.

I. After the tumor is excised, hypotension and hypoglycemia may occur because of the sudden fall in circulating catecholamines.

IV. Postoperative Care

A. The patient should be admitted postoperatively to an intensive care unit for continuous monitoring.
B. Postoperatively, check BS frequently and include dextrose in IV fluids.
C. The hemodynamic status usually stabilizes 24 to 48 hours after surgery.

HYPERTHYROIDISM

The most common causes of excess circulating thyroid hormones in children are (1) Graves' disease and (2) transient neonatal hyperthyroidism (see Table 18–4). Graves' disease (diffuse toxic goiter) has a peak incidence in adolescence and is five times more common in females. An autoimmune mechanism is important in the pathogenesis of Graves' disease. Transient neonatal hyperthyroidism results from transplacental transfer of maternal thyroid-stimulating immunoglobulins (TSAb). Clinical manifestations in the newborn are transient (1 to 2 months), because the half-life of the maternal immunoglobulin is short.

I. Clinical Manifestations

A. Common manifestations of hyperthyroidism include weight loss, tremors, muscle weakness, diarrhea, nervousness, and exophthalmos. The cardiovascular system is hyperdynamic, as manifested by sinus tachycardia/atrial fibrillation, increased cardiac output, hypertension, and low peripheral vascular resistance.
B. Most children have an enlarged, palpable thyroid gland.

TABLE 18–4. Common Thyroid Function Tests

	T$_4$	TSH
Primary hypothyroidism	↓	↑
Secondary hypothyroidism	↓	↓
Primary hyperthyroidism	↑	↓
Secondary hyperthyroidism	↑	↑

T$_4$, Thyroxine; *TSH*, thyroid-stimulating hormone; ↓, decreased; ↑, increased.

II. Preoperative Evaluation

A. Elective surgery should be postponed until the patient is rendered euthyroid with medical treatment. Preoperative goals include normal thyroid function tests, a normal resting heart rate, and a calm and sedated patient.

B. Antithyroid (propylthiouracil, potassium iodide) and beta-adrenergic blocking medications should be continued on the day of operation.

C. A large goiter should be evaluated with neck radiographs, magnetic resonance imaging (MRI), or computed tomography (CT) scan. Tracheal deviation or compression may occur.

III. Intraoperative Management

A. A higher cardiac output may result in a prolonged inhalation induction.

B. Thiopental is the IV induction agent of choice, since it possesses some antithyroid activity.

C. Adrenergic receptors may be sensitized by thyroid hormones. Drugs that stimulate the sympathetic nervous system (ketamine) or have sympathomimetic effects (pancuronium) should be avoided.

D. Hypotension should be treated with direct-acting vasopressors. Esmolol provides an effective and easily titrated treatment for tachycardia.

E. A deep level of anesthesia should be obtained before airway instrumentation or surgical stimulation.

F. Minimal alveolar concentration (MAC) requirements for inhaled agents are not increased with hyperthyroidism.

G. Cardiovascular function and body temperature should be closely monitored in the perioperative period.

H. Prominent eyes demand meticulous protection.

IV. Thyroid Storm

A. Thyroid storm, or uncompensated thyrotoxicosis, is extremely rare in children. It is characterized by an onset of acute hyperpyrexia, tachycardia, and hypotension. Prompt treatment should include hydration, cooling, beta-adrenergic blockade, propylthiouracil, sodium iodide, and correction of any precipitating cause.

B. Intraoperatively, the hypermetabolic state may be mistaken for malignant hyperthermia.

HYPOTHYROIDISM

Hypothyroidism is among the most common endocrine disorders in pediatric patients. Low production of thyroid hormones (triiodothyronine [T_3], thyroxine [T_4]) in children results from pituitary failure to produce thyroid-stimulating hormone (TSH) or from primary thyroid dysfunction (congenital or acquired). In the pediatric age-group, approximately one third of the hypothyroid cases present in infancy and two thirds in childhood.

I. Clinical Manifestations

A. Congenital hypothyroidism usually appears in infancy and presents with classic features, such as a large tongue, sluggish reflexes, puffy face, abnormal neurologic sequelae (cretinism), and large fontanelles.

B. In the older child, a generalized reduction in metabolic activity is manifested as lethargy, intolerance to cold, bradycardia, narrowed pulse pressure, and impaired growth.

C. Myxedema coma (profound hypothyroidism) is rare in children. Manifestations include impaired mentation, hypoventilation, hypothermia, hyponatremia, and congestive heart failure.

II. Preoperative Evaluation

A. Patients with uncorrected hypothyroidism should not undergo elective surgery. Gradual correction over a 2-week period is usually advised. Patients who are adequately treated have normal T_4 and TSH levels.

B. Children with severe hypothyroidism may have adrenal insufficiency that warrants stress dose steroid coverage (hydrocortisone, 2 mg/kg q6h).

C. Thyroid replacement medications should continue in the perioperative period.

III. Intraoperative Management

A. Patients with incompletely restored thyroid hormone levels are sensitive to the myocardial and respiratory depressant effects of inhalational and IV anesthetics. Agents must be titrated slowly.

B. Intravascular volume may be decreased 10% to 24%. Invasive hemodynamic monitoring may be warranted if a large blood loss or fluid shift is expected.

C. To guard against intraoperative hypoglycemia, fluids should contain dextrose.

D. Delayed gastric emptying may warrant precautions for a full stomach.

E. Ketamine as an induction agent is advantageous because of its sympathomimetic activity.

F. Decreased cardiac output may shorten inhalation induction time.

G. Hypothyroid infants and children are particularly sensitive to heat loss, and extra care should be taken to prevent hypothermia.

H. MAC requirements for inhaled agents are not changed with hypothyroidism.

IV. Postoperative Care

A. Slowed drug biotransformation and excretion, hypothermia, and respiratory depression may delay recovery from general anesthesia.

ADRENOCORTICAL INSUFFICIENCY

Adrenocortical insufficiency, although not common in childhood, may be the result of (1) a primary defect in the adrenal glands themselves or (2) pituitary or hypothalamic failure or suppression. Primary hypoadrenalism (Addison's disease) is associated with both glucocorticoid (cortisol) and mineralocorticoid (aldosterone) deficiency and is most commonly of autoimmune origin. Secondary hypoadrenalism from pituitary or hypothalamic failure is associated principally with glucocorticoid deficiency. Causes include pituitary resection, pituitary irradiation, or suppression of the hypothalamic-pituitary-adrenal axis from the use of synthetic glucocorticoids.

I. Clinical Manifestations

A. Progressive muscle weakness, anemia, hyponatremia, hypovolemia, hypotension, and hyperkalemia are salient findings in mineralocorticoid deficiency.

B. Hypoglycemia, nausea, vomiting, and fatigue are features of glucocorticoid deficiency.

C. Increased adrenocorticotropic hormone (ACTH), associated with Addison's disease, stimulates melanocyte receptors and produces cutaneous and mucosal hyperpigmentation.

II. Preoperative Evaluation

A. Glucocorticoid and mineralocorticoid replacement forms the basis for treatment of hypocorticism.

B. In a healthy patient, fever, acute illness, and surgery increase the secretion of cortisol from the adrenal glands. The patient with adrenal insufficiency (primary or secondary) cannot manifest an appropriate stress response and requires corticosteroid administration above the physiologic dose (stress dose) in the perioperative period. The administration of IV hydrocortisone (Hydrocortone, Solu-Cortef), 2 mg/kg/6 h, on the day of surgery is appropriate for most surgical procedures. For major surgery, the dose may be extended and then tapered over the following 3 to 5 days to maintenance levels.

C. It is generally accepted that patients with a history of high-dose steroid use for longer than 1 week in the year before surgery may have hypothalamic-pituitary-adrenal axis suppression. These patients should receive perioperative steroid supplementation.

III. Intraoperative Management

A. A heightened sensitivity to myocardial depressant agents and the propensity for hypotension should be considered in the selection and dosage of anesthetic agents.

B. Serum electrolytes and blood glucose concentrations should be monitored frequently in the perioperative period.

C. A peripheral nerve stimulator can help guide muscle relaxant titration in the patient with associated muscle weakness.

D. Trauma, infection, and surgery in the inadequately treated patient can precipitate adrenal crises (hypotension or possible shock, abdominal pain, nausea, vomiting, dyspnea, lethargy). Therapy includes (1) aggressive hydration with fluids, (2) glucocorticoids, and (3) hemodynamic support.

ADRENAL CORTEX HYPERSECRETION

Hypercorticism (Cushing's syndrome) is characterized by chronic, excessive corticosteroid hormone secretion. In infants and children, the cause is usually a functioning tumor of the adrenal cortex or prolonged exogenous administration of glucocorticoids. Cushing's disease is the result of excessive secretion of ACTH, resulting in elevated cortisol levels.

I. Clinical Manifestations

A. Moon facies and truncal obesity with thin extremities are prominent physical manifestations of excess adrenal cortex hormone secretion.

B. Hypertension (salt and water retention), osteoporosis, hyperglycemia, hypokalemic alkalosis, and muscle weakness are commonly present.

C. Impaired wound healing and an increased incidence of infection (immunosuppressive effects of glucocorticoids) are also seen.

II. Preoperative Evaluation

A. Evaluate and control hyperglycemia and hypertension perioperatively.

B. Correct hypokalemia.

III. Intraoperative Management

A. Cushing's syndrome does not alter drug metabolism, and the selection of specific anesthetic drugs is not affected by the diagnosis of hypercorticism.

B. Position the patient with care because of possible osteoporosis.

C. Muscle relaxant doses may need to be reduced because of hypokalemia and accompanying muscle weakness.

ADDITIONAL READINGS

Keon, T.P., & Templeton, J.J. (1993). Diseases of the endocrine system. In Katz, J., & Steward, D.J. (Eds.). *Anesthesia and uncommon pediatric diseases* (pp. 420–460). Philadelphia: W.B. Saunders.

Maxwell, L.G., Deshpande, J.K., & Wetzel, R.C. (1994). Preoperative evaluation of children. *Pediatric Clinics of North America*, 41(1), 93–109.

Maxwell, L.G., Zuckerberg, A.L., Motoyama, E.K., et al. (1996). Systemic disorders in pediatric anesthesia. In Motoyama, E.K., & Davis, P.J. (Eds.). *Smith's anesthesia for infants and children* (pp. 827–875). St. Louis: Mosby.

O'Riordan, J. (1997). Pheochromocytomas and anesthesia. *International Anesthesiology Clinics*, 35(4), 99–128.

Sheeran, P., & O'Leary, E. (1997). Adrenocortical disorders. *International Anesthesiology Clinics*, 35(4), 85–98.

19

Anesthesia for Pediatric Patients with Renal System Diseases

Mary Karlet, PhD, CRNA

I. Renal Physiology

A. Kidney's major functions.
   1. Regulation of the volume and composition of the body's extracellular fluids
   2. Excretion of waste products of metabolism, toxins, foreign chemicals
   3. Control of erythrocyte production
   4. Modulation of arterial blood pressure
   5. Metabolic activator of vitamin D activity

B. Full nephrogenesis is complete at 36 weeks' gestational age. By the time the normal full-term infant is 1 month old, the kidneys are approximately 70% mature.

C. Despite accounting for only 0.5% of the body weight, the kidneys receive 20% to 25% of the cardiac output. Renal blood flow (RBF) remains almost constant for a range of arterial blood pressure from 60 to 160 mm Hg, a phenomenon known as *autoregulation.*

D. Nerve supply to the kidneys is abundant. Sympathetic vasoconstrictor fibers originate from the T4 to L1 spinal segments. Pain fibers, mainly from the renal pelvis and upper ureter, are conveyed back to spinal cord segments T10 to L1.

E. Total body water content.
   1. Infants <6 months of age have a higher percentage of total body water (~75% of body weight) than older infants and children (~60% of body weight).

F. Glomerular filtration rate (GFR).
   1. In newborn infants the GFR is only 15% to 30% of normal adult values.
   2. The GFR reaches 50% of normal values by the fifth to tenth day of life.
   3. By 1 year of age an infant's GFR approximates normal adult values.

G. Concentrating and diluting mechanisms.

1. The full-term infant has limited ability to concentrate and dilute the urine. The concentrating ability reaches adult capacity by 1 to 3 years of age.
2. The diuretic response to a water load is sluggish in all infants and increases the risk of overzealous administration of water.

H. Urine output is very similar in all ages (1–2 ml/kg/h).

II. Laboratory Evaluation of Renal Function in Children

A. Creatinine clearance is the most reliable laboratory indicator of GFR. A creatinine clearance of 25 to 50 ml/min/1.73 m^2 indicates early evidence of renal failure. Patients with a creatinine clearance <20 ml/min/1.73 m^2 will manifest more severe symptoms of renal failure and are often on dialysis.

B. Blood urea nitrogen (BUN) and plasma creatinine are valuable indices of GFR. Normal serum creatinine values increase every year until the end of puberty. Plasma creatinine varies inversely with GFR. A doubling of the plasma creatinine generally is associated with a 50% reduction in GFR.

C. The kidney's inability to concentrate the urine is often an early sign of disease. A specific gravity of 1.018 or more following an overnight fast suggests that concentrating ability is intact.

III. Children at Risk for Acute Renal Failure in the Perioperative Period

Acute renal failure (ARF) is a sudden decrease in renal function resulting in the loss of the kidneys' ability to excrete nitrogenous and other wastes. ARF can be classified as arising from prerenal (renal hypoperfusion), intrinsic, or postrenal (obstructive uropathy) causes. Common risk factors associated with perioperative ARF in surgical pediatric patients include

A. Decreased preoperative renal reserve or renal insufficiency

B. Cardiac dysfunction (poor cardiac output reduces RBF and increases the potential for renal vasoconstriction and ischemic injury)

C. Patients undergoing vascular or cardiac surgery

D. Inadequate intravascular volume

E. Patients with multiple organ system trauma, sepsis, or burns (involve systemic hemodynamic derangements, myoglobin release, and inflammatory mediator–induced renal vasoconstriction)

F. An episode of severe rhabdomyolysis (muscle ischemia, trauma, malignant hyperthermia)

G. Exposure to nephrotoxic agents (see Table 19–1)
H. Hemolysis (transfusion reactions, sickle cell anemia)
I. Hepatic disease (bilirubin)

IV. Interventions to Avoid Acute Renal Failure in the Perioperative Period

A. Limit the magnitude and duration of renal ischemia. Provide optimal hydration to maintain adequate intravascular volume and promote solute excretion.
B. Optimize preload and cardiac output.
C. Monitor urine output.
   1. A urine flow rate of <0.5 ml/kg/h (oliguria) is a sign of renal impairment due to dehydration or renal disease.
D. Employ "renal protective" drugs during select cases in the adequately hydrated patient.
   1. Mannitol (0.25–0.5 g/kg) promotes renal vasodilation, protects against hemoglobin- or myoglobin-induced ARF, prevents tubular obstruction, and reduces renal cellular swelling.
   2. Dopamine increases RBF, GFR, and urine output at dosages of 1 to 4 µg/kg/min.
   3. Furosemide (1–2 mg/kg) increases RBF and GFR and promotes tubular flow.
E. Avoid, if possible, concurrent use of potentially nephrotoxic drugs.
F. In some cases, invasive hemodynamic monitoring may be required to guide intraoperative fluid management.

TABLE 19–1. Nephrotoxins Associated with Acute Renal Failure

IMMUNOSUPPRESSANTS/ ANTINEOPLASTICS	ANTIBIOTICS
Methotrexate	Aminoglycosides
Acyclovir	Vancomycin
Gold salts	Amphotericin B
Cisplatin	Cephalosporins
Ifosfamide	Sulfonamide
Cyclosporin A	Penicillins
Azathioprine	
	MISCELLANEOUS
	Radiocontrast agents
NONSTEROIDAL ANTIINFLAMMATORY DRUGS	Carbamazepine
Aspirin	Cimetidine
Naproxen, ibuprofen	Angiotensin-converting enzyme (ACE) inhibitors
Indomethacin	Acetaminophen
Ketorolac	

TABLE 19–2. Causes of End-Stage Renal Failure in Children

Glomerulonephritis	Nephrotic syndrome
Obstructive uropathy	Hereditary interstitial nephritis
Reflux nephropathy	Retroperitoneal and renal tumors
Pyelonephritis	Amyloidosis of the kidney
Glomerular sclerosis	Hemolytic-uremic syndrome
Dysplastic or hypoplastic kidneys	Lupus nephritis
Medullary cystic disease	Anaphylactoid purpura
Polycystic disease	Obstructive uropathy

    G. Despite the early intervention of dialysis, the mortality for postsurgical ARF remains 25% to 65%.

V. Chronic Renal Failure

Chronic renal failure (CRF) is characterized by a permanent decrease in GFR with a rise in serum creatinine and azotemia. A 60% to 80% reduction in functional nephrons is required for clinical renal disease to be evident. Therefore history and physical examination are usually unremarkable early in the disease. In the United States, the incidence of pediatric end-stage renal disease (ESRD) has remained constant for the past 5 to 10 years at 11 children (0–19 years old) per 1 million child population. More than half these cases are due to congenital or hereditary disorders (see Table 19–2).

VI. Causes of Chronic Renal Failure in Children

    A. Glomerulonephritis
        1. Glomerulonephritis is the leading cause of acquired CRF during childhood.
        2. It is caused by inflammation of the glomerulus and thickening of the glomerular basement membrane, usually because of immunologic injury.
    B. Nephrotic syndrome
        1. Nephrotic syndrome is defined as massive proteinuria (>3.5 g/d), hypoalbuminemia, hyperlipidemia, and edema.
        2. It is characterized by intravascular volume depletion and decreased oncotic pressure.
    C. Aplastic, hypoplastic, and dysplastic kidneys
        1. Multicystic dysplastic kidney (MCDK) is the most common congenital renal anomaly and the most frequently diagnosed pediatric renal cystic disease.
    D. Tubulointerstitial diseases
        1. Tubulointerstitial diseases primarily affect the renal

tubules and interstitium, resulting in interstitial inflammation.

2. Common causes of tubulointerstitial disease are pyelonephritis (acute or chronic infection of the kidney) and hypersensitivity nephritis (an allergic reaction to drugs such as methicillin).

E. Hemolytic-uremic syndrome

1. Hemolytic-uremic syndrome is the most frequent cause of ARF in infants and young children and an important cause of stroke and CRF in children.

2. Ninety percent of childhood cases follow a diarrheal prodrome and are linked to enterohemorrhagic *Escherichia coli*. The pathogenic cascade begins with ingestion of enterohemorrhagic *E. coli* and culminates in thrombotic microangiopathy.

F. Obstructive uropathy

VII. Pathophysiologic Manifestations of Chronic Renal Failure

The clinical manifestations of CRF involve almost every organ. Preoperative assessment of the child with CRF must focus on volume status, acid-base, electrolyte, hemoglobin, and end-organ derangements (see Table 19–3).

A. Anemia

1. Most children with CRF develop a normochromic, normocytic anemia by the time their serum creatinine is

TABLE 19–3. Pathophysiologic Changes Associated with End-stage Renal Failure in Children

CARDIOVASCULAR SYSTEM	FLUIDS AND ELECTROLYTES	GASTROINTESTINAL SYSTEM
Increased cardiac output	Volume overload, edema	Delayed gastric emptying
Dysrhythmias	Hyperkalemia	Anorexia, nausea, vomiting
Hypertension	Hyperphosphatemia	Gastric ulcers, uremic colitis
Cardiomyopathy, cardiac failure	Hypocalcemia	
Pericarditis, pericardial tamponade	Hypermagnesemia	**NEUROLOGIC SYSTEM**
	Hyponatremia or hypernatremia	Peripheral and autonomic neuropathy
HEMATOLOGIC SYSTEM	Hyperglycemia	Fatigue, lethargy, somnolence
	Metabolic acidosis	
Anemia		**SKELETAL SYSTEM**
Platelet dysfunction		Osteodystrophy
Impaired immunologic competence		Growth retardation

>3 mg/dl or their GFR has decreased to between 20 and 35 ml/min/1.73 m². The hematocrit commonly stabilizes at 25% to 28%.

2. The primary cause of the anemia is decreased erythropoietin production. Gastrointestinal bleeding, weekly blood studies, nutritional deficiencies, and decreased red blood cell (RBC) survival from uremic toxins may be additional causes.

3. Compensation for the chronic anemia includes an increased heart rate, stroke volume, and cardiac index and increased RBC 2,3-diphosphoglycerate, with a resultant rightward shift in the oxygen-hemoglobin dissociation curve.

4. Recombinant human erythropoietin is of proven benefit in raising the hematocrit.

B. Coagulopathy

1. Qualitative platelet defects result in decreased platelet adhesion and prolonged bleeding times. Mild thrombocytopenia may be present, but platelet counts <100,000 × 10⁹ are unusual.

2. The prothrombin time (PT) and partial thromboplastin time (PTT) are usually normal.

C. Acid-base imbalance

1. Children produce about twice the amount of acid as adults. With a decrease in GFR to about 20 ml/min/1.73 m², retention of fixed acid occurs. A partial respiratory compensation usually minimizes pH changes.

2. Serum levels of HCO_3^- <15 mEq/L should be corrected preoperatively by dialysis, if time permits, or by the administration of sodium bicarbonate ($NaHCO_3$, 1 mEq/kg, can be expected to raise the serum HCO_3 by about 2 mEq/L). Acidosis should be corrected slowly and cautiously and serum Ca^{2+} and K^+ monitored.

D. Renal osteodystrophy

1. Hypocalcemia and hyperphosphatemia induce secondary hyperparathyroidism and result in generalized bone demineralization and osteoclastic bone fractures. Renal osteodystrophy is more common in children than adults. The CRF patient should be positioned with care.

2. Many of these children also receive long-term steroid therapy with resultant osteodystrophy.

E. Electrolyte imbalance

1. Children with CRF may be hyponatremic or hypernatremic.

   a. Children with polycystic kidneys or severe pyelonephritis (tubular damage > glomerular damage) are more likely to be salt wasters.

    b. Children with glomerulonephritis (glomerular damage > tubular damage) are prone to salt retention and associated edema and hypertension.

  2. Hyperkalemia is the result of decreased excretion of K^+ and the displacement of K^+ from intracellular sites by excess H^+.

    a. A preoperative serum K^+ <5.5 mEq/L is generally considered safe unless hyperkalemic electrocardiogram (ECG) signs, such as peaked T waves, decreased P wave amplitude, or widened QRS, are present.

    b. Hyperkalemia's most serious effects are seen on the heart and become dangerous as K^+ levels approach 6 to 7 mEq/L. Effects may include

      (1) Decreased force of contraction

      (2) Impaired conduction

      (3) Increased dysrhythmogenicity

    c. Sudden increased serum K^+ (succinylcholine, sepsis, increased acidosis) creates a risk for circulatory instability and cardiac arrest.

    d. In an emergency, K^+ can be lowered rapidly.

      (1) Calcium gluconate 10% reverses cardiotoxicity by antagonizing the membrane effects of hyperkalemia.

      (2) Hyperventilation abruptly increases the urinary excretion of K^+.

      (3) $NaHCO_3$ 8.4% (1–2 mEq/kg by intravenous [IV] bolus) drives K^+ into cells within minutes, irrespective of acid-base status.

      (4) Glucose (0.3–0.5 g/kg, as a 10% IV glucose solution) with regular insulin (1 unit for every 3–4 g of glucose) facilitates the transfer of K^+ from the serum into the intracellular compartment; onset is about 30 minutes.

      (5) If potassium levels >6.5 mEq/L persist despite aggressive therapy, acute dialysis is indicated, particularly in the presence of ECG abnormalities.

  3. Uremia-induced anorexia, nausea, and vomiting aggravate water, electrolyte, and acid-base imbalance.

F. Hypervolemia and hypertension

  1. Hypertension may result from fluid and sodium overload or be renin mediated.

    a. Renin-mediated hypertension is more recalcitrant to treatment.

b. The patient's antihypertensive therapy should be continued into the preoperative period.

2. Incipient heart failure.
   a. The negative inotropic effects of electrolyte derangements and acidosis predispose to congestive cardiac failure. Increased cardiac output to meet O_2 transport requirements in the presence of anemia or an arteriovenous (AV) fistula contributes to the failure.
   b. Hypertension further stresses the left ventricle.

G. Pulmonary congestion
   1. Decreased plasma proteins (decreased plasma oncotic pressure), sodium and water retention, and left ventricle failure contribute to decreased diffusion capacity and mild restrictive defects ("uremic lung"). The low colloid oncotic pressure promotes the formation of interstitial and pulmonary edema.

H. Neuropathy
   1. Peripheral and autonomic neuropathies are common.
   2. Autonomic neuropathy delays gastric emptying time and produces a labile neurovascular response.
   3. Central nervous system (CNS) changes, which vary from lethargy to severe encephalopathy, may be the result of hypertension, uremia, or a defective blood-brain barrier. Most manifestations of encephalopathy are controlled with regular dialysis.

VIII. Anesthetic Considerations for the Child with Chronic Renal Failure

Elective surgical procedures should be delayed until the patient's hydration, electrolyte, metabolic, and nutritional status is optimized. Serum levels of electrolytes and creatinine, BUN, and hematocrit values should be obtained in the immediate preoperative period.

A. Dialysis.
   1. A well-functioning renal transplant results in the best quality of life for children with ESRD, but dialysis serves as a critical bridge to care for these patients until they can receive transplants.
   2. In North America, 65% of children with ESRD undergo long-term renal replacement via peritoneal dialysis, whereas 35% receive hemodialysis. Peritoneal dialysis is less hemodynamically destabilizing, especially in children.
   3. Children with ESRD should be dialyzed at least 24 hours before surgery. The child's dialysis schedule and any problems during dialysis should be determined.

4. For children on hemodialysis, locate, assess, and protect shunt or fistula patency. Thrombosis is the most common reason for loss of vascular access.
   a. Avoid pressure on the involved limb.
   b. Monitor shunt patency continually, and chart it.
   c. Avoid hypotension.
   d. Do not use the involved limb for blood pressure monitoring or arterial or IV lines.
   e. Keep the involved limb warm.
5. Goals of dialysis include maintenance of a euvolemic state with normal acid-base, metabolic, and electrolyte status; improved platelet function; and improved growth and development.
6. Dialysis does not rectify renin-dependent hypertension, anemia, impaired immunity, hypoproteinemia, and gastrointestinal ulceration.

B. The patient's medication history should be detailed.
C. Low O_2-carrying capacity.
   1. Chronic anemia is generally well tolerated. Assess the patient's level of activity at his or her usual hemoglobin level.
   2. If a patient is well compensated and hematocrit values are >18%, preoperative RBC transfusion is generally not indicated.
   3. Preoxygenate and use generous F_{IO_2} to maximize O_2 transport.
D. Hemostasis may be impaired as a result of defective platelet function or a heparin effect following hemodialysis. Dialysis, cryoprecipitate, and desmopressin (DDAVP) improve the thrombocytopathy.
E. The child may demonstrate a low resistance to infection because of impaired white blood cell function or long-term steroid use.
   1. Infection is the major cause of death in patients with CRF.
   2. Maintain scrupulous attention to the details of asepsis.
F. The chronic and debilitating nature of the disease may result in psychosocial maladjustment or low pain tolerance. Psychologic support and empathetic communication can help allay anxieties and minimize discomfort.
G. Up to 55% of patients receiving hemodialysis are hepatitis B or C antigen carriers. Transmission can occur with mucosal as well as percutaneous exposure to infected secretions or blood.
H. Altered pharmacokinetics and pharmacodynamics produce enhanced or prolonged drug effects.

1. The acid pH may result in a higher percentage of nonionized (active) drug.
2. Decreased plasma proteins (proteinuria) result in increased bioavailability of protein-bound drugs.
3. A defective blood-brain barrier may be associated with increased sensitivity to CNS depressants, reducing the requirements for sedation by up to 50%.
4. The loss of effective nephrons decreases excretion of drugs or their metabolites.
5. An increased volume of distribution of certain agents prolongs their elimination half-life.

I. Children with CRF quickly develop hypothermia. Diminish heat losses by insulation of body parts and warming inspired gases and fluids.

IX. Anesthetic Techniques

A. Local anesthesia/monitored anesthesia care
1. For short, superficial procedures in the cooperative patient, local anesthesia without epinephrine should be considered.
B. Regional anesthesia
1. Before proceeding with regional anesthesia, the patient's coagulation status should be determined and the presence of uremic neuropathy documented.
2. Spinal anesthesia and epidural anesthesia depress renal function proportional to the magnitude of sympathetic block. If the blood pressure is maintained, GFR and renal hemodynamics are only minimally altered.
3. Avoid epinephrine in local anesthetic solutions because of alpha-adrenergic effects and the potential for decreased RBF.
C. General anesthesia
1. Growth impairment and reduced muscle mass can make standard calculation of equipment size, fluids, and medications based on age unreliable.
2. Myocardial depressants, including volatile anesthetics, are associated with an increase in renal vascular resistance to maintain blood pressure and a decrease in RBF and GFR.
3. The same degree of preoperative hyperventilation should be maintained intraoperatively.
4. The risk of regurgitation and aspiration during induction of and emergence from anesthesia is increased. Rapid sequence induction should be considered.

X. Specific Anesthetic Medications

A. As a general rule, decrease the initial dose of IV anesthetic medications by 25% to 50% and titrate to effect

B. Premedicate only if necessary, and decrease sedative doses by 25% to 50%

C. Induction medications

1. Thiopental and etomidate are protein-bound medications and have greater bioavailability in the hypoalbuminemic patient. The defective blood-brain barrier and acidemia further reduce requirements. Decrease the initial dose by one third to one half the normal dose, and titrate.

2. Propofol's CNS effects are not prolonged with standard bolus doses.

3. Ketamine is not affected by renal failure, but its use may be limited by its hypertensive side effect.

D. Narcotics

1. Fentanyl and alfentanil are metabolized in the liver but are highly protein bound. Their duration and effect may be moderately increased in chronic renal disease. Small to moderate doses are well tolerated. Sufentanil has greater variability in clearance and elimination half-life with renal disease.

2. Remifentanil does not rely on the kidneys for metabolism or excretion.

3. Avoid meperidine and morphine because metabolites accumulate.

E. Inhalational agents

1. Advantages

a. Inhalational agents are minimally dependent on the kidneys for their excretion. They also control hypertension and allow a higher F_{IO_2} and lower muscle relaxant dosage.

2. Disadvantages

a. All decrease renal blood flow. Maintenance of systemic blood pressure and preoperative hydration lessen the effect on renal function.

b. A theoretic concern regarding the nephrotoxicity of enflurane (inorganic F^-) or sevoflurane (inorganic F^- and compound A) in patients with renal dysfunction exists.

F. Muscle relaxants

1. For patients who are at significant risk for regurgitation and whose recent serum potassium is in the normal range (<5 mEq/L), the use of succinylcholine, with its rapid onset of action, is justified. The duration of a bolus dose is

not significantly prolonged. Succinylcholine normally increases the serum K^+ by 0.5 to 0.7 mEq/L after a single bolus dose.

2. Atracurium, mivacurium, and cisatracurium rely least on renal excretion, and their actions are minimally affected by renal disease.
3. Rocuronium and vecuronium rely 20% to 30% on renal excretion, and their durations are slightly to moderately prolonged in the CRF patient. Pancuronium is approximately 40% excreted unchanged by the kidney, and prolonged effects are observed with renal disease.
4. Patients are often given antibiotics in the perioperative period that enhance neuromuscular blockade. Hypercalcemia and hypermagnesemia also potentiate the muscle relaxation.
5. Because dosing requirements may vary, the use of a neuromuscular blockade monitor is recommended.
   G. Reversal agents
1. Cholinesterase inhibitors (pyridostigmine, edrophonium, neostigmine) rely on the kidneys for elimination, and their effects are prolonged with CRF.
2. The kidneys similarly eliminate the anticholinergic agents atropine and glycopyrrolate, and their effects are prolonged with CRF.
3. Because the two classes of drugs are used in concert for muscle relaxant reversal, dosage adjustment is not indicated.

XI. Volume Status and Fluid Administration

Preoperative evaluation of fluid status is essential. Children with renal disease are intolerant of rapid fluid shifts and cannot compensate for incorrect Na^+ and water administration. Fluid management must consider preoperative fluid status, basal fluid requirements, intraoperative losses, and fluid shifts associated with translocation into third-space compartments. Children with ESRD are likely to be at the extremes of fluid volume, either having recently undergone dialysis and being hypovolemic, or awaiting dialysis and being hypervolemic.
   A. Comparison of the present weight with the postdialysis "dry" weight helps to estimate the child's current fluid volume.
   B. It is important to determine the individual child's pattern of abnormal Na^+ and water excretion; this will influence perioperative fluid management and determine the selection of perioperative replacement fluids.

C. Proceed cautiously with fluid administration, and avoid overhydration and underhydration.

D. Ensure adequate blood volume for satisfactory blood pressure, adequate perfusion, and function of AV fistula or shunt. Avoid using potassium-containing solutions (e.g., lactated Ringer's solution).

  1. Insensible losses and maintenance fluids are commonly replaced with 5% dextrose and 0.45% sodium chloride. Urine output is replaced with IV fluid milliliter for milliliter.

  2. Small blood losses can be replaced with maintenance fluids.

  3. Significant blood losses can be replaced with packed, washed RBCs.

E. Antidiuretic hormone increases with surgical stimulation and may further impair the ability to excrete a water load or concentrate urine.

F. For major cases a central venous catheter or pulmonary artery catheter may help guide fluid management. Postoperative dialysis may be required.

ADDITIONAL READINGS

Andrew, M., & Brooker, L.A. (1996). Hemostatic complications in renal disorders of the young. *Pediatric Nephrology*, 10, 88–99.

Blowey, D.L., Shlomit, B.D., & Koren, G. (1995). Interactions of drugs with the developing kidney: pediatric nephrology. *Pediatric Clinics of North America*, December, 1415–1431.

Cramolini, G.M. (1993). Diseases of the renal system. In Katz, J., & Steward, D.J. (Eds.). *Anesthesia and uncommon pediatric diseases* (pp. 214–287). Philadelphia: W.B. Saunders.

Dabbagh, S., Ellis, D., & Gruskin, A.B. (1996). Regulation of fluids and electrolytes in infants and children. In Motoyama, E.K., & Davis, P.J. (Eds.). *Smith's anesthesia for infants and children* (pp. 105–132). St. Louis: Mosby.

Frink, E.J., Green, W.B., Brown, E.A., et al. (1996). Compound A concentrations during sevoflurane anesthesia in children. *Anesthesiology*, 84(3), 566–571.

Maxwell, L.G. (1997). Preoperative evaluation in children: preoperative evaluation in an era of cost containment. *Problems in Anesthesia*, 9(2), 235–240.

Milner, L.S., Al-Mugeiren, M., & Kaplan, B.S. (1992). Therapeutic agents and the kidney: pharmacokinetics and complications. In Yaffe, S.J., & Aranda, J.V. (Eds.). *Pediatric pharmacology* (pp. 510–523). Philadelphia: W.B. Saunders.

Other Conditions

V

20

Malignant Hyperthermia

Denise Martin-Sheridan, EdD, CRNA

I. Definition

A. Malignant hyperthermia (MH) is a hypermetabolic disorder of skeletal muscle and a rare, life-threatening, pharmacogenetic disease that may be triggered in susceptible individuals by commonly administered anesthetic agents.

B. If MH is not treated, the mortality is nearly 80%. Death ensues from cardiac arrest, brain damage, internal hemorrhaging, or failure of other body systems.

C. Although MH events may occur at any age, 53% of cases reported to the Malignant Hyperthermia Association of the United States (MHAUS) were 15 years old or younger. MH occurs in approximately 1 in 15,000 anesthetics in children.

II. Pathophysiology

A. MH is a genetic disorder of skeletal muscle that may go undetected in the absence of triggering agents.

B. When susceptible individuals are exposed to triggering agents, a receptor (ryanodine receptor) mediated release of calcium from the sarcoplasmic reticulum occurs.

C. The elevation in myoplasmic calcium activates the troponin/tropomyosin complex associated with actin and allows the interaction of actin and myosin, an essential step in producing skeletal muscle contraction.

D. Increase in myoplasmic calcium is thought to be the result of a defect in the intracellular calcium–regulating processes or a defect in the permeability of the sarcolemma.

E. Associated disorders include Duchenne's or Becker's muscular dystrophy, central core disease, King-Denbrough syndrome, myotonia congenita, and myoadenylate deaminase deficiency.

III. Diagnostic Testing

A. Testing is recommended for susceptible individuals who have suspicious MH episodes, relatives (first line) of a family member who has a documented episode, and individuals with risk factors.

   B. Halothane-caffeine muscle contracture test.
      1. Muscle biopsy is performed, and the specimen is tested for a contracture response to halothane and caffeine.
      2. MH-positive muscle will develop a contracture at a lower concentration than normal.
      3. A limited number of centers are available for testing.

IV. Anesthetic Agents

   A. The commonly administered anesthetic agents have been identified as triggering and nontriggering agents for MH and are listed in Table 20–1.

V. Manifestations

   A. Manifestations of the syndrome may vary widely across the population of susceptible individuals.
   B. Since MH is an inherited disorder, prior history of a family member who has experienced an anesthetic death should place the patient at high risk.

TABLE 20–1. Anesthetic Agents

TRIGGERING AGENTS
Inhalation anesthetics
  Halothane
  Isoflurane
  Desflurane
  Enflurane
  Sevoflurane
Depolarizing muscle relaxants: succinylcholine

NONTRIGGERING AGENTS
Local anesthetics, both amides and esters
Nitrous oxide
Barbiturates
Opioids
Ketamine
Etomidate
Propofol
Nondepolarizing muscle relaxants
Cholinesterase inhibitors (neostigmine, edrophonium, pyridostigmine)
Anticholinergic agents (atropine, glycopyrolate)
Antidysrhythmic agents (calcium channel blockers should be avoided in the event dantrolene administration is required)

TABLE 20–2. Clinical Manifestations of Malignant Hyperthermia

EARLY SIGNS
Unexplained tachycardia
Hypertension
Tachypnea
Rapid increase in end-tidal carbon dioxide level
Prolonged masseter muscle rigidity

LATER SIGNS
Decreased oxygen saturation
Rapidly developing fever
Dysrhythmias
Increased muscle tone
Metabolic and respiratory acidosis
Hyperkalemia, hypercalcemia, lactacidemia
Myoglobinemia
Mottling of the skin
Disseminated intravascular coagulation (DIC)
Myoglobinuric renal failure

    C. Classic signs of the MH syndrome are a hypermetabolic state characterized by hypercarbia, skeletal muscle rigidity, and hyperthermia.
    D. Symptoms of MH are listed in Table 20–2.
    E. The early symptoms may be attributed to insufficient levels of anesthesia.

VI. Preparation for the Known or Suspected MH Patient

The best method to manage the known or suspected MH-susceptible patient is to develop a departmental plan or protocol before the situation arises. Most anesthesia departments have an MH cart with all necessary supplies and drugs readily available. Ready access to the items listed under treatment is critical to successful patient outcome. MHAUS recommends that 36 vials of dantrolene be stocked in a readily accessible area. Dantrolene has a shelf life of 3 years from the date of manufacturing and costs approximately $50.00 per vial.

    A. Anesthesia equipment
        1. If possible, a "clean" anesthesia machine with vaporizers removed should be available for use in case an MH event occurs. If vaporizers are not removed, they should be drained and disconnected.
        2. If a clean machine is not practical, drain vaporizers and flow O_2, 10 L/min, through the circuit for a minimum of 20 minutes before use.

   3. All circuits should be changed to disposable hoses, including those to the machine ventilator.

B. Cooling equipment
1. A cooling blanket should be placed on the table.
2. Ice and cold intravenous (IV) solutions should be readily available if needed.

C. Drugs
1. An adequate supply of dantrolene sodium (Dantrium) must be available. Dantrolene is supplied in a vial containing 20 mg of dantrolene and 3 g of mannitol. Each vial must be mixed with 60 ml of sterile distilled water.
2. Since dantrolene may be stocked and go unused for long periods, vials must be checked for expiration date on a regular basis.

D. Anesthetic technique
1. Avoidance of triggering agents is essential.
2. General or regional anesthetic techniques may be used.
3. Some providers prefer spinal, epidural, regional, or local anesthetic technique whenever possible.
4. Avoid administration of agents that may produce similar symptoms to MH:
  a. Atropine can cause fever or flushing.
  b. Butyrophenones and phenothiazines can cause neuroleptic malignant syndrome.
5. The routine prophylactic administration of dantrolene is controversial.
6. Postoperative management.
  a. If the anesthetic course is uneventful, observe the patient for 2 to 4 hours postoperatively.
  b. If the patient is to be discharged on the same day, observe him or her for a minimum of 4 hours postoperatively.
  c. If an MH event occurs, follow guidelines listed in the next section.

VII. Treatment

When an MH event is suspected during the course of an anesthetic, the following actions should be taken:

A. Call for assistance. It is essential to have additional help available to assist with mixing the dantrolene (20 mg in 60 ml of sterile distilled water) and the other tasks for successful treatment. Have MH cart brought into the room.
B. Notify all persons involved in patient care management. If possible, contact the MH Hotline at 1-800-644-9737 for consultation.

C. Discontinue administration of volatile inhalation anesthetics.

D. Discontinue succinylcholine.

E. Secure the airway with an endotracheal tube. Hyperventilate patient with 100% oxygen at a flow of ≥10 L/min.

F. Administer IV dantrolene sodium, 2.5 mg/kg, rapidly; repeat up to 10 mg/kg bolus until signs of MH have abated.

G. Monitor temperature, electrocardiogram (ECG), oxygen saturation, end-tidal carbon dioxide, arterial blood gas (ABG) values, and urine output.

H. Consider invasive monitors as indicated by the patient's condition. A central venous or pulmonary artery catheter can be used for monitoring and mixed venous blood gas determinations. An arterial line is inserted for blood pressure monitoring and serial laboratory determinations.

I. Monitor ABG values, and treat metabolic acidosis with bicarbonate (1–2 mEq/kg increments as indicated by ABG values).

J. Take steps to cool the hyperthermic patient. This includes lavage of the stomach, bladder, rectum, and open cavities with cold saline. Use ice and a cooling blanket to surface cool.

K. Treat hyperkalemia with hyperventilation, bicarbonate, IV glucose (50 ml of 50%), insulin (10 units), and calcium.

L. Treat dysrhythmias with standard antidysrhythmic agents, avoiding administration of calcium channel blockers.

M. Promote urine output of greater than 2 ml/kg/h. This may be accomplished with administration of IV fluids, furosemide (Lasix, a loop diuretic, 1 mg/kg for four doses), and mannitol (an osmotic diuretic).

N. Monitor serial laboratory work to evaluate coagulation profile, electrolytes, oxygenation, and carbon dioxide.

O. Creatine kinase (CK) elevations may not occur until 6 to 10 hours after the acute onset of MH.

P. Myoglobinuria usually occurs within 4 hours of the acute MH episode.

Q. Complete the form for reporting an MH episode to the North American MH Registry. (This form is available from MHAUS.)

VIII. Post-MH Treatment

A. The MH event can recur without reexposure to a triggering agent. Patients should be managed in an intensive care unit (ICU) or comparable setting for a minimum of 24 hours so that immediate treatment may be instituted if required.

B. Administer dantrolene IV, 1 to 2 mg/kg every 4 to 6 hours for 24 to 36 hours followed by a course of oral therapy, 4 mg/kg for 7 days.

C. Serial laboratory work is monitored to evaluate coagulation profile, electrolytes, oxygenation, carbon dioxide elimination, CK, and urine for myoglobin.

D. Close monitoring of body and core temperature as well as all other organ systems is essential. Disseminated intravascular coagulation (DIC) and myoglobinuric renal failure are complications associated with an acute MH episode.

E. Family counseling and referral services are available through the Malignant Hyperthermia Association at 32 S. Main Street, P.O. Box 1069, Sherburne, NY 13825. The phone number is 1-800-MHHyper.

ADDITIONAL READINGS

Karlet, C.K. (1997). Musculoskeletal pathophysiology and anesthesia. In Nagelhout, J.J., & Zaglaniczny, K.L. (Eds.). *Nurse anesthesia* (pp. 955–968). Philadelphia: W.B. Saunders.

Malignant Hyperthermia Association of the United States. (1997). *Clinical update 1997/98: Managing malignant hyperthermia.* Sherburne, NY: The Association.

Malignant Hyperthermia Association of the United States. (1997). *Preventing malignant hyperthermia, an anesthesia protocol.* Sherburne, NY: The Association.

Rosenberg, H., Fletcher, J.E., & Seitman, D. (1997). Pharmacogenetics. In Barash, P.G., Cullen, B.F., & Stoelting, R.K. (Eds.). *Clinical anesthesia* (3rd ed., pp. 489–517). Philadelphia: Lippincott-Raven.

21

Anesthetic Management of the Pediatric Burn Patient

Cormac T. O'Sullivan, MSN, CRNA

I. Introduction

A. Thermal injury results in the hospitalization of more than 25,000 pediatric patients per year.

B. Toddlers present with scald burns from contact with hot fluids, whereas older children present with flame burns from playing with matches.

C. Toddlers' burns involve the chest (43%), arms (34%), legs (28%), and face (27%). Flame burns can occur anywhere on the older child.

D. Child abuse, sunburn, electricity, chemicals, radiation, and frostbite are other causes of thermal injury in children.

E. Competent anesthesia care for the pediatric burn patient requires an appreciation of physiologic and pharmacologic alterations and a working knowledge of the physiologic differences of the pediatric patient.

II. Physiologic Changes in Burn Injury

A. Altered pulmonary function
 1. Burn injuries produce direct or indirect airway damage.
 2. Direct injury results from the inhalation of hot gases, steam, or other by-products of combustion.
  a. The inhalation of these materials produces direct tissue damage as the upper airways attempt to cool these gases by absorbing their heat before they reach the lower airways.
  b. Extensive tissue edema and destruction compromise upper airway patency, necessitating emergency airway management.
 3. Indirect injury results from inhaling cooler but noxious by-product gases of combustion and carbon monoxide (see Table 21-1).
 4. Circumferential burns of the chest or abdomen will produce a tourniquet effect, reducing thoracic compliance

316 PART V *Other Conditions*

TABLE 21–1. Toxic By-products of Combustion Commonly Produced During Home and Automobile Fires

Sulfur or nitrous oxides + lung H_2O	Corrosive acids
Burning wood ⟶	CO
Cotton or plastics combustion ⟶	Aldehydes causing protein denaturation and cellular damage
Polyvinylchloride ⟶	Chlorine and HCl released
Polyethylene ⟶	Hydrocarbons, ketones, and other acids
Polyurethane ⟶	Cyanide gas

From Lieh-Lai, M., & Rotta, M. (1995). Smoke inhalation and surface burns. In Lieh-Lai, M, Asi-Bautista, M., & Ling-McGeorge, K. (Eds). *The pediatric acute care handbook* (p. 190). Boston: Little, Brown, & Co. With permission.

with reductions in functional residual capacity (FRC) and minute ventilation and consequent ventilation-perfusion mismatch, hypoxemia, and hypercarbia.
  5. Massive volume fluid resuscitation may produce secondary respiratory distress syndrome (RDS).
  6. Pneumonitis and tracheal stenosis may follow prolonged endotracheal intubation.
 B. Altered cardiovascular function
  1. Cardiac output is dramatically reduced following the initial injury after the loss of circulating volume and tissue extravasation.
  2. Cardiac output may be compromised by decreased venous return produced by a tourniquet effect of circumferential burns of the chest and abdomen.
  3. Direct myocardial depression results from the release of endotoxins from burned tissue despite appropriate central venous pressure (CVP) readings.
  4. Increased cardiac output (three to five times normal) secondary to a hypermetabolic state follows the initial burn injury beginning 3 to 5 days after injury and continuing for weeks or months.
  5. Concurrent injuries, underlying pathologic conditions, and gram-negative sepsis contribute to reduced cardiac output and complicate management.
  6. Organ perfusion depends on satisfactory fluid resuscitation and may be guided by CVP monitoring.
 C. Altered renal function
  1. Decreased glomerular filtration rate (GFR) secondary to hypovolemia and hypotension, myoglobinuria (electrical

burn), and hemoglobinuria after large body surface area burns predispose to renal insufficiency and failure.

2. Increased GFR secondary to an increased cardiac output begins in 3 to 5 days, producing postburn diuresis.
3. Burns in excess of 40% produce renal tubular dysfunction.
4. Burn patients may not respond to antidiuretic hormone and aldosterone.
5. Accordingly, adequate hydration may not be inferred from urine output.
6. Hypertension can occur secondary to increases in renin or catecholamines.

D. Altered hepatic function
1. Hepatic injury follows hypoxemia and hypotension secondary to hypovolemia and decreased cardiac output during early burn management.
2. Injury may also occur from inhaled or absorbed toxins from the burn injury or from drug toxicity during treatment of infections and complications associated with the injury.
3. Hepatitis and other blood-borne diseases may be transmitted via blood and blood product transfusions received during the initial injury and many debridement and reconstructive surgeries.
4. Drug toxicity is more likely once cardiac output increases and more drugs are delivered to the liver for detoxification.
5. Enzyme induction from multiple drugs affects metabolism, as does liver blood flow, size of the burn, and time since the injury (see section on pharmacologic changes).

E. Altered neurologic function
1. Initial fluid resuscitation may produce cerebral edema or increased intracranial pressure (ICP) and should be treated with elevation of the head 30 degrees, hyperventilation, and intravenous (IV) mannitol.
2. Encephalopathy, seizures, hallucinations, and coma may follow.

F. Altered hematologic function
1. Blood viscosity increases because of initial fluid losses resulting in elevated hemoglobin and hematocrit values from hemoconcentration.
2. Fluid resuscitation lowers hemoglobin and hematocrit concentrations and further decreases plasma concentrations of coagulation factors and plasma proteins.
3. Initial thrombocytopenia results from platelet aggregation and trapping of platelets in the lungs.

4. Platelet counts increase for 10 to 14 days after injury and remain elevated for the long term.

5. Persistent hemolytic anemia suggests the hematopoietic system is adversely affected by burn injury. A sepsis work-up for unexplained thrombocytopenia is recommended.

G. Altered gastrointestinal and metabolic function

1. Gastric and intestinal ileus results in decreased gastrointestinal function for 48 to 72 hours after burn injury and requires appropriate venting to avoid pulmonary aspiration of gastric contents.

2. Early enteral feeding provides needed resuscitation calories, attenuates the hypermetabolic response, prevents gluconeogenesis, and may decrease the development of stress (Curling) ulcers.

3. Current recommendations for treatment of stress ulcers include H_2 receptor antagonists, antacids, and frequent oral feedings. Parenteral feedings are necessary if enteral feedings are not tolerated.

4. Hyperalimentation may alter metabolism, oxygen consumption, and carbon dioxide production, necessitating adjustments in ventilation in children mechanically ventilated.

5. Fluid and electrolyte status should be monitored frequently and adjustments in parental formulas made.

6. Plasma glucose must be closely monitored during the administration of and following the abrupt discontinuation of hyperalimentation solutions.

H. Altered integumentary function

1. Large body surface burns destroy the ability to thermoregulate, maintain fluid and electrolyte homeostasis, and fight infection.

2. Children have greater body surface area/weight ratios than adults (see Figure 21–1 and Table 21–2) so these effects are magnified.

3. Methods to keep the child's core temperature at an appropriate level and minimize heat loss include
   a. Prewarmed operating room (as high as 85–90°F)
   b. Radiant warmer
   c. Forced air warmer
   d. Fluid warmers
   e. Active or passive respiratory humidifiers

4. Scar formation may restrict airway and IV access as treatment progresses.

5. Monitors may not function correctly on burned or grafted tissue.
   a. Disposable pulse oximetry probes may be applied to a

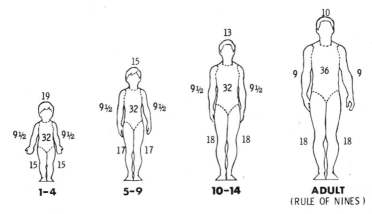

FIGURE 21–1. Alterations in body surface area percentages with age. (From Carvajal, H.J., & Goldman, A.S. [1975]. Burns. In Vaughn, V.C., III, McKay, R.J., & Nelson, W.E. [Eds.]. *Nelson's textbook of pediatrics* [p. 281]. Philadelphia: W.B. Saunders.)

nonburned pulsatile bed (finger, toes, ear lobe), or a reflectance pulse oximetry probe may be applied to the forehead or bridge of the nose.

    b. Extensive burns may prohibit the use of gelled electrocardiogram (ECG) electrodes. Subcutaneously placed needles may be substituted.

6. Table 21–3 summarizes physiologic changes associated with burn injuries.

III. Pharmacologic Changes in Burn Injury

A. General principles

1. Burn injury produces acute and chronic alterations in fluid and electrolyte homeostasis and multiple organ physiologic changes that alter drug pharmacokinetics.

2. Acutely, burn injury causes *a decrease in circulating albumin*, increasing the plasma free fraction of protein-bound drugs, such as benzodiazepines and barbiturates.

3. There is *an increase in alpha$_1$-acid glycoprotein (AAG)* that results in a decrease in the plasma free fraction of drugs such as analgesics and nondepolarizing muscle relaxants that bind to these proteins.

4. Volume of distribution, plasma clearance, and free fraction are all dynamic in the burn patient, producing unpredictable pharmacologic responses.

5. Judicious administration and close observation are war-

TABLE 21-2. Lund and Browder Chart Used at Baltimore Regional Burn Center to Calculate the Extent of Injury

Area	Percent of Burn					Severity of Burn		Total Percent
	0–1 Year	1–4 Years	5–9 Years	10–15 Years	Adult	2°	3°	
Head	19	17	13	10	7			
Neck	2	2	2	2	2			
Ant. Trunk	13	17	13	13	13			
Post. Trunk	13	13	13	13	13			
R. Buttock	2½	2½	2½	2½	2½			
L. Buttock	2½	2½	2½	2½	2½			
Genitalia	1	1	1	1	1			
R.U. Arm	4	4	4	4	4			
L.U. Arm	4	4	4	4	4			
R.L. Arm	3	3	3	3	3			
L.L. Arm	3	3	3	3	3			
R. Hand	2½	2½	2½	2½	2½			
L. Hand	2½	2½	2½	2½	2½			
R. Thigh	5½	6½	8½	8½	9½			
L. Thigh	5½	6½	8½	8½	9½			
R. Leg	5	5	5½	6	7			
L. Leg	5	5	5½	6	7			
R. Foot	3½	3½	3½	3½	3½			
L. Foot	3½	3½	3½	3½	3½			
					Total			

From Pearson, K.S., & Furman, W.R. (1998). Anesthesia for patients with major burns. In Longnecker, D.E., Tinker, J.H., & Morgan, G.E., Jr. (Eds.). *Principles and practice of anesthesiology* (2nd ed., p. 2167). St. Louis: Mosby.

TABLE 21–3. A Summary of the Systemic Effect of Burn Injury During Acute and Latent Phases of Treatment

System	Early	Late
Cardiovascular	↓ CO caused by decreased circulating blood volume, myocardial depressant factor	↑ CO caused by sepsis ↑ CO 2–3 times over baseline for months (hypermetabolism) Hypertension
Pulmonary	Upper airway obstruction caused by edema Lower airway obstruction caused by edema, bronchospasm, particulate matter ↓ FRC ↓ Pulmonary compliance ↓ Chest wall compliance	Bronchopneumonia Tracheal stenosis ↓ Chest wall compliance
Renal	↓ GFR secondary to 1. ↓ Circulating blood volume 2. Myoglobinuria 3. Hemoglobinuria Tubular dysfunction	↑ GFR secondary to ↑ CO Tubular dysfunction
Hepatic	↓ Function caused by ↓ circulating blood volume, hypoxia, hepatotoxins	Hepatitis ↑ Function caused by hypermetabolism, enzyme induction, ↑ CO ↓ Function caused by sepsis/drug interaction
Hematopoietic	↓ Platelets ↑ Fibrin split products, consumptive coagulopathy, anemia	↑ Platelets ↑ Clotting factors Possible AIDS, hepatitis
Neurologic	Encephalopathy Seizures ↑ ICP	Encephalopathy Seizures ICU psychosis
Skin	↑ Heat, fluid, electrolyte loss	Contractures, scar formation
Metabolic	↓ Ionized calcium	↑ Oxygen consumption ↑ Carbon dioxide production ↓ Ionized calcium

Table continued on following page

TABLE 21–3. A Summary of the Systemic Effect of Burn Injury During Acute and Latent Phases of Treatment
Continued

System	Early	Late
Pharmacokinetics	Altered volume of distribution Altered protein binding Altered pharmacokinetics Altered pharmacodynamics	↑ Tolerance to narcotics, sedatives Enzyme induction, altered receptors Drug interaction

↓, Decrease in; ↑, increase in; *AIDS,* acquired immunodeficiency syndrome; *CO,* cardiac output; *FRC,* functional residual capacity; *GFR,* glomerular rate; *ICP,* intracranial pressure; *ICU,* intensive care unit.

From Szyfelbein, S.K., Martyn, J.A.J., & Coté, C.J. (1993). Burn injuries. In Coté, C.J., Ryan, J.F., Todres, I.D., & Goudsouzian, N.G. (Eds.). *A practice of anesthesia for infants and children* (2nd ed. p. 367). Philadelphia: W.B. Saunders.

ranted. Alterations of drug dosages depend on the fluid status, metabolic state, and myocardial, renal, and hepatic function.

B. Opioid and nonopioid analgesics
1. Pain control is paramount for the burned child.
2. Multiple pharmacokinetic and pharmacodynamic factors are responsible for alterations in analgesic effects.
3. The burned child will exhibit tolerance to opioids and require increased dosages as treatment progresses.
4. Adjunctive agents, such as the benzodiazepines, are suggested to assist with anxiolysis and achieve synergy with the analgesics administered.
5. A baseline infusion of a long-acting opioid (morphine, methadone) or oral morphine sulfate (MS Contin) and supplemental oral acetaminophen may provide steady effective plasma concentrations. The plasma half-life of morphine in the burned child is less than one third of the half-life in a similar child without burn injury.
6. As treatment progresses the child will undergo less painful procedures and opioid needs will decrease.

C. IV induction agents
1. The choice of induction agent for the burned child does not matter as much as the dose of agent given.
2. Drug free fraction is increased secondary to decreased albumin levels.
3. Increased circulating fluid volume following fluid resusci-

tation may dilute the administered dose so as to decrease the concentration at the receptor site.

4. The induction dose of sodium pentothal in the *normovolemic* burned child is 7 or 8 mg/kg and remains elevated for 1 year after injury.

5. Propofol as well as etomidate is appropriate, keeping in mind the need for careful titration to effect.

6. Ketamine is a popular choice of some practitioners because it possesses cardiac stimulating properties, provides intense postoperative analgesia, and can be administered intramuscularly. Disadvantages of ketamine include a rapid tolerance, increased salivation, and emergence hallucinations.

D. Skeletal muscle relaxants

1. Depolarizing muscle relaxants
    a. Succinylcholine must not be used in a burn patient from 24 hours after injury until 2 years after injury.
    b. The depolarizing action produces hyperkalemia, which may lead to cardiac arrest.
    c. Contemporary nondepolarizing agents are available for the rapid securing of the airway, negating the required use of succinylcholine.

2. Nondepolarizing muscle relaxants (NDMRs)
    a. Burn patients require increased doses of NDMRs to achieve appropriate receptor site concentrations to produce blockade because of increased AAG proteins.
    b. The dose of NDMR necessary to achieve blockade is two to five times the dose needed in nonburn patients when the burn is greater than 20% of body surface area.
    c. With the increased potential for renal failure in these patients, NDMRs such as atracurium or cis-atracurium that do not undergo renal metabolism should be considered.
    d. Some practitioners advocate the use of rapidly acting NDMRs for rapid sequence intubations. However, the increased dose of NDMR agent required to achieve ideal intubating conditions in 1 minute results in a very prolonged duration of muscle relaxation and may lead to complications if the airway cannot be secured.

E. Anxiolytics

1. Benzodiazepines have an important role in the treatment of burn patients purely as anxiolytics and because of the synergy they produce when administered with opioids.

2. The free fraction of active drug at the receptor site is increased secondary to decreased plasma albumin.

3. Diazepam, which undergoes significant phase I hepatic metabolism, will have an increased duration of action, whereas lorazepam, which is metabolized during phase II reactions, shows increased clearance and therefore shorter duration of action.

F. Exogenous catecholamines

1. Epinephrine or phenylephrine (Neo-Synephrine) soaked gauze sponges are used to cover debridement and graft harvest sites to produce vasoconstriction and reduce blood loss. Epinephrine may be absorbed with this application.

2. Dysrhythmias are uncommon with use of epinephrine, but elevated blood pressure may be seen with both epinephrine and phenylephrine absorption.

3. This falsely elevated blood pressure may lead the anesthetist to underestimate the blood loss and result in serious hypotension when the effect of the catecholamines dissipates.

G. Antibacterials

1. Classification.
   a. Beta-lactams: aztreonam, ceftazidime, imipenem, piperacillin, ticarcillin
   b. Aminoglycosides: amikacin, gentamicin, tobramycin
   c. Quinolones: ciprofloxacin, enoxacin
   d. Glycopeptides: vancomycin, teicoplanin

2. Drug clearance of these antibacterials is renal dependent.

3. The aminoglycosides in particular are very nephrotoxic and may impact the choice of anesthetic agents.

H. Stress ulcer prophylaxis

1. Burn patients are at risk for the development of stress ulcers.

2. Pharmacologic prophylaxis may include H_2-receptor antagonists, such as cimetidine, ranitidine, famotidine, or nizatidine.
   a. Cimetidine inhibits the cytochrome P450–catalyzed oxidative drug metabolism pathway and reduces hepatic blood flow.
   b. This may lead to increased pharmacologic effects of drugs that depend on this pathway for metabolism, such as warfarin, phenytoin, metoprolol, labetalol, quinidine, caffeine, lidocaine, theophylline, alprazolam, diazepam, triazolam, flurazepam, chlordiazepoxide, carbamazepine, ethanol, tricyclic antidepressants, metronidazole, calcium channel blockers, and sulfonylureas.

IV. Initial Stabilization and Resuscitation: The First 24 Hours After Burn

A. Initial management and stabilization of the burned child focus on Airway management, maintenance of Breathing, and establishment of IV access to allow fluid resuscitation and ensure Circulation

B. Information about the burn scene will suggest evaluation for injuries not yet discovered. This is especially important in the pediatric patient who may be scared and unwilling to talk to health care providers

C. Airway management and maintenance of breathing

1. Airway management must begin with careful assessment and inspection of the oropharyngeal and nasopharyngeal cavities.

2. Perioral burns, sooty or carbonaceous sputum, or history of fire in an enclosed space should alert the anesthetist to the possibility of airway compromise from swelling and edema as resuscitation proceeds.

3. Signs and symptoms of impending airway collapse include coughing, wheezing, tachypnea, dyspnea, hypoxia, hypercarbia, rales, and rhonchi.

4. Endotracheal intubation is a necessity in children with upper airway burns.

5. Delay in airway management may lead to total airway obstruction and the need for emergent tracheostomy.

6. Mortality approaches 100% in pediatric burn patients receiving tracheostomies. Accordingly, tracheostomy is reserved for extreme situations when intubation is technically impossible.

7. Supplemental O_2 is administered to treat carbon monoxide (CO) poisoning.

   a. CO is produced during combustion of fuel particles and combines with hemoglobin with an affinity 250 times more readily than oxygen, producing tissue hypoxia and death.

   b. Carboxyhemoglobin (COHb) is interpreted as saturated hemoglobin by pulse oximetry and results in falsely elevated pulse oximetry (Sp_{O_2}) determinations.

   c. Small COHb levels shift the oxyhemoglobin dissociation curve to the left.

   d. COHb levels are determined via an arterial blood sample in the laboratory with a co-oximeter.

   e. In adults, the half-life of COHb when breathing room air is 4 hours but decreases to 1 hour when spontaneously breathing 100% O_2 and 30 minutes when mechanically ventilated with 100% O_2.

    f. Additional treatment of CoHb poisoning may include hyperbaric oxygenation to decrease CoHb binding from the cytochrome system.

  8. Supplemental oxygen therapy is recommended for all burn victims.

D. Fluid resuscitation

  1. Establishing adequate large-bore intravenous (IV) access is crucial to establish fluid resuscitation.

  2. Large volumes of crystalloid, colloid, and/or blood products are needed to maintain fluid homeostasis.

  3. IV access should be initiated in a noninjured extremity but can be placed through burned tissue if necessary.

  4. Predisposition to infection mandates strict aseptic technique during IV access.

  5. IV access should be avoided in circumferential extremity burns.

    a. With accumulated tissue edema a tourniquet effect will obstruct IV flow in that extremity.

    b. If this occurs, new access is needed because additional fluid in that extremity may lead to a compartment syndrome.

  6. Isotonic fluid resuscitation should begin with 20 ml/kg/h until replacement calculations can be completed.

  7. Fluid resuscitation is based on the amount of body surface burned and the severity of the burn.

  8. The two most widely used formulas for calculating fluid requirements are the Parkland Memorial Hospital and the Brooke Army Medical Center formulas (see Table 21–4). Both formulas are designed to deliver normal daily maintenance fluid requirements plus resuscitation fluid requirements.

  9. These formulas underestimate the fluid requirements for children weighing less than 10 kg; thus normal hourly fluid maintenance requirements should be added to the fluid volumes calculated from the Parkland or Brooke formulas for these children.

  10. Regardless of the formula used, one half the fluid calculated is infused over the first 8 hours after burn injury. The remaining half is infused over the next 16 hours followed by the administration of calculated maintenance fluids.

  11. All formulas are guidelines, and adjustments are made after evaluation of the child's physiologic response, as

TABLE 21–4. Three Commonly Accepted Formulas for Calculating Fluid Resuscitation Requirement for the Burn Patient

Formula	First 24 Hours	Second 24 Hours
BROOKE		
Crystalloid	2 ml lactated Ringer's per percent burn per kilogram of body weight Half in first 8 h Half in next 16 h	D_5W maintenance
Colloid	None	0.5 ml per percent burn per kilogram of body weight
PARKLAND		
Crystalloid	4 ml lactated Ringer's per percent burn per kilogram of body weight Half in first 8 h Half in next 16 h	D_5W maintenance
Colloid	None	0.5 ml per percent burn per kilogram of body weight
MGH		
Crystalloid	1.5 ml lactated Ringer's per percent burn per kilogram of body weight Half in first 8 h Half in next 16 h	Not specified
Colloid	0.5 ml per percent per kilogram of body weight None in first 4 h Half in second 4 h Half in next 16 h	Not specified

NOTE: For children weighing less than 10 kg, add hourly maintenance fluid calculated via the 4-2-1 rule to these burn fluid calculations.

From Pearson, K.S., & Furman, W.R. (1998). Anesthesia for patients with major burns. In Longnecker, D.E., Tinker, J.H., & Morgan, G.E., Jr. (Eds.). *Principles and practice of anesthesiology* (2nd ed., p. 2173). St. Louis: Mosby.

determined by hemodynamic monitoring and laboratory results.

12. Early colloid infusion reduces the amount of edema in nonburned tissue and maintains circulating blood volume more suitably than crystalloids.

13. However, long-term outcomes have not been shown to be affected significantly by choice of fluids administered.

14. Appropriate clinical end points during fluid resuscitation include normal values for heart rate for the age of the child, systolic blood pressure, CVP, arterial oxygenation, and pH. Urinary output should be at least 0.5 ml/kg/h.

E. Estimation of burn size in the pediatric patient
   1. The *rule of nines* estimates burn size in the adult patient but is not adequate for the pediatric patient because of differences in percentages of body surface area.
   2. The percentages of body surface area change throughout childhood until about 14 years of age when the rule of nines may be used. Figure 21–1 lists the estimation of the percentage of burns for pediatric and adult patients.

F. Management of other injuries
   1. Obtain as much information about the "accident" scene as possible, and assess for additional injuries.
   2. If the child is not responding to resuscitative efforts as expected, review the available information and reassess for additional injuries.
      a. Reassess A, B, C, D, and E of trauma management. (See Chapter 22.)
      b. Check for pneumothorax that occurred after establishing positive pressure ventilation.
      c. Exsanguination from a previously tamponaded bleeder is possible now that circulation is reestablished.

V. Latent Phase: Wound Debridement and Tissue Grafting (24 hours to 2 years)

A. Depending on the size of their burn, children will return to the operating room numerous times for debridement and tissue grafting. This may be as frequently as every other day for 2 to 3 weeks after burn injury

B. Airway management and maintenance of breathing
   1. Intubation may be complicated by oral or facial burns; by scar tissue around the airway or neck resulting in decreased range of motion; by airway edema from prior intubations and fluid resuscitation regimens; and occasionally by surgical implants such as tissue expanders in the head and neck region.
   2. Airway management should begin with a thorough assessment (see Chapter 6).
   3. If potential difficulties are predicted, awake fiberoptic intubation is the safest technique for securing the airway.
   4. Once the child is intubated, securing the endotracheal tube may require suturing or wiring depending on the site of

surgery, condition of the facial tissues, and surgeon and anesthetist preference.

5. Wire-reinforced endotracheal tubes should be available but may not be usable in the small child.

6. Multiple intubations over the course of treatment may lead to the development of subglottic stenosis, vocal cord granuloma, or polyp.

7. Recording the tube size, the presence of a cuffed endotracheal tube, and the amount of air required to produce minimal cuff pressure will guide successive anesthetic management.

8. Over time the child may require a smaller endotracheal tube and may need diagnostic bronchoscopy to evaluate the airway.

C. Fluid management during debridement procedures

1. Burn wound debridement consist of tangential and fascial excision.

2. Blood products must be available before incision.

3. Depending on the extent and degree of burn injury, blood transfusion initiated before incision may be appropriate since blood loss can exceed the child's blood volume.

4. Tangential excision consists of eschar removal in repeated layers (shaved off) until briskly bleeding tissue is reached. This style of excision and grafting can result in massive, rapid blood loss up to 4 ml/cm^2.

5. During fascial excision all tissue, including lymph vessels and the accompanying fat layer, is removed to the muscle fascia. The loss of all underlying tissue leads to a less cosmetically appealing result. Blood loss estimation is approximately 1.5 ml/cm^2.

6. Epinephrine or phenylephrine soaked gauze sponges are placed over the debrided areas.

   a. This reduces blood loss and allows local control of bleeding before graft placement.

   b. However, absorption of these catecholamines may lead to normotension in the face of hypovolemia until their effects wear off.

   c. Absorption of epinephrine may lead to increased incidence of dysrhythmias in children anesthetized with halothane.

7. Anesthetic management should include the following:

   a. Clear communication with the surgical team

   b. Anesthesia provider familiarity with burn excision procedures

   c. Possible need for early transfusion of blood products

     d. Liberal use of direct application of catecholamine soaked gauze sponges to debrided areas

     e. Agreement between the anesthetist and the surgical team as to predetermined stopping points in the surgical procedure

       (1) Excising no greater than 15% of body surface area per surgical procedure

       (2) Limiting excision time to less than 2 hours

       (3) Limiting excision to a 4-unit blood loss

8. Frequently monitored laboratory values are the best way to assess adequacy of oxygen carrying capacity. Serial arterial blood gases, hemoglobin, hematocrit, platelet count, coagulation profile, potassium, and ionized calcium levels should be checked frequently.

9. Large volumes of citrated blood products and/or IV calcium administration should be administered through peripheral IV lines to avoid high concentrations of citrate and calcium in the central circulation.

ADDITIONAL READINGS

Harris, M.M., & Berry, F.A. (1988). Pediatric trauma patients. In Grande, C.M. (Ed.). *Textbook of trauma anesthesia and critical care*. St. Louis: Mosby.

Jaehde, U., & Sorgel, F. (1995). Clinical pharmacokinetics in patients with burns. *Clinical Pharmacokinetics*, 29(1), 15–28.

Leih-Lai, M., & Rotta, M. (1995). Smoke inhalation and surface burns. In Leih-Lai, M., Asi-Bautista, M., & Ling-McGeorge, K. (Eds.). (1995). *The pediatric acute care handbook*. Boston: Little, Brown & Co.

Palmisano, B.W. (1994). Anesthesia for plastic surgery. In Gregory, G.A. (Ed.). *Pediatric anesthesia* (3rd ed.). New York: Churchill-Livingstone.

Pearson, K.S., & Furman, W.R. (1998). Anesthesia for patients with major burns. In Longnecker, D.E., Tinker, J.H., Morgan, G.E., Jr. (Eds.). *Principles and practice of anesthesiology* (2nd ed.). St. Louis: Mosby.

Sartain-Spivak, E. (1998). Anesthesia for the burn patient. In Nagelhout, J.J., & Zaglaniczny, K.L. (Eds.). *Nurse anesthesia*. Philadelphia: W.B. Saunders.

Szyfelbein, S.K., Martyn, J.A.J., & Cote, C.J. (1993). Burn injuries. In Cote, C.J., Ryan, J.F., Todres, I.D., & Goudsouzian, N.G. (Eds.). *A practice of anesthesia for infants and children* (2nd ed). Philadelphia: W.B. Saunders.

22

Pediatric Trauma

Karen Zaglaniczny, PhD, CRNA

I. Introduction

A. Trauma is the leading cause of death and disability in the pediatric population.

B. Motor vehicle accidents (MVAs) resulting in either pedestrian or passenger injuries are the most common cause of trauma.

C. The rise in violent crimes, especially for the adolescent population, has resulted in an increase in blunt and penetrating injuries.

D. Children are more likely to sustain multisystem injuries versus single organ damage.

E. Traumatic injuries are twice as common among males as females.

F. There are different patterns of injury for the different age-groups:
1. Toddlers and preschoolers: burns, drownings, falls, poisonings, and child abuse
2. School-age children: falls, MVAs, bicycle accidents
3. Adolescents: MVAs; bicycle, diving, and motorcycle accidents; gunshot wounds

G. Other factors associated with trauma include the environment, family influences, child abuse, and drug and alcohol abuse.

II. Initial Treatment

A. The initial care of the patient is organized systematically and is based on the pediatric advanced life support (PALS) and advanced trauma life support (ATLS) protocols.

B. Care of these patients is based on their anatomic and physiologic characteristics, which differ from adults' characteristics. Pediatric patients have a smaller body mass, a larger head size, abdominal organs that are closer to the surface, and a skeleton that is more flexible, which alters their patterns of injury (see Chapter 1).

C. The primary and secondary survey priorities of management follow the pneumonic *ABCDE:* *A*irway, *B*reathing, *C*irculation, *D*isability, and *E*nvironment.

1. Airway and breathing: Support oxygenation and ventilation.
   a. Children have a higher oxygen consumption and develop hypoxemia more rapidly than adults.
   b. Assess adequacy and quality of respiration.
   c. Administer oxygen therapy with humidification.
   d. Correct airway obstruction; if necessary, ventilate and intubate (see Chapter 6).

2. Circulation: Control bleeding; recognize and treat shock.
   a. It is essential to know the vital sign distribution for the various age ranges and what is the lowest acceptable level (70 mm Hg + 2 × child's age in years).
   b. Children maintain a normal blood pressure even with 25% to 30% blood loss. They compensate with an increase in heart rate and systemic vascular resistance. Tachycardia is the primary symptom associated with hypovolemia. When bradycardia develops, cardiac arrest is usually imminent.
   c. When the blood pressure does decrease, there is subsequent decompensation and cardiovascular collapse.
   d. Assessment of other clinical signs, such as skin color, peripheral perfusion, capillary refill, central and distal pulses, level of consciousness, activity level, and adequacy of urine output, facilitates diagnosis and treatment.
   e. Correction of hypovolemia is a priority of care and is guided by the patient history, clinical evidence of poor perfusion, tachycardia, and response to fluid challenge.
   f. Usually at least two intravenous (IV) sites are initiated. If there is difficulty in securing peripheral lines, the intraosseous route and central lines may be placed. The intraosseous route is recommended for children under 6 years of age in which peripheral access has not been established within 60 to 90 seconds.
   g. An initial bolus of 15 to 20 ml/kg of either lactated Ringer's or normal saline is administered and can be repeated up to four times.
   h. Physiologic parameters are reassessed, and if necessary blood therapy is initiated at 5 to 15 ml/kg.

      i. Monitor for the occurrence of hypoglycemia and hypocalcemia with acute volume loss.

      j. Although the usual response to trauma is hyperglycemia, hypoglycemia may occur as a result of higher metabolism and low glycogen stores. Glucose levels are monitored, and replacement therapy is administered as needed.

      k. Calcium levels are usually maintained; however, hypocalcemia may occur. Replace with calcium chloride (10%) or calcium gluconate (10%).

      l. Treatment with sodium bicarbonate is restricted to severe metabolic acidosis (pH <7.1).

      m. Resuscitation guidelines are listed in Appendix C.

3. Disability: Assess neurologic status, and perform neurologic examination.

      a. Head injury is more prevalent in pediatric patients and is associated with better outcomes than adults.

      b. The Glasgow Coma Scale, which accounts for the physiologic age responses in infants and toddlers, may be used (see Table 22–1).

      c. A quick assessment tool (AVPU) can also be used for level of consciousness: A: *a*lert and responsive; V: responds to *v*erbal stimuli; P: responds to *p*ainful stimuli; and U: *u*nresponsive.

      d. Examination of pupils (size, reactivity, and symmetry), eye movements, and reflexes is performed.

      e. Priorities are to control intracranial pressure (ICP), maintain adequate cerebral perfusion pressure (CPP), and prevent hypoxia.

      f. Therapy may include administration of steroids, hyperventilation, head elevation to 30 degrees, and ICP monitoring.

      g. Spinal cord injuries can occur without radiographic abnormality (SCIWORA). Young children are prone to high cervical spine (C1 to C2) injuries, whereas in adolescents lower cervical spine injuries are more common.

4. Exposure: Establish presence of visible injuries and prevent hypothermia.

      a. Complete examination (head to toe) is done to determine extent and severity of injuries.

      b. Pediatric patients are prone to hypothermia because of anatomic and physiologic differences. They have a larger body surface area in relation to their body mass

TABLE 22-1. Glasgow Coma Score for Infants and Children

EYE OPENING (E)

Opens spontaneously	4
Opens to voices	3
Opens to pain	2
None	1

BEST MOTOR RESPONSE (M)

Spontaneous (obeys verbal command)	6
Localizes pain	5
Withdraws from pain	4
Abnormal flexion to pain (decorticate posture)	3
Abnormal extension to pain (decerebrate posture)	2
No response	1

VERBAL RESPONSE (V)

Oriented or social smile; oriented to sound; follows objects; cooing; jargon; converses; interacts appropriately with environment	5
Confused/disoriented or consolable cries; aware of environment; uncooperative interactions	4
Inappropriate words or inappropriate persistent cries; moaning; inconsistently aware of environment/inconsistently consolable	3
Incomprehensible sounds or agitated; restless; inconsolable cries; unaware of environment	2
No response	1

E + M + V = COMA SCORE OF 3 TO 15

From Rubenstein, J.S., and Hageman, J.R. (1988). Monitoring of critically ill infants and children. *Critical Care Clinics,* 4(3), 634.

and less subcutaneous tissue for heat insulation. Hypothermia can attenuate successful resuscitation because of an increased oxygen demand and peripheral vasoconstriction.

c. Methods should be initiated early to attenuate hypothermia and include the use of overhead radiant lights, warming blankets, IV fluid and blood warmers, humidification of gases, and increasing the ambient temperature.

III. Trauma Scoring Score

Trauma scores are used to facilitate rapid assessment, triage, and prediction of outcome of the patient. The pediatric trauma score is listed in Table 22–2.

IV. Other Areas of Injury

A. Thoracic injuries
1. Thoracic injuries usually occur with blunt trauma and include pulmonary contusions, pneumothorax, and hemothorax.
2. In penetrating traumatic injuries single organ damage to the heart or lung may occur.

B. Abdominal injuries
1. The most frequent abdominal injuries involve the spleen and liver.
2. If the patient is stable, observation and nonsurgical treatment may be selected.

C. Extremity injuries
1. Closed or open extremity fractures may occur that can require surgical intervention.

D. Pelvic and genitourinary injuries
1. These injuries usually occur with multiple injuries and pelvic fractures.
2. Significant bleeding may be present that requires immediate resuscitation of the patient.

TABLE 22–2. Pediatric Trauma Score

Component	+2	+1	−1
Weight	>20 kg	10–20 kg	<10 kg
Airway	Normal	Maintainable Oxygen mask or nasal cannula	Unmaintainable Intubated
Systolic blood pressure	>90 mm Hg	50–90 mm Hg	<50 mm Hg
	Good peripheral pulses, perfusion	Carotid/femoral pulses palpable	Weak or no pulses
Consciousness	Awake	Obtunded or unconscious	Comatose Unresponsive
Skeletal injury	None	Single, closed fracture	Open or multiple fractures
Cutaneous injury	None	Contusion, abrasion	Major or penetrating
		Laceration <7 cm	Any gunshot wound or stab wound

Adapted from Tepas, J.J. III, Molitt, D.L., Talbert, J.L., et al. (1987). The pediatric trauma score as a predictor of injury severity in the injured child. *Journal of Pediatric Surgery*, 22, 15.

V. Preoperative Assessment

A. The condition of the patient and the urgency of the surgery may limit the time available for preoperative evaluation.

B. A rapid and complete evaluation of the patient and emergency department treatment is essential. Information can be obtained from the parents or family members, the chart, and other health care providers.

C. Pertinent details of the child's past health, medical, and surgical history; allergies; current medications; immunizations; time of last meal; and prior anesthetic experiences are included.

D. The pneumonic *AMPLE* can be used for quick assessment: *A*llergies, *M*edications, *P*ast medical and surgical history, *L*ast meal, and *E*vents leading to the injury.

E. The extent of injuries, degree of physiologic disturbance, and planned medical and surgical treatments are determined.

F. Communication of the proposed plan and informed consent are provided to the parents.

VI. Preparation

A. All necessary equipment and supplies must be available in the operating room with consideration of the variations in size requirements for the different ages of patients.

B. Appropriate airway supplies, fluid and blood warmers, warming blankets, monitoring equipment, and drug therapy are matched for the pediatric age-group of the patient.

C. Most institutions have pediatric carts readily available and stocked that can facilitate rapid setup and save valuable time.

D. The anesthesia machine, ventilator, cardiac monitor, pulse oximeter, capnograph, temperature monitor, noninvasive blood pressure machine, and suction are prepared for the pediatric patient.

E. Additional monitoring equipment for arterial and central venous pressures is readily available.

F. Drugs for induction and maintenance are drawn up and prepared.

G. Resuscitative drugs and equipment are immediately accessible.

VII. Monitoring

A. Standard monitoring equipment for blood pressure, heart rate and rhythm, temperature, carbon dioxide, and pulse

oximeter is applied as soon as the patient arrives in the operating room.
   B. Invasive monitoring of arterial and central venous pressures may be warranted and depends on the patient's condition.
   C. Arterial lines can be started with 22- or 24-gauge angiocaths (depending on patient's size and age) in the radial artery of the nondependent arm.
   D. Urine output is monitored through a Foley catheter.
   E. Serial laboratory value determinations are performed as indicated by the patient's condition.

VIII. Temperature Control
   A. Pediatric trauma patients can become hypothermic quickly as a result of exposure, cold operating rooms, and infusion of cold IV fluids and blood.
   B. Application of warming methods is essential to maintain or increase body temperature.

IX. Anesthetic Selection and Induction
   A. Selection of induction agents and techniques depends on the proposed procedure, hemodynamic status of the patient, and severity of injury.
   B. General anesthesia is most commonly selected although local and regional anesthesia techniques can be used for minor procedures.
   C. Critically injured patients will need immediate resuscitation with minimal anesthetic agents until hemodynamic stability is restored.
   D. Rapid sequence induction is advocated because all trauma patients have a "full stomach."
      1. Induction agents can include thiopental, ketamine, or propofol with consideration of the hemodynamic status, neurologic condition, and severity and location of the patient's injury.
      2. Muscle relaxants to facilitate tracheal intubation include either succinylcholine or rocuronium. Although other nondepolarizing agents may be used, their onset of action is not as rapid.
      3. The use of agents for aspiration prophylaxis is controversial for the various age-groups.

X. Maintenance
   A. Administration of anesthetic agents is based on the patient's condition. Patients who are hypotensive and hypovo-

lemic will require insignificant amounts of anesthesia until bleeding is controlled and hemodynamic stability is achieved.

1. Inhalation agents (sevoflurane, desflurane, isoflurane) can be administered in low concentration with observation of hemodynamic effects. These agents are easily titratable and provide rapid alterations in anesthetic depth.

2. Narcotic agents (fentanyl) and benzodiazepines (midazolam) can be administered in small incremental doses.

B. The patient's physiologic parameters and pattern and severity of injury guide fluid and blood therapy (see Chapter 7).

C. Other goals of optimal management include the correction of acid-base abnormalities, prevention and treatment of hypothermia, and implementation of resuscitation protocols as indicated.

D. Management of the emergence from anesthesia and extubation depends on the patient's condition, severity of injury, and type of surgical procedure.

1. Children who have sustained severe injuries, have undergone prolonged operating room procedures, or have unstable hemodynamic or neurologic parameters are ventilated and transported to the intensive care unit (ICU) or postanesthesia care unit (PACU).

2. Children who are stable can be extubated when awake with adequate return of their reflexes.

XI. Postoperative Care

A. Close monitoring and ongoing assessment of the patient continue in the PACU.

B. Adequate pain control is initially achieved through administration of IV medications.

C. Warming methods are continued in the PACU or ICU, usually through the use of a forced air warming blanket.

D. Emotional support and counseling may be necessary for the patient, parents, and other family members.

ADDITIONAL READINGS

Berman, J.M., & Grande, C.M. (Eds.). (1994). Pediatric trauma anesthesia. *International Anesthesiology Clinics, 32*(1).

Buttain, W.L. (Ed.). (1995). *Management of pediatric trauma.* Philadelphia: W.B. Saunders.

Kapklein, M.J., & Malhadeo, R. (1997). Pediatric trauma. *Mount Sinai Journal of Medicine, 64*(4–5), 302–310.

Nichols, K. (1996). Quick reference guide for pediatric trauma care. *International Journal of Trauma Nursing,* (2), 56–58.

Pascucci, R., & Walsh, J. (1991). Evaluation and management of the injured child. In Capan, L.M., Miller, S.M., & Turndorf, H. (Eds.). *Trauma anesthesia and intensive care* (pp. 567–598). Philadelphia: J.B. Lippincott.

23

Latex Allergy

Brent Sommer, CRNA, MPHA

I. Introduction

A. Etiology and background

1. Latex allergy is an immunologic reaction to natural rubber latex (NRL) processed from the *Hevea brasiliensis* tree indigenous to Central and South America.

2. Although definitive etiologic proof of latex allergy remains to be presented, most theories suggest that sensitization may occur from early, constant, or intense and repeated exposure to products containing rubber, such as through multiple surgeries, diagnostic procedures, and clinical examinations.

3. Increasing information regarding latex allergy has continued to be presented since the first reported case of an allergic reaction to rubber appeared in the medical literature in 1933. In 1979 the first reported immunoglobulin E (IgE) mediated reaction to a rubber product resulted in a documented urticarial response.

4. The lone definitive therapy to treat latex allergy is avoidance of such exposures, but this is difficult to ensure because of the ubiquity of latex in most medical environments.

B. Population at risk

1. Pediatric case reports of anaphylactic episodes attributable to latex continue to increase, and albeit rare, fatal outcomes have resulted. Latex covered or "dipped" enema tips have been responsible for the majority of reported fatalities.

2. Pediatric patients remain a significant high-risk population subject to latex allergy and require individual consideration and evaluation before care that involves exposure to latex.

3. Various populations are thought to possess distinct immune-specific properties that contribute to their particular response in both degree and incidence of exposure.

4. Pediatric patient populations sensitized to latex have exhibited a fourfold increase in histories of rhinoconjunc-

tivitis, asthma, or atopic eczema when compared to those who were not previously exposed.

5. Although adult populations reflect an increased incidence of latex allergy in females, the pediatric population continues to reflect a more even distribution relative to gender. Historically females have shown a greater incidence of perioperative anaphylaxis than males at a ratio of approximately 1.6:1.

C. Incidence

1. The incidence of latex allergy throughout the general population is estimated to be 2% to 6%, but certain pediatric populations may experience an incidence as high as 73% (spina bifida and related pathologic conditions).

2. The sudden appearance and recognition of latex allergy are attributable to the increased use of latex gloves by health care professionals to prevent the transmission of blood-borne pathogens.

   a. Latex can trigger respiratory symptoms when it becomes airborne, usually in cornstarch powder particles used to coat gloves that are then inhaled, or through contact with mucosal membranes.

   b. Clinical areas where powdered gloves are present in significant concentrations, such as operating rooms (ORs), have exhibited high levels of latex allergen because of this mode of exposure.

   c. Scientific investigation has proven that as the amount or concentration of substances that cause allergic reactions increases, sensitized persons experience reactions that increase proportionately. In addition, continued and repeated skin exposure to latex during the presence of dermatitis will increase the likelihood of a more serious preexisting allergic reaction.

   d. Recent studies have shown that powdered latex gloves produce atmospheric contamination with latex particles and may contribute to sensitization of health care providers as well as patients.

3. IgE from latex-sensitized individuals may react with various proteins other than latex; therefore antigens that are structurally related to latex may also be antigenic to the individual with IgE antibody to latex.

II. Clinical Presentation

A. An allergic reaction occurs when an antigen (foreign substance) is introduced and binds with an antibody. The immune system elicits a response that becomes excessive or inappropriate and is classified as varying degrees of hypersensitivity.

B. Anaphylactic (allergic) drug reactions are profound, immediate hypersensitivity reactions produced by an immunologic mechanism presenting clinically as urticaria, wheezing, dyspnea, syncope, and cardiovascular collapse. This immunologic reaction involves the interaction of antigens, antibodies, and a specific effector cell (usually mast cells and basophils) that is reproducible when the subject is again challenged with the specific antigen.

C. Type I reactions.
   1. Patients exhibit an immediate or IgE antibody–mediated allergic hypersensitivity. This is potentially the most serious form of allergic reaction.
   2. This type of reaction can result in a full spectrum of symptoms ranging from localized pruritus and urticaria to wheezing and cardiovascular collapse.
   3. In general, IgE mediates reactions in individuals who have had previous exposure to the foreign substance (i.e., latex).
   4. Conjunctivitis, sneezing, and rhinitis result from an aerosolized or more direct facial exposure and contact familiar to most as an initial allergic reaction.
   5. Those patients possessing a greater degree of sensitivity display a more dramatic systemic reaction, which can include bronchospasm, laryngospasm, and hypotension.
   6. A life-threatening reaction is seldom the first sign of latex allergy.
   7. The specific amount of exposure needed to initiate the sensitization or symptoms is unknown. Exposures that have occurred at very low levels have been shown to have triggered allergic reactions in some sensitized individuals.

D. Type IV reactions.
   1. Contact dermatitis (delayed hypersensitivity) is a poison ivy–like rash and is classified as a type IV sensitivity.
   2. Presentation begins 12 to 48 hours following contact with latex, and symptoms differ from those exhibited with type I reactions.
   3. Contact dermatitis is usually the result of sensitization by chemicals added during rubber processing and does not appear to be increasing in the latex allergic population.
   4. Skin lesions usually present as a patchy and diffuse skin

eczema and tend to be very irritating although not life threatening.

E. Recognition of allergic response to latex can initiate a reaction and intervention that can prevent a drastic outcome. Table 23–1 compares the most common signs and symptoms of allergic reactions to latex in both the *awake* patient and the *anesthetized* patient.

III. Diagnosis

A. A complete and thorough medical history remains the most reliable screening test to predict the likelihood of an anaphylactic reaction

B. Pediatric patients most likely to exhibit a sensitivity to latex that may result in varying degrees of reactivity include children with

   1. A known or suspected allergy to latex by having

TABLE 23–1. Signs and Symptoms of Allergic Reactions to Latex

Symptoms usually occur within 30 min following anesthesia induction; however, the actual onset can range from 10 to 290 min.

AWAKE PATIENT
Itchy eyes
Generalized pruritus
Shortness of breath
Feeling of faintness
Feeling of impending doom
Unexplained restlessness and crying
Agitation
Nausea
Vomiting
Abdominal cramping
Diarrhea
Wheezing

ANESTHETIZED PATIENT
Tachycardia
Hypotension
Wheezing
Bronchospasm
Cardiorespiratory arrest
Flushing
Facial edema
Laryngeal edema
Urticaria

exhibited an allergic or anaphylactic reaction, positive skin testing, or positive IgE antibodies against latex

2. A documented history of intraoperative anaphylaxis of unknown etiology
3. A history of neural tube defects
   a. Spina bifida
   b. Myelomeningocele or meningocele
   c. Lipomyelomeningocele
4. A history of multiple operations, particularly as a neonate
5. Chronic bladder catheterizations as a result of
   a. Spinal cord trauma
   b. Exstrophy of the bladder
   c. Neurogenic bladder
6. Some history of atopy and multiple allergies, including food products. Particular allergies to fruits and vegetables, including banana, avocado, celery, fig, chestnut, papaya, and passion fruit, are most significant
7. Children with a strong or confirmed allergy to bananas should be considered to be allergic to latex
8. Those who have experienced a high degree or repeated exposure to latex products are more likely to develop a latex allergy. These situations may include treatment that involved
   a. Repeat surgical procedures
   b. Surgical procedures involving mucosal membranes
   c. Repeated placement of ventriculoperitoneal shunts (i.e., cerebral palsy)
   d. Repeated or chronic intravenous (IV) and urinary catheterizations

C. Although information regarding these at-risk pediatric populations continues to proliferate, confirmatory data are necessary to establish a definite diagnosis. A strong suspicion should be elicited when a history reflects information described above. The exact amount or degree of latex exposure required to elicit an allergic reaction has not been determined. Efforts to reduce the amount of exposure to latex have been associated with an apparent decrease in both symptoms and sensitization exhibited following such exposures

D. Laboratory diagnosis
   1. Diagnosis of latex allergy is best accomplished by a complete and thorough medical history. Reliable information, including time and length of exposure to NRL products and related residue (i.e., gloves, powder), is

paramount to establishing a confirmatory diagnosis and correlation of latex sensitivity and allergy.

2. Clinically diagnostic confirmation of latex allergy can be established by blood tests available and approved for use by the U.S. Food and Drug Administration (FDA) that are capable of detecting latex antibodies.

3. Less reliable yet confirmatory diagnostic methods, including (a) standardized glove exposure use tests and (b) skin response to liquid latex proteins applied following an intentional skin prick or scratch exposure, further establish an allergy. A definitive skin testing system has not been approved yet because of varying degrees of reliability.

4. Radioallergosorbent (RAST) testing is designed to detect IgE antibodies but will not predict the chance or severity of a particular reaction. This test is easily accomplished and poses no immediate physiologic threat to the child.

5. A skin patch test that uses latex additives is available; however, it confirms a positive contact dermatitis to latex as opposed to an actual allergy. It is important that any confirmatory testing that equates latex sensitivity and allergy is conducted by experienced and qualified practi-

---

Pediatric Latex/Rubber Questionnaire

1. Does the child have asthma, hay fever, or eczema?
2. Does the child play with latex or rubber products, such as balloons, regularly?
3. Has the child ever had itching, swelling, hives, or a runny nose after playing with a balloon or rubber ball?
4. Has the child ever had hives, asthma, or shock following surgery?
5. Does the child have spina bifida, cerebral palsy, quadriplegia, or other congenital medical problems?
6. Has the child had any abdominal, genitourinary, or orthopedic surgeries or neurosurgical (shunt) procedures? How many?
7. Does the child itch, swell, or have trouble breathing after eating any of these foods: banana, kiwi, avocado, chestnut, papaya, hazelnut, sesame seeds, or other fruits and vegetables?

tioners because it may precipitate an anaphylactic reaction. More reliable and predictive laboratory testing to confirm latex allergy is forthcoming.

6. Each suspected case of latex allergy should be individually evaluated by experienced practitioners qualified to manage such situations. There remains no substitute for a complete and thorough medical history in establishing a positive latex allergy.

7. The box on page 345 gives a sample pediatric latex/rubber questionnaire to be completed by parents and children (when appropriate) to assist in establishing an allergic suspicion or confirmatory diagnosis. A positive response to any of these questions would warrant further investigation.

IV. Prevention

A. Preventive measures to avoid latex allergic responses require considerable efforts and resources using a multidisciplinary approach.

B. Initial efforts to identify an at-risk population include all infants and children that are characterized by identified categories and documented positive histories.

C. Once a child is thought to possess any degree of risk for latex sensitivity or allergy, systems operations should be initiated to protect that child throughout all aspects of care.

D. Home health agencies are rapidly establishing procedures and protocols to manage latex allergic patients both before and after their care in health care facilities such as hospitals and clinics.

V. Pretreatment

A. Debate regarding the efficacy and usefulness of premedication to treat patients with confirmed latex allergy remains controversial.

B. Individual consideration for each patient undergoing elective operation or diagnostic and therapeutic procedures requiring anesthesia services should be undertaken.

C. Premedication with steroids, antihistamines, and H_2 blockers before general anesthesia or deep sedation may be preferred for children with a known and documented latex allergy. These agents will not prevent an allergic reaction, but they may attenuate the severity of the reaction.

D. Medication regimens representative of several recom-

TABLE 23–2. Current Pretreatment Recommendations for Latex Allergy

---

1. No premedication is recommended for the neonate.
2. For a child 1–12 y of age:
Prednisone	1 mg/kg PO q6h	Maximum dose 40 mg
Hydroxyzine	0.7 mg/kg PO q6h	Maximum dose 50 mg
3. For a child >12 y of age:
Prednisone	1 mg/kg PO q6h	Maximum dose 40 mg
Loratadine	10 mg PO at bedtime the evening before the procedure	
4. For a child who is unable to take oral medications:
Methylprednisolone	1 mg/kg IV q6h	Maximum dose 60 mg
Hydrocortisone	4 mg/kg IV	
Diphenhydramine	1 mg/kg IV q6h	Maximum dose 50 mg
5. The following H_2 blockers may be added:
Ranitidine	2 mg/kg PO or 1 mg/kg IV q6h	Maximum dose 150 mg
Cimetidine	4 mg/kg PO or 2 mg/kg IV q6h	Maximum dose 300 mg
6. A modified approach would consist of one dose each H_2 blocker and corticosteroid 1 h before the procedure.
7. Postoperative pharmacologic management would ideally continue such protocols up to 12 h postoperatively.

---

mended approaches currently used by pediatric care institutions throughout the United States are listed in Table 23–2.

VI. Perioperative Management

A. The traditional perioperative environment contains a considerable degree of latex in furniture, equipment, and supplies.

B. Table 23–3 lists a variety of items that frequently contain latex or NRL polymers and are commonly found in the perioperative area.

C. Current thoughts and recommendations in managing patients with a known or suspected latex allergy have demanded considerable forethought, planning, and accommodation by the perioperative team members. The anesthetist must maintain a constant vigilance to recognize and treat the sudden and frequently unexpected latex allergy as well as accommodate patients with a suspected or known allergy.

TABLE 23–3. Common Latex Medical Devices Used in Perioperative Areas

Mattresses on stretchers
Rubber gloves
Adhesive tape (porous)
Urinary catheters and drainage systems
Electrode pads
Wound drains
Eye shields
Stomach and intestinal tubes
Chest tubes and drainage systems
Condom urinary collection devices
Protective sheets
Enema tubing kits
Dental dams
Surgical drapes
Instrument pads
IV solutions and tubing systems
Fluid circulating thermal blankets
Hemodialysis equipment
Ambu (bag-valve) masks
Medication syringes
Bulb syringes
Elastic bandages, wraps
Medication vial stoppers (multidose)
Stethoscope tubing
Band-Aids and other similar bandage products
Gloves, examination and sterile
Patient-controlled analgesia syringes
Tourniquets

D. Anesthesia equipment and products that contain latex are listed in Table 23–4.
E. Planning for the known latex allergic patient should begin with substitution of any product that is known to contain latex. If the provider is unsure regarding the latex content of a product, it should not be used. FDA standards to require explicit labeling of products regarding latex content are forthcoming.
F. An organized and clearly defined approach to treat each known latex allergy patient should become an institutional routine.
G. Primary providers (i.e., allergists, pediatricians) will routinely consult and provide specific patient-oriented recommendations. An established referral system and appropriate consultation and educational resources should be a depend-

able and integral piece of the institutional latex allergy management program.

VII. OR Preparation

A. A *latex-free* OR should be the responsibility of all persons involved in the patient's care, including the departments of anesthesia, surgery, nursing, and environmental services.

B. The following plan for OR preparation should be adopted:

1. Identify the case as "latex precautions" or "latex safe" at the time it is scheduled.
2. Communication is paramount to successful orchestration of these efforts.
3. Appropriate identification should be maintained throughout the hospitalization and perioperative period. Distinctive signs, labels, and identification (ID) bands that provide clear warning should be consistently utilized.
4. Continuous efforts to advertise and promote the prevention program are important.
5. All interactive departments should be notified of the

TABLE 23–4. Anesthesia Equipment and Products Containing Latex

Stethoscope tubing
Rubber masks
Electrode pads (e.g., electrocardiogram, peripheral nerve stimulator, contact pads)
Head straps
Rubber tourniquets, Esmarch bandages
Rubber oral or nasal pharyngeal airways
Teeth guards, eye shields, bite-blocks
Blood pressure cuffs (inner bladder and tubing)
Breathing circuits containing rubber
Reservoir breathing bags, disposable oxygen masks, nasal cannulae
Rubber ventilator hoses and bellows
Rubber endotracheal tubes
Latex cuffs on plastic endotracheal tubes
Latex injection ports on IV tubing, stopcocks
Certain epidural catheter injection adapters
Multidose vial stoppers
Patient-controlled analgesia syringes
Rubber suction catheters, specimen traps
IV solutions and tubing systems (injection ports)

planned procedure and respond according to institutional policy and procedure to best accommodate the patient throughout all phases of care.

6. Remove all latex products from the OR.
   a. Remove all stock items and latex examination and sterile gloves.
   b. Notify central supply and ancillary departments to ensure that articles containing latex are not included in sterile trays.
   c. Provide nonlatex alternatives for all participants to use.
7. Place "latex precautions" or "latex free" notices on doors of OR and recovery areas.
8. Use a latex-free cart if available.
9. Cover the band on the black reservoir bag of the anesthesia machine if it contains latex. Replace latex-containing ventilator bellows, or use a known latex-free machine and ventilator.
10. Use latex-free IV setup and delivery systems, invasive monitors, and so on.
11. Cover all rubber injection ports with tape. *Do not inject or withdraw fluid through any rubber ports.*
12. Use a disposable or any heating blanket that is not latex or rubber.
13. Have an emergency O_2 tank, with an appropriately prepared apparatus with which to administer positive pressure ventilation.

VIII. Anesthesia Management

A. Anesthesia-related preparation to sustain a latex-free environment should include the following:
   1. Maintain latex-free perianesthesia areas, including the preoperative area, OR suite, and recovery area. Remove all latex-containing furniture, equipment, and supplies. Many institutions use a latex-free cart that contains all necessary substitutional products that contain no latex and can be used to accommodate known and suspected latex allergy cases.
   2. Any items that cannot be replaced with a latex-free substitution should be covered (i.e., Stockinette or Webril) to avoid direct skin contact.
   3. IV sets should have stopcocks and no rubber injection ports. (Place tape over rubber injection ports if they are present.)
   4. Avoid rubber Heplocks or T-connectors in the IV system.

5. Use latex-free stethoscopes and temperature and esophageal monitoring probes.
6. Cover any rubber mattress or stretcher pads, armboards, or bumpers with cloth or tape.
7. Maintain a sufficient supply of all latex-free products health providers might need in caring for the allergic patient (i.e., gloves, masks, oxygen, delivery supplies).

IX. Medication Administration

A. Contamination of medications contained in a multidose vial with a latex stopper may act as a trigger to initiate a reaction.
B. Latex particles may be "cored" from the rubber stopper following repeated passes with a needle through the rubber stopper. This practice should be avoided.
C. Medications should be managed as follows:
   1. All medications should be drawn immediately before use and should not be kept in a syringe for a prolonged time.
   2. Single-dose vials should be used whenever possible, and every attempt should be made to use a new vial of medication for each high-risk patient. Preparations that contain rubber parts should be transferred to a latex-free system before administration (i.e., tube injection services).
   3. The black rubber in the syringes is hardened and should not contribute to leaching of latex particles into the solution. Timing remains important.

X. Presentation, Emergency Response, and Treatment

A. It is essential to remember that premedication will not prevent an allergic reaction resulting from exposure to latex.
B. Signs and symptoms of an allergic reaction to latex can occur at any time in patients possessing the highest risk factors aforementioned.
C. These responses may not be observed because of limitations imposed by the operative field and procedure or masked by general anesthetics or deep sedation.
   1. The first indication that an allergic reaction is transpiring is frequently reflected by an acute hypotensive episode and oxygen desaturation
   2. Emergency response to a suspected latex allergic reaction should include an organized and dedicated plan. Prompt intervention and treatment of a latex allergy emergency can result in quality outcomes

3. Protocol for management
   a. Removal of all latex-containing products and agents if possible. Do not delay immediate emergency therapy.
   b. Inform the surgical team to stop treatment or abort the procedure.
   c. Assess and sustain ABCs of resuscitation (airway, breathing, circulation).
   d. Maintain the airway, and administer 100% oxygen.
   e. Discontinue inhalational halogenated agents (they are cardiovascular depressants that sensitize the myocardium to catecholamines, which may be required for therapy).
   f. Start intravascular volume expansion with Ringer's lactate solution or normal saline (10–20 ml/kg if hypotension is present and the patient has no history of heart failure or any volume-related contraindication). Fluid resuscitation may require that large volumes be administered rapidly.
   g. Treat pharmacologically as indicated by presentation and clinical course.
   h. Administer epinephrine; start with a 0.5 to 1 μg/kg bolus (10 μg/ml dilution). Escalate to higher doses depending on the patient's response.
   i. If an IV line has not been established, epinephrine can be given subcutaneously in doses larger than would be administered intravenously (dose of 10 μg/kg). Endotracheal dosage may be necessary if IV access has not been established.
4. Secondary pharmacologic treatment
   a. Hydrocortisone, 0.25 to 1 g, or methylprednisolone, 1 mg/kg, IV (maximum dose 60 mg)
   b. Diphenhydramine, 0.5 to 1 mg/kg (maximum dose 50 mg)
   c. Epinephrine infusion, 2 to 4 μg/min or more (titrate to effect)
   d. Aminophylline, 5 to 6 mg/kg over 20 minutes for persistent bronchospasm
   e. Ranitidine, 0.5 to 2 mg/kg IV (maximum dose 150 mg)
   f. Sodium bicarbonate, 0.5 to 1 mEq/kg for persistent hypotension with acidosis diagnosed with laboratory confirmation
5. Nonpharmacologic considerations
   a. Obtain allergy, pulmonary, and pediatric consults as indicated.

      b. Draw and send a blood sample for IgE RAST testing and tryptase level (1 hour after reaction).

      c. Report incident to appropriate institutional entities (i.e., pharmacy, therapeutics, quality assurance) following departmental protocols.

      d. Document events thoroughly and succinctly to examine at morbidity and mortality review at a later date.

    6. Postreaction stabilization should include appropriate monitoring by dedicated providers well versed in managing postanaphylaxis patients. The pediatric intensive or special care area should be used when appropriate

XI. Institutional Program and Protocols

    A. Prevention of exposure to NRL is the ideal approach to best manage both latex sensitive and latex allergic patients.

    B. Given the nature of health care institutions and environmental sources, the best approach that can be expected is decreased use of NRL and products that contain latex.

    C. A latex-free environment should be the goal in providing optimal care for the patient with known, suspected, or documented allergy to latex or who possesses an appreciable risk from the aforementioned factors listed.

    D. Substitution of products and supplies requires considerable forethought, planning, and consistency. Resource listings have extensive lists of potential substitutional products and supplies that are available via Internet access.

    E. Medical gloves are a major source of latex; particular efforts and attention are required to plan comparable alternatives for health care providers to have readily available.

    F. Staff education and training are necessary to ensure consistency with program demands while making every effort to conserve costs and resources.

    G. A multidisciplinary approach to institutional latex management programs will best serve all patients.

    H. A reliable patient screening process should include both patient and support persons that interface with qualified providers who can counsel and manage the atopic or allergic patient and patients at potential risk for latex allergy.

    I. Medic Alert bracelet identification of children with documented latex allergy and those who have experienced clinical symptoms or anaphylaxis could easily alert both lay and professional responders during an emergency.

    J. Resources listed at the end of this chapter provide information to obtain a Medic Alert bracelet.

XII. Summary

A. The child with a latex allergy presents a unique challenge when procedures requiring anesthesia care are necessary. A thorough medical history, testing, and evaluation and detailed perioperative demands and management are necessary to afford the safest environment and intervention possible.

B. Constant vigilance and attention to detailed planning and orchestration are fundamental aspects required by the provider challenged with caring for the latex allergic patient.

C. An institution-wide program supported and maintained by all involved participants will best serve the latex allergic patient and support system participants.

BIBLIOGRAPHY

Birmingham, P.K., Dsida, R.M., Grayhack, J.J., et al. (1996). Do latex precautions in children with myelodysplasia reduce intraoperative allergic reactions? *Journal of Pediatric Orthopedics*, 16(6), 799–802.

Dormans, J.P., Templeton, J.J., Edmonds, C., et al. (1994). Intraoperative anaphylaxis due to exposure to latex (natural rubber). I. Children. *Journal of Bone and Joint Surgery [American Volume]*, 76, 1688–1691.

Freeman, G.L. (1997). Co-occurrence of latex and fruit allergies. *Allergy and Asthma Proceedings*, 18(II).

Kelly, K.J., Kurup, V.P., Reijula, K.E., & Fink, J.N. (1994). The diagnosis of natural rubber latex allergy. *Journal of Allergy and Clinical Immunology*, 93(5), 813–816.

Pasquariello, C.A., Lowe, D.A., & Schwartz, R.E. (1993). Intraoperative anaphylaxis to latex. *Pediatrics*, 91, 983–986.

Porri, F., Pradal, M., Lemiere, C., et al. (1997). Association between latex sensitization and repeated latex exposure in children. *Anesthesiology*, 86(3), 599–602.

Shaer, C., & Slater, J. (1993). Latex allergy in children. *Current Opinion in Pediatrics*, 5, 700–704.

Theissen, U., Theissen, J.L., Mertes, N., & Brehler, R. (1997). IgE-mediated hypersensitivity to latex in childhood. *Allergy*, 52, 655–669.

Turjanmaa, K., Alenius, H., Makinen-Kiljunen, S., et al. (1996). Natural rubber latex allergy. *Allergy*, 51, 593–602.

Vessey, J.A., McVay, C.J., Holland, C.V., et al. (1993). Latex allergy: a threat to you and your patients? *Pediatric Nursing*, 19, 517–520.

ADDITIONAL READINGS

American Association of Nurse Anesthetists, Occupational Safety and Hazard Committee. (1998). *Latex allergy protocol*. Obtainable from Practice Department, 222 So. Prospect Avenue, Park Ridge, IL 60068-4001. Phone 847-692-7050, ext. 3015.

Committee Report. (1993). Task force on allergic reaction to latex. *Journal of Allergy and Clinical Immunology*, 92, 16–18.

NIOSH alert: Preventing allergic reactions to natural rubber latex in the workplace. DHHS (NIOSH) Publication no. 97-135.

Pasquarellio, C.A., & Lowe, D.A. (1992). *Protocol for the management of patients with allergy and risk for allergy to latex products.* Philadelphia: Department of Anesthesia and Critical Care, St. Christopher's Hospital for Children.

Ylitalo, L., Turjanmaa, K., Palosuo, T., & Reunala, T. (1997). Natural rubber latex allergy in children who had not undergone surgery and children who had undergone multiple operations. *Journal of Allergy and Clinical Immunology,* 100(5), 606–612.

INTERNET RESOURCES

Cleveland Clinic Foundation Perioperative Interactive Linked Online Tutorials. (1997). Anesthetic management of the latex allergic patient, *http://gasnet.med.vale.edu./gta/latex/manage.html.*

To obtain a list of latex-free medical products, visit "alert@execpc.com."

PATIENT RESOURCE

Medic Alert (bracelet orders)
2323 Colorado Avenue
Turlock, CA 95382
Phone 1-800-432-5378

Anesthesia Considerations for Pediatric Patients

VI

24

Regional Anesthesia and Pain Management

Michael J. Kremer, DNSc, CRNA, and
Margaret Faut-Callahan, DNSc, CRNA, FAAN

I. Introduction

A. Pain is a multifaceted syndrome of behaviors that includes neuroanatomic and sensory perception with associated quantitative factors and emotional, motivational, and affective factors.

B. Pain management has historically been a challenge for clinicians. Until the 1980s, researchers still questioned the need for analgesia and anesthesia in premature infants, term infants, and children. Early research findings supported the contention that complete nerve myelination was necessary for nerve tract function. The ensuing widespread assumption was that infants either did not experience or did not perceive pain as acutely or meaningfully as adults or perhaps did not experience pain at all. It is now clear that even neonates experience pain. Morbidity and mortality are reduced when pain is adequately treated.

II. Pathophysiology

A. Acute and chronic pain, or pain resulting from tissue damage or disruption, is associated with an increase in small fiber activity and a decrease in large fiber activity. The perception of pain acutely is a protective mechanism that has the benefits of allowing the avoidance or interruption of injury.

B. Chronic pain consists of both physical and psychologic pain.
   1. The physical component involves the actual neuroanatomic and physiologic transmission of painful stimuli throughout a complex system of pain pathways.
   2. The psychologic component is influenced by the following factors: context of the pain; prior experience with pain; cultural beliefs; individual pain threshold; anxiety level of child and parents; birth order; and gender.

359

III. Reasons for the Undertreatment of Pediatric Pain

A. Some reasons that pain has been undertreated in pediatric patients are
   1. Infants and preverbal children cannot describe why they are in pain. Children will not always cry when they are experiencing pain.
   2. The response of the older child to pain is different from that of the adult. Often these children will be quiet and withdrawn.
   3. When postoperative intramuscular narcotic injections were prevalent, children often feared the injection more than the pain. Because of this fear, some pediatric patients suffered in silence, perpetuating the myth that children felt pain less than adults.
   4. Clinicians have been uncertain regarding the safety of analgesics in infants. It had been stated that infants are exquisitely sensitive to the respiratory depressant effects of morphine, leading to ultraconservative prescribing practices.
   5. Many physicians, especially junior house staff to whom the responsibility for pain management often was delegated, were unsure of the correct dosage of analgesics for pediatric patients.
   6. Nurses have also tended to underestimate pain while overestimating the danger of the child becoming overly sedated or addicted to potent analgesics.
B. With greater understanding of developmental physiology and pharmacology, there is no reason why any infant or child should be denied adequate analgesia.
C. Evidence suggests inadequate analgesia may have detrimental consequences beyond the obvious concern for compassionate care.
D. Neuroendocrine responses, tissue catabolism, and postoperative pulmonary function are favorably altered by various techniques that provide postoperative analgesia.

IV. Assessment of Pain in Children

A. Children 7 years of age and older can often use a visual analog scale or numeric rating scale; however, assessing pain and the adequacy of therapy in younger children is challenging.
B. A self-assessment scale is preferable to an observer's objective assessment and should be used whenever possible because pain is a subjective experience.

C. Younger school-age children can often use a numeric rating scale, although it may be easier to explain if the scores are reversed. Children associate high scores with good grades in school and a desirable outcome: a score of 10 is better interpreted as no pain and 0 as the worst pain imaginable.

D. Reviewing pain assessment tools with patients and their families preoperatively enables them to better use the pain scale postoperatively.

E. Preverbal children must be assessed by an objective observer, and no fully adequate system has been devised.

F. All objective rating systems rely on physical signs of autonomic arousal coupled with behavioral assessments. If one believes that pharmacologic management has been adequate, an attempt should be made to comfort the child with behavioral interventions. If these measures are not successful, then additional analgesia should be provided.

G. In infants, the level of pain is assessed using both physiologic and behavioral indices:
1. Physiologic indices include tachycardia, tachypnea, increased blood pressure, and sweating.
2. Behavioral indices: facial expression may be the most reliable, but cry characteristics and body movement (especially flexion of the limbs) are also useful.

V. Management of Postoperative Pain

A. Both the chronologic age and the neurodevelopmental age of a patient need to be considered when planning postoperative analgesia

B. Older children with significant developmental delay may require a management technique appropriate for their developmental age

C. Premature or young infants
1. May have problems with central respiratory drive and benefit from a technique that avoids opioids and central respiratory depression
2. Suggested management techniques
   a. Infiltration of the wound edges with local anesthetics, peripheral nerve blocks, or regional blockade are especially useful.
   b. Regional blockade can be achieved by single-shot or continuous-catheter techniques using low concentrations of bupivacaine (0.25% to 0.1%), which cause little motor blockade.
   c. Acetaminophen, 15 mg/kg orally repeated every 4 hours or 20 to 30 mg/kg rectally, repeated every

6 hours can be a useful adjunct because it has a large therapeutic window and few untoward effects.

    d. Opioids are not contraindicated, but careful observation and monitoring are necessary to detect respiratory depression, especially in premature infants or term infants less than 1 month of age.

D. Older infants and toddlers

  1. In addition to the measures above, this age-group may benefit from continuous opioid infusions or neuraxis opioids in low to moderate doses.

  2. Behavioral techniques such as play therapy and the presence of a comforting parent can augment whatever pharmacologic modalities are used.

  3. A painless and nonthreatening induction technique and the presence of a parent or familiar adult during induction and emergence can alleviate much of the anxiety and fear that may accompany the immediate postoperative period.

E. Preschool and school-age children

  1. These children have greater fears and better understanding of the postoperative experience than do their younger counterparts. They need to be reassured that postoperative pain is transient and that it will be treated effectively.

  2. Children older than approximately 7 years are often able to understand the concept of patient-controlled analgesia (PCA). This technique may be helpful in giving a sense of control back to the child during a period when all other aspects of control are removed.

  3. Regional techniques are excellent for providing analgesia, especially in children who are easily nauseated or disturbed by dysphoria that may accompany opioids.

F. Adolescents

  1. In this population the issues of control and dependency assume greater importance.

  2. Allowing the adolescent to participate in decision making will contribute to the success of any analgesic technique.

VI. Classification of Modalities Useful for Pain Management

A. Pharmacologic

  1. This modality includes the administration of opioids, sedatives, antidepressants, and anticonvulsants.

  2. Dosing regimens can be either intermittent or continuous infusions.

  3. Patient-controlled analgesia (PCA) is an option in older children.

4. Regional anesthetic techniques, local anesthetic infiltration, and topical application are also viable pharmacologic choices.

B. Diagnostic and therapeutic nerve/plexus blocks
1. Include the administration of epidurals (caudal, lumbar, thoracic), which can all be used in pediatric patients.
2. Brachial plexus blocks can be used, although techniques relying on paresthesia may be distressing.
3. Both bolus and continuous infusion techniques are applicable here.

C. Nonpharmacologic
1. Psychologic techniques such as distraction, relaxation and music, or behavioral modification approaches may be effective.
2. Family or individual psychotherapy may be warranted in some situations.
3. Hypnotherapy, physical therapy, and massage therapy can provide significant nonpharmacologic pain relief.

VII. Acute Pain Management

A. Concern about opioid addiction in children has been cited as a reason for avoiding opioids for acute or chronic pain relief. The fear of addiction may be attributable to confusion between the concepts of physical dependence and addiction
1. Physical dependence refers to an altered physiologic state that occurs after repeated drug administration and results in the manifestation of withdrawal symptoms on discontinuation of the drug.
2. Addiction is a behavior pattern involving compulsive drug use and obsession with attaining a drug supply.
3. Dependence is common with repeated administration of opioids but can be controlled when necessary through gradual tapering in the hospital. The question of opioid dependence should be irrelevant for terminally ill children with pain.
4. When using PCA in patients with cancer, basal infusion rates should be considered routine to avoid the peak and trough effects and provide analgesic blood levels of the selected opioid.

B. Oral medications
1. A variety of analgesics are available for oral administration.
2. Nonopioid agents, such as acetaminophen, aspirin, and other nonsteroidal antiinflammatory drugs (NSAIDs), are useful for treating mild to moderate pain.

3. Acetaminophen, the most widely used analgesic, has a high therapeutic index in children.
4. Aspirin, although especially useful in inflammatory pain, has a statistical association with Reye syndrome and side effects of gastritis and platelet dysfunction.
5. The NSAIDs inhibit prostaglandin synthetase and have side effects similar to aspirin.
6. Naproxen (Naprosyn) (maximum daily dose 15 mg/kg/d) and ibuprofen (maximum dose 40 mg/kg/d) have been approved by the U.S. Food and Drug Administration for use in children.

C. Recommended dosing techniques
1. Intramuscular injections should be avoided whenever possible. Absorption is highly variable as compared to oral or intravenous administration.
2. The opioids produce excellent analgesia but include other physiologic effects, such as sedation, respiratory depression, pruritus, nausea, vomiting, decreased gastric motility, miosis, biliary spasm, vasodilation, and cough suppression.
3. Suggested starting doses for postoperative analgesia with opioids
   a. Continuous intravenous (IV): morphine 0.02 to 0.03 mg/kg/h, or fentanyl 0.5 to 3 µg/kg/h
   b. Intermittent IV: morphine 0.05 to 0.1 mg/kg q2h, or meperidine 0.5 to 1 mg/kg q2h
   c. Oral: codeine 0.5 to 1 mg/kg q4h, or morphine 0.2 to 0.4 mg/kg q4h.
4. Meperidine has an active metabolite, normeperidine. With prolonged use, neurobehavioral changes and seizures can result from normeperidine accumulation.
5. Doses in infants younger than 3 months of age are given in increments of one third to one half of the above doses because there is some evidence of increased risk of respiratory depression.
   a. Neonates have reduced plasma concentrations of albumin and alpha-acid glycoprotein compared with older children.
   b. Accordingly, less opioid is bound, and therefore there is greater availability of active drug at receptor sites.
6. Ibuprofen may be given orally and has been found to be effective in reducing postoperative opioid requirements. Ibuprofen may cause gastrointestinal upset and inhibits platelet aggregation, increasing the potential for bleeding.

7. Ketorolac is another NSAID with analgesic effects similar to those of morphine without respiratory depressant effects.
   a. When given after surgery, ketorolac, 0.9 mg/kg IV, appears to provide postoperative analgesia comparable to morphine, 0.1 mg/kg.
   b. It inhibits platelet aggregation and is not recommended where bleeding may be a problem.
   c. Other serious, albeit uncommon potential side effects include gastrointestinal hemorrhage, interstitial nephritis, and acute renal failure (ARF). ARF occurs as a result of the inhibition of prostaglandin synthesis, which is important to maintain afferent arteriole dilation.
D. Transmucosal drug administration
   1. Opioids are traditionally effective in the management of acute and chronic pain. Transmucosal opioids are alternatives to needles for administration.
   2. The limitations of this route include unpredictable absorption, nausea and vomiting, and sedation.
   3. This transmucosal route has been used to provide sedation and analgesia for minor procedures, such as lumbar puncture or bone marrow biopsy.

VIII. General Considerations for Regional Blockade

A. Regional blockade with the administration of local anesthetics or opioids modulates the transmission of afferent nociceptive impulses and provides pain relief with minimal side effects.
B. The main disadvantage of regional anesthesia is that some pain may occur during placement of the block. Many of these regional techniques are used in combination with general anesthesia. Most children do not tolerate the insertion of an epidural or spinal needle when awake or without IV sedation.
C. Regional techniques often provide more complete relief of pain, and the patient can have a higher functional activity level.
D. Local anesthetic blockade can be accomplished with local infiltration, individual peripheral nerve blocks, and plexus blockade at the brachial or lumbar levels.
E. Epidural analgesia, whether caudal, lumbar, or thoracic, is probably the most versatile regional technique, either by single injection, repeated injections, or continuous infusion through a catheter with a local anesthetic or opioid.

1. The epidural space can be approached at any level, but the lumbar or caudal level is commonly used in children.
2. The caudal approach is most commonly used in young infants.
3. Local anesthetics can be useful when postoperative immobilization or regional sympathetic blockade will result in surgical benefits.
4. The addition of opioids results in activation of the opioid receptors in the dorsal horn of the spinal cord, producing regional analgesia without anesthesia.
5. Hypotension is unlikely with local anesthetics, especially in younger children.
6. Motor blockade is rarely a problem, especially if the patient is not yet ambulatory.
7. Fentanyl by continuous epidural infusion may be inadvisable in neonates, especially if there is a history of prematurity. A higher incidence of respiratory depression is noted with fentanyl compared with epidural morphine and is dose related.

F. Regional techniques for postoperative pain control in children.
   1. Wound infiltration for suture of laceration, skin tag removal, central line insertion
   2. Wrist block for removal of extra digits
   3. Penile block for circumcision, hypospadias repair
   4. Ilioinguinal/iliohypogastric block for inguinal hernia repair
   5. Axillary block for repair of Colles fracture and plastic surgery procedures
   6. Femoral block for midshaft femur fracture
   7. Intercostal block for thoracotomy, nephrectomy
   8. Caudal epidural for inguinal herniorrhaphy, complex hypospadias repair, clubfoot repair, ureteral reimplantation
   9. Lumbar epidural for orchiopexy, urologic recontruction
   10. Thoracic epidural for thoracotomy, thoracic or abdominal surgery in patients with severe lung disease
   11. Spinal anesthesia is useful for small infants, especially the ex-preterm infant with residual lung disease who has a hernia or lower abdominal surgical pathology
   12. Epidural analgesia may be a suitable alternative to general anesthesia in some older children (e.g., those with cystic fibrosis) and may then be continued into the postoperative period

13. IV regional anesthesia (Bier block) can be used for some older children having superficial surgery to lesions on the distal limbs
14. The possibility of using regional or local infiltration analgesia should be considered for any minor procedure in a high-risk patient (e.g., a skeletal muscle biopsy in a child with cardiomyopathy or a lymph node biopsy in a patient with a mediastinal mass)

G. Considerations for regional analgesia administration.
1. Calculate the allowable dose of the local analgesic agent for each child, and do not exceed this dose.
2. Use appropriate aseptic technique.
3. Avoid intravascular injections; test by aspirating frequently.
4. Plan ahead and allow adequate time for the block to have effect before allowing the surgeon to approach the patient.
5. Considerations for use of local anesthetics in infants and young children are listed on page 368.
6. Always be prepared to deal with the complications of regional analgesia. Drugs and equipment to induce general anesthesia, secure the airway, and ventilate the patient must be immediately available.
7. Anticipate that unsatisfactory regional analgesia may require administration of general anesthesia to permit completion of the surgical procedure.
8. Apply EMLA cream over the site if possible at least 60 to 90 minutes before initial needle insertion.
9. Supplement the regional technique with age-appropriate sedation.
   a. For neonates, a pacifier with a few drops of 50% dextrose may suffice.
   b. Oral midazolam can be used in age-appropriate doses.
   c. Analgesics, such as fentanyl, or hypnotics, such as propofol, can be administered.
   d. Distractions such as a Walkman and earphones may facilitate cooperation.

H. The suggested maximum doses of local anesthetic drugs are listed in Table 24–1.

IX. Spinal Anesthesia for Infants
A. This technique is most commonly used for surgery at or below the umbilicus but has also been used for upper abdominal surgery in small infants with a history of respiratory disease.

Considerations for the Use of Local Anesthetics in Infants and Children

1. Absorption of drugs is rapid. The cardiac output and regional tissue blood flows are higher. The epidural space contains less fat tissue to buffer uptake. Drugs sprayed into the airway are very rapidly absorbed.
2. The volume of distribution of the drug is larger. The greater volume of distribution also extends the elimination half-life.
3. The extent of protein binding is less. Serum albumin and alpha$_1$-acid glycoprotein levels are low in the neonate. Bilirubin may further reduce the potential for protein binding. Caution must be exercised when local anesthetics are used in the jaundiced neonate.
4. The rate of metabolism of local anesthetics is reduced in very young infants.
   a. Plasma cholinesterase activity is lower, and metabolism of the ester type of drugs may be prolonged; for example, the plasma half-life of procaine or chloroprocaine is extended in the neonate.
   b. The hepatic pathways for the conjugation of the amide local anesthetics are immature. The neonate has a reduced capacity to metabolize mepivacaine or bupivacaine. By 1 to 6 months of age, the latter is cleared as rapidly as in adults. Older infants and children metabolize drugs more rapidly because of their relatively large liver size.
5. The metabolism of prilocaine can result in methemoglobinemia. This may be more significant in infants, because their levels of the enzyme methemoglobin reductase may be reduced.

B. It avoids the need for intubation and ventilation with the risks of further airway damage or repeated ventilator dependence.
C. Minimal alterations in blood pressure occur in infants or children following spinal block.
D. Postoperative apnea of the ex-preterm infant may be less common after spinal analgesia.
E. Special considerations.
   1. The spinal cord may extend as low as L3 in the infant versus L1–2 in the older child or adult (see Fig. 24–1).

TABLE 24–1. Local Anesthetics for Pediatric Regional Anesthesia

Drug	Technique	Concentration	Dose*	Duration (min)*
Bupivacaine (Marcaine)	Epidural/caudal	0.25%	2.5 mg/kg or 0.5–1 ml/kg	120–240 120–240
	Spinal†	Hyperbaric: 0.5% in 8% dextrose	<5 kg: 0.5 mg/kg 5–15 kg: 0.4 mg/kg >15 kg: 0.3 mg/kg	30–60
	Brachial plexus	0.25%	0.7 ml/kg up to 50 kg	150–360
Mepivacaine (Carbocaine)	Brachial plexus	0.5%–2.0%	5 mg/kg (maximum 8 mg)	60–90
	Caudal	0.5%–1.5%	0.5 mg/kg	120–360
Lidocaine (Xylocaine)	Epidural/caudal	1%–2%	5 (7)	30–60
	Brachial plexus	0.5%–2.0%	5 (7)	45–160
	Spinal	5% with 7.5% dextrose	2 mg/kg	Variable
Tetracaine (Pontocaine)	Spinal†	0.5% in 10% dextrose	<5 kg: 0.4 to 0.8 mg/kg 5–15 kg: 0.4 to 0.8 mg/kg >15 kg: 0.3 mg/kg	60–90 60–90 60–90

*Without (with epinephrine).
†Indications: Patient <60 weeks' postconceptual age, high risk for apnea and bradycardia.

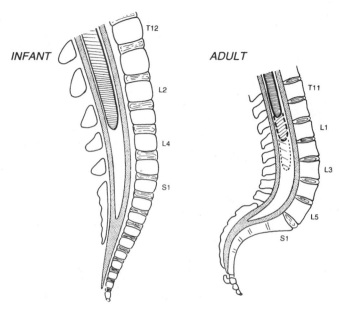

FIGURE 24–1. Anatomic differences between adults and children that affect the performance of spinal and epidural anesthesia; an infant's sacrum *(left)* is flatter and narrower than an adult's *(right)*. Note that the tip of the spinal cord in a neonate ends at L3 and does not achieve the normal adult position (L1–2) until approximately 1 year of age. (From Coté, C.J., Ryan, J.F., Todres, I.D., & Goudsouzian N.G. [Eds.]. [1993]. *A Practice of anesthesia for infants and children* [2nd ed.]. Philadelphia: W.B. Saunders.)

    2. It is best to perform lumbar puncture at L4–5.
    3. The dural space extends to S3–4 in the neonate.
    4. The volume of cerebrospinal fluid (CSF) is relatively higher in infants (4 ml/kg) than in adults (2 ml/kg).
  F. Contraindications to spinal anesthesia.
    1. Sepsis or infected lumbar puncture site
    2. Coagulopathy
    3. Lack of parental consent
  G. Anesthesia management.
    1. Preoperative considerations
      a. The patient should receive nothing by mouth (NPO), as for general anesthesia.
      b. No premedication is necessary for small infants.
    2. Perioperative considerations
      a. Observe all special precautions for infants, both term

and preterm. Prepare the anesthesia machine, endotracheal tubes, and so on.
   b. A sweet-tasting pacifier can be used to comfort the infant.
   c. The use of ketamine negates the advantages of spinal anesthesia.
   d. Establish a reliable IV infusion.
3. Administration of the spinal block
   a. Instruct assistant to gently but firmly restrain the patient in the chosen lateral or sitting position (see Fig. 24–2).
   b. Avoid neck flexion, which may compromise the airway.
   c. Prepare and drape the patient.
   d. Infiltrate the skin over the L4–5 interspace with 1% lidocaine.
   e. Prepare a neonatal spinal needle, 22 gauge × 1 inch.
   f. Prepare a syringe containing 0.4 to 0.6 mg/kg of 1% tetracaine mixed with an equal volume of 10% dextrose (the final solution is tetracaine 0.5% and detrose 5%), plus a volume of this mixture equal to the dead space of the needle (approximately 0.2 ml). For upper abdominal surgery, tetracaine, 1 mg/kg, has been used.
   g. Insert the needle at L4–5 with the bevel facing laterally until CSF is obtained.
   h. Slowly inject the local anesthesia solution.
   i. Turn the patient to a supine horizontal position.
   j. Some clinicians may choose to apply the IV catheter and oximeter probe to one leg and the blood pressure cuff to the other, minimizing disturbance of the infant (see Fig. 24–3). Motor function in lower limbs usually ceases immediately.
   k. Do not allow the patient's legs to be raised (e.g., to apply the cautery pad), or an excessively high block may result (see Fig. 24–4).
   l. The duration of surgical anesthesia is usually about 1 to 1½ hours.
   m. Total spinal anesthesia in infants is heralded by apnea with little change in blood pressure.
   n. Treatment consists of intubation with controlled ventilation and support of hemodynamic parameters until recovery occurs.
4. Postoperative considerations

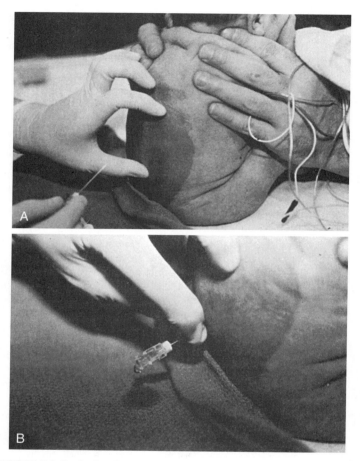

FIGURE 24–2. **A,** Lumbar puncture in a neonate or infant is generally performed in the sitting position. Note that the head is maintained in the neutral position to prevent airway obstruction. **B,** After local infiltration of 1% lidocaine with a 25- to 27-gauge needle, lumbar puncture is performed with a 22-gauge 1½-inch *styletted* needle at the L4–5 or L5–S1 interspace. Entrance into the subarachnoid space is confirmed by free flow of cerebrospinal fluid.

      a. Continue to care for the patient in the horizontal position until motor function in the legs returns.

      b. Monitor the ex-preterm infant carefully for apnea. Apnea is less common after regional anesthesia but may occur.

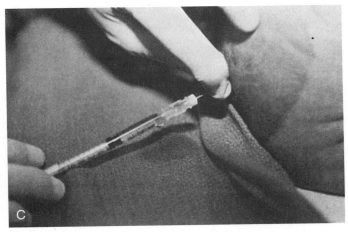

FIGURE 24–2 *Continued.* **C,** Local anesthetic is injected with a tuberculin syringe. Be careful not to inject rapidly, or a high level of blockade might result. (From Coté, C.J., Ryan, J.F., Todres, I.D., & Goudsouzian, N.G. [Eds.]. [1993]. *A practice of anesthesia for infants and children* [2nd ed.]. Philadelphia: W.B. Saunders.)

X. Caudal Block

A. This is a useful block in infants and children, providing good postoperative analgesia following lower abdominal and perineal surgery.

B. Caudal analgesia has also been used as an alternative to spinal anesthesia for lower abdominal surgery in infants.

C. In young patients the contents of the epidural space offer little resistance to the spread of local anesthetic solutions. In this age-group, epidural analgesia is accompanied by very little change in blood pressure or cardiac output.

D. Continuous caudal catheters have been used intraoperatively for more extensive surgical procedures, and they may be advanced cephalad in infants for procedures involving thoracic dermatomes.

E. They are not generally favored for postoperative use because of the risk of infection.

F. Occlusive dressings can be carefully applied to isolate the catheter site from contamination by urine and feces.

G. Drug and volume to be injected.
   1. Bupivacaine 0.25% with epinephrine 1:200,000 can be used. Total dose should not exceed 2.5 mg/kg.

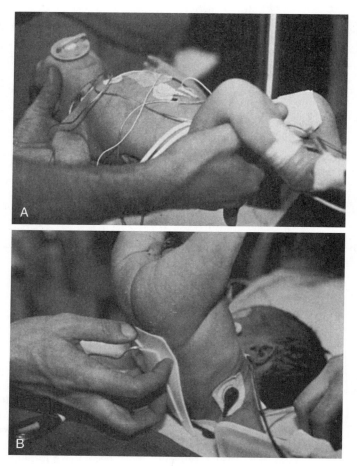

FIGURE 24–3. A, The proper method of applying an electrocautery pad. The infant's entire body is elevated while maintaining the *horizontal* position to avoid excessively high spread of subarachnoid blockade. **B,** Improper method of applying an electrocautery pad in a neonate after subarachnoid administration of local anesthetic; the legs should never be elevated. (From Coté, C.J., Ryan, J.F., Todres, I.D., & Goudsouzian, N.G. [Eds.]. [1993]. *A practice of anesthesia for infants and children* [2nd ed.]. Philadelphia: W.B. Saunders.)

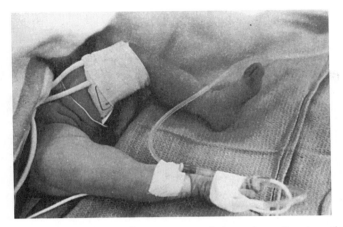

FIGURE 24–4. Placement of intravenous catheter and monitors in patients receiving spinal anesthesia. After spinal anesthesia is initiated, the IV catheter and oximeter probe are applied to one leg and the blood pressure cuff is applied to the other. The infant is thus allowed to remain undisturbed. (From Coté, C.J., Ryan, J.F., Todres, I.D., & Goudsouzian, N.G. [Eds.]. [1993]. *A practice of anesthesia for infants and children* [2nd ed.]. Philadelphia: W.B. Saunders.)

      a. Perineal surgery (e.g., hypospadias repair): 0.5 ml/kg
      b. Lower abdominal surgery (e.g., orchiopexy): 1 ml/kg
  2. Bupivacaine 0.125% may be adequate for perineal surgery and may minimize the risk of urinary retention.
H. Preferred technique.
  1. For postoperative analgesia, the block should be performed after general anesthesia is induced but before surgery begins. This allows the block to become well established during surgery.
  2. The child is placed in a lateral position with the hips flexed (see Fig. 24–5).
  3. The landmarks should now be identified.
  4. The tip of the coccyx is the midline, and the sacral cornua is bound by the sacral hiatus.
  5. The sacral hiatus lies at the apex of an inverted equilateral triangle, the base of which is a line drawn between the posterosuperior iliac spines.
  6. The patient is carefully prepared and draped, and the operator wears gloves.
  7. A skin nick is made of the sacral hiatus using an 18-gauge needle.

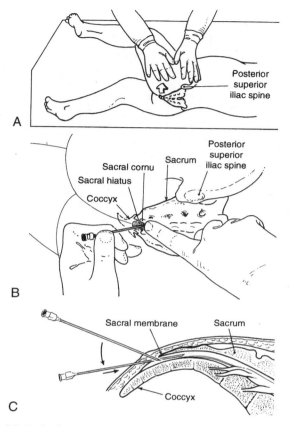

FIGURE 24–5. Performing a caudal block. **A,** The patient is placed in a lateral position. **B,** The posterosuperior iliac spines are located and the sacral cornu palpated; an IV needle, an IV catheter, or a Crawford needle of appropriate size is advanced at an angle of approximately 45 degrees until a distinct pop is felt as the needle pierces the sacrococcygeal ligament. **C,** The angle of the needle with the skin is reduced to 30 degrees, and the needle or IV catheter is advanced into the caudal canal.

8. Through this a 20- or 22-gauge Angiocath is advanced cephalad at a 45-degree angle to the skin with the bevel facing anteriorly.
9. A distinctive sudden loss of resistance is felt as the needle passes through the sacrococcygeal membrane. At this point the angle of the needle can be lowered slightly.

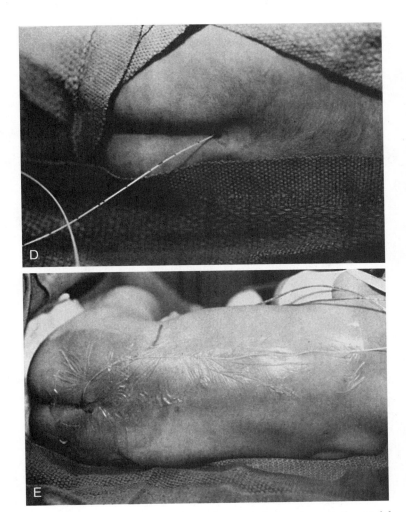

FIGURE 24–5 *Continued.*   **D,** If a continuous technique is used, the caudal catheter is advanced to the midlevel of the surgical incision (it usually readily passes in children less than 5 years), and the introducing needle or catheter is withdrawn. **E,** The catheter is secured with an occlusive dressing. (From Coté, C.J., Ryan, J.F., Todres, I.D., & Goudsouzian, N.G. [Eds.]. [1993]. *A practice of anesthesia for infants and children* [2nd ed.]. Philadelphia: W.B. Saunders.)

10. The needle is withdrawn while the catheter is advanced. This is done to minimize dural puncture by the needle tip.
11. The catheter is carefully aspirated, determining the absence of blood or CSF, and a small test dose of the chosen local anesthetic may be administered.
12. If there is no indication of intravascular injection (bradycardia, tachycardia, or peaking of T waves), incremental injection of the selected local anesthetic is undertaken.
13. During the injection a finger should be placed over the sacrum to detect inadvertent subcutaneous injection.
14. The use of an IV catheter rather than a needle diminishes the risk that movement during injection will result in intravascular administration.

XI. Lumbar Epidural Block

A. Lumbar epidural block has been widely used for postoperative pain relief in children.
B. The technique used is similar to that used in adults; the loss of resistance with saline is used to identify the epidural space.
C. In children weighing more than 10 kg, the distance from the skin to the epidural space in millimeters is approximately numerically similar to the child's weight in kilograms (e.g., the distance in a 20 kg child is about 20 mm).
D. A 19-gauge Tuohy needle and a 21-gauge catheter can be used in children younger than 5 years of age.
E. Above this age, an 18-gauge Tuohy needle and 20-gauge epidural catheter can be used.
F. Dose requirements for local anesthetic solutions are less predictable when the lumbar route as opposed to the caudal route is used.
G. Epidural block is associated with few changes in hemodynamic parameters.
H. Drug dosages: Bupivacaine 0.25% with epinephrine 1:200,000, 0.5 ml/kg (0.75 ml/kg for infants), supplemented with doses of 0.2 ml/kg, can be used to achieve the block level required.

XII. Intercostal Nerve Block

A. Intercostal nerve blocks may be performed to relieve pain following thoracotomy or some upper abdominal procedures. In infants this is best performed by the surgeon before closure of the wound.

B. Systemic absorption of local anesthetics from the vascular intercostal space may be rapid, with the commensurate risk of toxic effects. It is important not to exceed a total bupivacaine dose of 2 ml/kg.

C. The risk of pneumothorax is high, especially in small children, where the distance from the intercostal nerve to the pleura is small.

D. The intercostal nerves are sheathed in a dural layer posteriorly. Injection near their origin can result in subarachnoid administration with consequent spinal anesthesia.

E. Technique.

    1. In infants and small children, the nerve in the intercostal space can be more precisely approached by angling the needle posteromedially, so that it lies almost parallel to the rib rather than at right angles to it.

XIII. Ilioinguinal and Iliohypogastric Nerve Blocks

A. This nerve block provides skin analgesia over the inguinal region and is useful for providing postoperative analgesia after herniorrhaphy.

B. The block should preferably be performed immediately after induction of general anesthesia, before the operation begins.

C. The nerves run beneath the internal oblique muscle just medial to the anterosuperior iliac spine and may be blocked by a fan-shaped infiltration of the abdominal wall in this region.

D. Bupivacaine 0.25% or 0.5% up to 2 mg/kg may be used. More complete analgesia may be obtained by using the 0.5% solution, but occasionally this concentration produces a transient motor block of the femoral nerve, with leg weakness.

XIV. Penile Block

A. The paired dorsal nerves pass inferior to the pubic bones on either side of the midline and supply the dorsal aspect of the penis and foreskin.

B. A block of these nerves provides pain relief after a circumcision but does not provide adequate analgesia after hypospadias repair.

C. Epinephrine-containing solutions should not be used, because vasoconstriction might result in damaging ischemia.

D. Bupivacaine 0.25% without epinephrine, up to 2 mg/kg, to a maximum dose of 1 ml in a small child and 6 ml in a large child is suggested.

XV. Brachial Plexus Block

A. The axillary approach is recommended because of its simplicity and lack of serious complications (e.g., pneumothorax).

B. It is easy to perform if the patient can abduct the arm and is further simplified by placing the hand behind the head.

C. This block is useful for forearm fractures, plastic surgery procedures, and insertion of dialysis shunts.

D. Performance of the block does not include anesthesia to the area of the upper arm and the area supplied by the musculocutaneous nerves. A supplemental block can be used to administer local anesthesia to this area.

E. Suggested local anesthetics.
   1. Lidocaine 1% with epinephrine 1:200,000, 0.3 to 0.5 ml/kg
   2. Bupivacaine 0.25%, 0.5 ml/kg

F. For the older child, a maximum volume of 20 ml is usually satisfactory.

G. Technique.
   1. With careful asepsis, after skin analgesia, advance a 1-inch long 25-gauge small vein needle cephalad, at a 45-degree angle to the skin, alongside and parallel to the axillary artery.
   2. A slight give or pop should be felt as the neurovascular sheath is entered.
   3. Support the needle gently, and connect plastic extension tubing with attached syringes of the local anesthetic.
   4. Aspirate and then inject the local anesthetic with periodic aspiration.
   5. Apply pressure distally over the axillary artery, which may promote proximal spread of the local anesthesia and a more complete block.
   6. The use of a nonstick material (Teflon)–coated block needle and nerve stimulator will more precisely direct needle placement in the brachial plexus by attaining distal (e.g., finger) twitches at a current intensity of <0.5 mA (see Fig. 24–6).

XVI. Intravenous Regional Anesthesia (Bier Block)

A. The Bier block may be useful in older children having limb lesions such as ganglions excised.

B. This technique involves insertion of a small IV catheter in the hand or foot.

C. A reliable double pneumatic tourniquet is necessary.

D. The success of the block is related to adequate limb exsanguination, which is achieved by elevation and wrap-

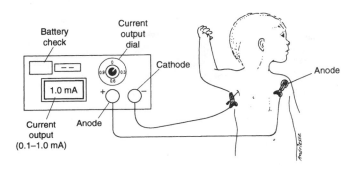

A

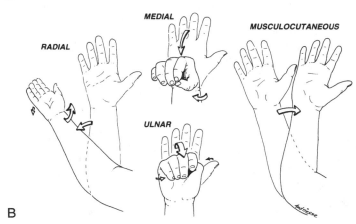

B

FIGURE 24–6. Performing an axillary block with a nerve stimulator. **A,** A nerve stimulator may be used to locate a nerve in a child who is anesthetized or who is too young to report the presence or absence of a paresthesia. In this example, the brachial plexus is sought in the axilla. Note that the appropriate muscle response to nerve stimulation is elicited at 0.5 mA current and should continue to respond with 0.2 mA current. **B,** Characteristic movements of the fingers, wrist, and elbow in response to nerve stimulation. (**A** from Coté, C.J., Ryan, J.F., Todres, I.D., & Goudsouzian, N.G. [Eds.]. [1993]. *A practice of anesthesia for infants and children* [2nd ed.]. Philadelphia: W.B. Saunders. **B** from Cousins, M.J., Bridenbaugh, P.O. [Eds.]. [1988]. *Neural blockade in clinical anesthesia and management of pain* [2nd ed., p. 406]. Philadelphia: J.B. Lippincott.)

ping with an Esmarch bandage before injection of the local anesthetic.

E. Inflate the proximal cuff, and inject the local anesthetic solution.

F. Do not exceed the following dose: 0.2% to 0.4% of preservative-free lidocaine 3 mg/kg.

G. Bupivacaine should never be used for an IV block because of its marked potential for cardiotoxicity.

H. When the block is established (usually within 5 minutes), inflate the distal cuff and deflate the proximal cuff.

I. It is recommended not to release the remaining cuff until at least 30 minutes have passed, even if the operation is finished sooner.

ADDITIONAL READINGS

Alifimoff, J.K., & Coté, C.J. (1993). Pediatric regional anesthesia. In C.J. Coté, J.F. Ryan, I.D. Todres, & N.G. Goudsouzian (Eds.). *A practice of anesthesia for infants and children* (2nd ed., pp. 429–450). Philadelphia: W.B. Saunders.

Berry, F.A., & Steward, D.J. (Eds.). (1993). *Pediatrics for the anesthesiologist.* New York: Churchill Livingstone.

Dobbins, P., & Hall, S.M. (1997). In J.J. Nagelhout & K.L. Zaglaniczny (Eds.). *Nurse anesthesia* (pp. 333–349). Philadelphia: W.B. Saunders.

Kart, T., Walther-Larden, S., Svejborg, T.F., et al. (1997). Comparison of continuous epidural infusion of fentanyl and bupivacaine with intermittent epidural administration of morphine for postoperative pain management in children. *Acta Anaesthesiologica Scandinavica, 41,* 461–465.

Polaner, D.M., & Berde, C.B. (1993). Postoperative pain management. In C.J. Coté, J.F. Ryan, I.D. Todres, & N.G. Goudsouzian (Eds.). *A practice of anesthesia for infants and children* (2nd ed., pp. 451–470). Philadelphia: W.B. Saunders.

Rogers, J., & Moro, M. (1994). Acute postoperative and chronic pain in children. In D.K. Rasch, & D.E. Webster (Eds.). *Clinical manual of pediatric anesthesia* (pp. 291–308). New York: McGraw-Hill.

Shayevitz, J.R., Merkel, S., O'Kelly, S.W., et al. (1996). Lumbar epidural morphine infusions for children undergoing cardiac surgery. *Journal of Cardiothoracic and Vascular Anesthesia* 10(2), 217–224.

Steward, D.J. (Ed.). (1995). *Manual of pediatric anesthesia* (4th ed., pp. 119–136 and 177–188). New York: Churchill Livingstone.

25

Postoperative Care

Theresa L. Culpepper, PhD, CRNA

I. Admission to Postanesthesia Care Unit

A. Transport from the operating room to the postanesthesia care unit (PACU) is a critical time in the emergence from anesthesia. Patients should be transported in the head down, lateral position to facilitate the management of the airway and to decrease the risk of aspiration. A minimum of a precordial stethoscope should be used in monitoring the patient in transit. Other monitoring modalities should be used based on the patient's condition and procedure performed.

B. The PACU nursing staff should be given a complete report about the patient before care is relinquished and the anesthesia provider's responsibility to that patient is completed. A report to the PACU nurse should include the following information:

1. Brief, concise history
   a. Drug allergies
   b. Preexisting diseases
   c. Long-term medications
   d. Premedication

2. Intraoperative information
   a. Procedure
   b. Type of anesthetic, agents used, and doses
      (1) Muscle relaxants and reversal status
      (2) Nonanesthetic drugs
   c. Status of fluid management plan
   d. Estimated blood loss
   e. Urine output
   f. Unexpected surgical or anesthetic events

3. Postoperative instructions
   a. Acceptable vital sign ranges
   b. Expected pain and plan for management
   c. Anticipated problems
   d. Responsible anesthesiologist or physician (where applicable)

II. Principal Goals of Recovery

A. Ventilation and oxygenation

1. Priority should be given to patency of the airway and adequacy of ventilation and oxygenation. Respiratory effort (chest excursion, retractions, nasal flaring), evidence of mechanical obstruction (stridor, wheezing, retractions), and presence or absence of cyanosis should be immediately evaluated.

2. Children are at increased risk for hypoxia secondary to decreased functional residual capacity (FRC), higher closing volumes, and greater oxygen consumption.

3. The chest should be auscultated and oxygen saturation determined immediately by pulse oximetry.

4. Measures to maintain or reestablish the airway should be undertaken if ventilation is not adequate.

5. Supplemental oxygen should be administered to maintain adequate oxygenation (see Table 25–1).

B. Return to conscious state

1. Return of a conscious state is determined by the redistribution of central nervous system (CNS) depressant drugs (anesthetic drugs) to sites away from the brain, to sites of metabolism and excretion.

2. The result is a return of cardiorespiratory reflexes—the gag and cough reflex to protect the airway, the baroreceptor reflexes to support perfusion, and the chemoreceptor responses to hypercarbia and hypoxia. Facial grimacing and opening of the eyes indicate wakefulness and a level of consciousness that will allow the appropriate assessment of pain.

C. Normothermia

1. Maintenance of normothermia is a challenge during and after any anesthetic, but it is an especially serious challenge in the infant and neonate. *Hypo*thermia and *hyper*thermia are common problems in this patient population.

2. The inability to regulate body temperature under general anesthesia; cold, dry anesthetic gases; cold operating rooms; and larger body surface area for heat loss (proportional to body weight) are the major causes of hypothermia.

3. The child responds to hypothermia by attempting to raise his or her temperature by shivering; this response is not well developed in the infant and neonate. Moreover, shivering increases oxygen consumption by as much as

TABLE 25-1. Goals of Recovery

Goals	Indicators
Adequate ventilation	Patent airway
	Clear breath sounds by auscultation
	Good chest excursion
	No stridor, retractions, or nasal flaring
	No wheezing
	Normal respiratory patterns without apnea or periodic breathing
Oxygenation	Spo_2 >90% on room air
	Acyanotic
Recovery of wakefulness	Return of cardiorespiratory reflexes
	Ability to prevent soft tissue airway obstruction
	Ability to cough
	Presence of baroreceptor and chemoreceptor reflexes
	Conscious: responds to verbal stimuli
Achievement of normothermia	Temperature of 36°C to 37°C
Reversal of neuromuscular blockade	Return of muscle strength: assess by peripheral nerve stimulation or clinical indices
	Inspiratory force >−20 cm H_2O
	Vital capacity >15 ml/kg
	Ability to protrude tongue and lift head for more than 5 s
	Knee flexion in infants
Pain relief	Ablation of physiologic responses indicating pain (i.e., tachycardia, hypertension, nausea and vomiting, agitation)
Relief of nausea and vomiting	Possibility of raised intracranial pressure, swallowed blood after tonsillectomy, severe gastric distention
Reduction of psychologic stress	Pain relief
	Parental presence to eliminate separation anxiety

Adapted from Shapiro, J. (1991). The post anesthesia recovery room. In *The pediatric anesthesia handbook* (revised edition, pp. 119–128). With permission.

200% to 600%, and the vasoconstriction response (to reduce heat loss) can result in metabolic acidosis.

4. *Hyper*thermia is more common in pediatric patients than in adults. It can result from aggressive warming in the perioperative period, dehydration, or after atropine administration. Just as quickly as temperature can decrease in children, it can also increase to dangerous levels.

D. Reversal of neuromuscular blockade

1. Residual neuromuscular blockade can impair adequate ventilation and oxygenation. The techniques used to monitor neuromuscular blockade in adults (full train-of-four and 50 Hz tetanic stimulus for 5 seconds; inspiratory force greater than −25 cm H_2O; vital capacity of at least 15 ml/kg) can be reliable in the toddler and school-age child.

2. Brisk flexion of the hips and knees is a sign of adequate neuromuscular function in the infant.

III. Additional Goals

A. Pain control

1. Pain is a protective mechanism and is initially beneficial; however, pain that is allowed to persist can be detrimental to the child, both physiologically and psychologically. Pain experiences, from preterm infants to older pediatric patients, result in a stress response.

2. Preterm infants and full-term neonates who have undergone surgery with minimal anesthesia have demonstrated a marked stress response. This stress response was shown to contribute to an increased morbidity and mortality in these infants.

3. Critically ill children who experience pain may demonstrate a decrease in lung volume, an increase in oxygen consumption, a decrease in mobility, and depletion of energy.

4. Crying is not always indicative of pain. More reliable indicators are
   a. Tachycardia
   b. Hypertension
   c. Tachypnea
   d. Agitation
   e. Nausea and vomiting
   f. Sweating

5. Moderate to severe pain can be treated with an intravenous (IV) opioid or agonist/antagonist. Less severe pain

can be treated with an acetaminophen suppository (see Table 25–2).

B. Control of nausea and vomiting

1. The cause of nausea and vomiting postoperatively must be determined to facilitate adequate and successful treatment. The mechanisms may be central, such as after opioid administration; a specific gastrointestinal problem, such as ileus or gastric distention, blood that has entered the stomach after tonsillectomy; or the presence of severe pain. A more serious mechanism is increased intracranial pressure.

2. Drugs commonly used to treat nausea and vomiting include droperidol, metoclopramide, phenothiazine drugs, and ondansetron (see Table 25–3).

C. Psychologic stress and emergence delirium

1. Anxiety associated with parental separation and disorientation from the residual effects of the anesthesia contribute to physiologic as well as behavioral problems after a surgical procedure. Manifestations include

   a. Restlessness
   b. Disorientation
   c. Crying
   d. Combative behavior
   e. Difficulty in communication

2. This has been shown to be more common after premedication with atropine, scopolamine, and barbiturates; pure inhalational anesthetics; or ketamine. Comfortable, gentle restraints; kinesthetic stimulation (stroking, handling); and such measures as warm blankets and a familiar toy may be reassuring.

TABLE 25–2. Pain Relief

Degree of Pain	Drugs	Techniques of Administration
Moderate to severe	Morphine, 0.1–0.2 mg/ kg IV Demerol, 1–2 mg/kg IV Fentanyl, 1–2 µg/kg IV Codeine, 0.5–1 mg/kg IV Butorphanol, 0.5–1 mg IV	Start with one fourth of dose, and titrate to effect Monitor for 30 min after administration
Moderate	Acetaminophen (per rectum), 20–40 mg/kg	Onset in approximately 30 min

IV, Intravenously.

TABLE 25–3. Treatment of Nausea and Vomiting

Drug	Dose
Droperidol	50–100 μg/kg IV or IM
Diphenhydramine	0.75–1 mg/kg IV or IM
Promethazine (Phenergan)	0.25–0.5 mg/kg IM
suppository	12.5–25 mg (total dose) PR
Metoclopramide	0.1–0.15 mg/kg
Ondansetron	0.15 mg/kg (max. 4 mg) IV
Prochlorperazine (Compazine suppository)	2.5–5 mg/kg (total dose) PR

IV, Intravenously; *IM*, intramuscularly; *PR*, rectally.

3. It is important to determine if this anxiety or delirium results from hypoxia, pain, or possibly hypoglycemia before assuming that the behavior is due to emergence from premedication or anesthesia.
4. Some institutions allow parents to be present in the PACU when the patient is stable. This policy is usually institution specific.

IV. Complications
A. Laryngospasm
1. Laryngospasm is more likely to occur in patients who have secretions or blood in the pharynx. On inspiration, the secretions touch the vocal cords, resulting in a spasm of the larynx.
2. Continuous positive pressure (5–10 cm H_2O) ventilation with bag and mask can successfully resolve the obstruction.
3. Intubation may be necessary, and pulmonary edema (postobstructive) could result. If this occurs, it should be treated with continued positive pressure ventilation and appropriate pharmacologic interventions.
B. Stridor
1. Stridor can occur from a partially obstructed airway or after the use of a large endotracheal tube or a traumatic laryngoscopy.
2. Conservative intervention consists of humidified oxygen and IV administration of dexamethasone (to reduce subglottic edema).
3. More aggressive therapy includes racemic epinephrine aerosol inhalation, and in the most severe instances, reintubation may be necessary.

C. Bronchospasm
1. Bronchospasm can occur as children are emerging from anesthesia, especially in children with a history of hyperactive airway disease and long-term treatment with bronchodilators (i.e., asthmatic patients).
2. The usual treatment is with albuterol (a beta$_2$-agonist), 0.25 mL in 2.5 mL saline delivered via face mask over 10 minutes.
3. Additional treatments may be administered in 30 minutes.
D. Pulmonary edema
1. Pulmonary edema can result from relative fluid overload in a child with poor cardiac reserve, absolute fluid overload in a healthy child, or complete airway obstruction and a strong attempt at inspiration (i.e., postobstructive pulmonary edema).
2. The standard treatment is to provide supplemental oxygen and positive pressure ventilation (reintubate if necessary). Administering diuretics, opioids, or sedatives may be necessary in certain cases. Furosemide, 1 mg/kg, and morphine sulfate, 0.05 mg/kg, are the recommendations of several experts.
3. If there are no underlying cardiovascular problems, the edema should abate within a few hours.
E. Aspiration
1. If vomiting occurs in the PACU and the child is somnolent from residual anesthesia, sedation, or pain management, aspiration is a very real risk.
2. The risk of this serious complication of recovery can be decreased by following several basic tenets:
   a. Proper positioning of recovering and sedated patients on their side to prevent vomitus from entering the pharynx
   b. Maintaining a strict NPO policy
   c. Suctioning the stomach after induction and before extubation
   d. Extubating patients with airway reflexes intact
3. If aspiration is suspected, a chest x-ray, oxygen saturation by pulse oximetry, and arterial blood gases (ABGs) should be obtained as a baseline.
4. If there are no symptoms of aspiration and there are no changes in the chest x-ray or ABGs within 4 hours, it can be safely determined that aspiration did not occur.
5. If major aspiration did occur, supportive therapy, such as intubation of the airway and mechanical ventilation of the lungs, should be instituted.

6. In less extreme cases, supplemental oxygen and possibly chest physiotherapy are all that is needed.

F. Hypotension

1. Hypotension, although rare in the pediatric patient, is usually the result of depleted intravascular volume. The exception to this may be the child with congenital heart disease.

2. The usual signs of hypovolemia (tachycardia, decreased pulses, decreased capillary refill, decreased urine output) could all be evidence of hypotension.

3. Fluid boluses of an isotonic crystalloid, albumin, or hetastarch, 5 to 10 ml/kg, can be used if the hematocrit is satisfactory. If the patient's hematocrit is low, red blood cells may be needed.

G. Hypertension

1. Pain is the most common cause for hypertension in the PACU. When pain is managed appropriately, blood pressure will usually decrease.

2. The manifestation of hypertension can also be a result of fluid overload. Diuretics may be needed, and, in the most extreme cases, dialysis may be necessary to decrease the vascular volume.

H. Dysrhythmias

1. Cardiac dysrhythmias are uncommon in children in the PACU except for children with congenital heart disease.

2. Tachycardia is usually a result of pain, hypercarbia, hypovolemia, emergence delirium, or atropine.

3. Bradycardia occurs with hypoxia, but vagal stimulation may also precipitate bradycardia.

4. Dysrhythmias that result from hypoxia or metabolic disturbances will abate with correction of the underlying problem.

5. Cardiac monitoring in the PACU is necessary only when there is documented need, such as in the child with congenital heart disease (repaired or unrepaired) or if other significant cardiovascular problems arise.

V. Criteria for Discharge

A. Recovery from anesthesia can be determined and decisions to discharge from the PACU can be made using a scoring system. Tables 25–4 and 25–5 show two scoring systems that assess a specific number of identified criteria and assign a point value to each.

B. The Aldrete scoring system (see Table 25–4), although oriented toward the adult population, is used in children,

TABLE 25–4. Aldrete Recovery Score

Criterion	Score
ACTIVITY	
Moves four extremities voluntarily or on command	2
Moves two extremities voluntarily or on command or moves weakly	1
Does not move any extremities voluntarily or on command	0
RESPIRATION	
Able to deep breathe, cough, or cry	2
Dyspneic or limited in breathing	1
Apneic	0
CIRCULATION	
BP ±20% of preanesthetic value	2
BP ±20%–50% of preanesthetic value	1
BP ±50% of preanesthetic value	0
CONSCIOUSNESS	
Fully awake	2
Arousable to stimuli	1
Unresponsive	0
COLOR	
Pink	2
Pale, dusky, blotchy, other	1
Cyanotic	0

BP, Blood pressure.

From Aldrete, J., & Kroulik, D. (1970). A postanesthetic recovery score. *Anesthesia and Analgesia, 49,* 924. With permission.

as well as the scoring system developed by Steward, (see Table 25–5).

1. There is no minimal length of time required before discharge from a physiologic perspective.
2. General criteria for patients being discharged to the care of another care unit
   a. Stable vital signs
   b. Patent airway with intact airway reflexes
   c. Awake or arousable state
   d. Acceptable level of activity
3. Before discharge to home in the care of a responsible adult, the following criteria should be met:
   a. Stable or near normal vital signs for that child
   b. Normal cough, gag, and swallow reflexes
   c. Normal coordination

TABLE 25–5. Steward Recovery Score

Criterion	Score
CONSCIOUSNESS	
Awake	2
Responding to stimuli	1
Not responding	0
AIRWAY	
Coughing on command or crying	2
Maintaining good airway	1
Airway requires maintenance	0
MOVEMENT	
Moving limbs purposefully	2
Nonpurposeful movement	1
Not moving	0

From Steward, D. (1975). A simplified scoring for the post-operative recovery room. *Canadian Anaesthesia Society Journal, 22*, 111. With permission.

   d. Controlled nausea without vomiting
   e. Alert, oriented, and comfortable patient
4. Taking fluids by mouth is not required before discharge. Outcomes are not affected if fluid deficits are addressed and adequate maintenance fluids were administered intraoperatively.
5. A requirement for voiding is not necessary, unless the urinary tract has been the site of the surgical procedure.

VI. Anesthesia Follow-up and Postanesthesia Visit

A. A postanesthesia visit should be done after the patient has been discharged to the unit to evaluate the condition of the patient and to document any postanesthetic complications.
B. A notation of this visit should be made in the patient's chart.
C. In the outpatient setting, the patient and parents should be given discharge instructions, and notation of any postanesthetic complications should be made in the patient's medical record.
D. A follow-up telephone call should be made to the patient or parents the following day to evaluate the patient's postanesthesia course.

ADDITIONAL READINGS

Aldrete, J., & Kroulik, D. (1970). A postanesthetic recovery score. *Anesthesia and Analgesia, 49*, 924.

Badgwell, J.M. (Ed.). (1997). *Clinical pediatric anesthesia.* Philadelphia: Lippincott-Raven.

Gregory, G. (1994). *Pediatric anesthesia* (3rd ed., Vol. 23). New York: Churchill Livingstone.

Ryan, J. (Ed.). (1993). *A practice of anesthesia for infants and children* (2nd ed.). Philadelphia: W.B. Saunders.

Shapiro, J. (1991). The post anesthesia recovery room. In Bell, C., & Kain, Z.N. (Eds.). *The pediatric anesthesia handbook* (revised edition, pp. 119–128). St Louis: Mosby.

Steward, D. (1975). A simplified scoring for the post-operative recovery room. *Canadian Anaesthesia Society Journal, 22,* 111.

26

Neonatal Anesthesia

Theresa L. Culpepper, PhD, CRNA

I. Introduction

Anesthesia for the neonate (0–4 weeks of age) often is required because of a life-threatening illness that requires surgical intervention. Except under extraordinary circumstances, all neonates require anesthesia for surgery. Physiologic development is in a transitional state, and congenital anomalies may be present. There is a tenfold incidence of intraoperative morbidity and mortality in neonates when compared to other age-groups of pediatric patients.

II. Preoperative Evaluation

A. Prenatal history
   1. Critical to the determination of the physiologic development of the neonate are the *gestational age* and *postconceptual age*.
      a. Gestational age is the actual number of weeks that the baby was in utero.
      b. Postconceptual age is the gestational age plus the chronologic age of the neonate. These ages indicate the functioning of the various organ systems.
      c. Newborns less than 26 weeks' gestational age have a higher mortality than infants born at 30 weeks' gestation.
   2. Delivery records reflect the difficulty of the delivery and the effect on the infant.
   3. The need for ventilatory and circulatory support is important in planning the intraoperative management of the neonate in need of surgery.

B. Initial evaluation: The preanesthetic assessment and neonatal anesthetic implications are listed in Table 26–1

C. Central nervous system
   1. Cortical activity is present, as documented by normal electroencephalogram (EEG) activity.
   2. Neonates hear, see, smell, and feel pain as early as 7 weeks' gestation.
   3. Myelination of sensory nerves is complete at birth;

TABLE 26–1. Preanesthetic Assessment and Neonatal Anesthetic Implications

System	Characteristics	Anesthetic Implications
CENTRAL NERVOUS	Incomplete myelination	Judicious use of muscle relaxants
	Lack of cerebral auto-regulation	Cerebral perfusion pressure control
	Cortical activity	Pain relief; adequate level of anesthesia
	Retinopathy of prematurity	Oxygen saturation (94%–98%)
RESPIRATORY		
Mechanical	↓ Lung compliance	Assist or control ventilation during general anesthesia
	↓ Elastic recoil	
	↓ Rigidity of chest wall	
	↓ V̇/Q̇ due to lung fluid	
	↑ Fatigue of respiratory muscles	
	↓ Coordination of nose and mouth breathing	Do not obstruct nasal passages
Anatomic	Large tongue	Consideration of airway management techniques
	Position of larynx, epiglottis, vocal folds, subglottic region	
Biochemical	Response to hypercapnia not potentiated by hypoxia	Avoid hypoxia Maintain normothermia
Reflex	Hering-Breuer reflex	Apnea/no desaturation/stimulation
	Periodic breathing	
	Apnea	Stimulation/airway support
CARDIOVASCULAR	↓ Myocardial contractility/↓ myocardial compliance	Maintain adequate volume
	CO rate dependent	Maintain heart rate
	Vagotonic	Use vagolytic agent
	Limited sympathetic innervation	
	Reactive pulmonary vasculature	Avoid hypoxemia resulting in ↓ pulmonary blood flow and possible shunting
	PDA/FO shunting	

Table continued on following page

TABLE 26-1. Preanesthetic Assessment and Neonatal Anesthetic Implications *Continued*

System	Characteristics	Anesthetic Implications
RENAL	↓ GFR	Maintain vascular volume/CO
	↓ Tubular function	Avoid overhydration
	Low glucose threshold	Avoid excess glucose (0.5–1 g/kg)
HEPATIC	Depressed hepatic enzymes	Judicious use of drugs metabolized by liver
	↓ Metabolism and clearance of drugs	
	Altered (decreased) protein binding	
	Hypoglycemia due to ↓ glycogen stores	
	Low prothrombin levels	Vitamin K (1 mg) before surgery
HEMATOLOGIC	Fetal hemoglobin (does not readily release O_2 to tissues)	Avoid hypoxia
	Oxyhemoglobin curve shifted left	

↓, Decreased; ↑, increased; $\dot{V}/\dot{Q}$, ventilation/perfusion ratio; *CO*, cardiac output; *PDA*, patent ductus arteriosus; *FO*, foramen ovale; *GFR*, glomerular filtration rate.

however, motor nerve myelination is not complete until 2 years of age.
4. Anesthetic and opioid doses and effects can differ because of alterations in the blood-brain barrier.
5. Lack of cerebral autoregulation increases the incidence of intraventricular hemorrhage with changes in cerebral perfusion pressure.
6. Retinopathy of prematurity is a risk in neonates less than 35 weeks' postconceptual age and weighing less than 2 kg when these neonates are exposed to high concentrations of oxygen for extended periods.
D. Respiratory system
1. Mechanical differences
a. The lungs are less compliant and have less elastic recoil.
b. The soft chest wall does not provide stability for an

opposing force to the descent of the diaphragm during inspiration or the maintenance of functional residual capacity (FRC).

c. The respiratory muscles are more prone to fatigue in the presence of increased airway resistance and increased work of breathing, making the neonate vulnerable to respiratory failure.

d. There is a ventilation-perfusion mismatch at birth because of lung fluid. However, this becomes more equal during the first few hours of life.

e. A deficiency of lung surfactant results in uneven distribution of ventilation, reduced compliance, and increased work of breathing.

f. Converting from nasal to oral breathing may be difficult if the nasal passages are obstructed.

2. Anatomic differences in the neonatal airway compared with the adult airway

a. Tongue: relatively large in proportion to oral cavity

b. Position of the larynx: C3–4 versus C4–5; "higher" in the neck

c. Epiglottis: longer, narrower, omega shaped, angled away from axis of trachea

d. Vocal folds: lower attachment anteriorly than posteriorly

e. Subglottic region: narrowest portion of infant's airway versus rima glottis in the adult

3. Ventilatory/biochemical control

a. Neonates' response to hypercapnia is not potentiated by hypoxia.

b. The response of the neonate to hypoxia is biphasic. There is a period of increased ventilation followed by a depressed ventilation.

c. Cool environmental temperatures will result in respiratory depression in the presence of hypoxia.

4. Reflex control of ventilation

a. The Hering-Breuer reflex (induced apnea in response to lung inflation) is present during the first few weeks of life.

b. Periodic breathing (apnea without desaturation, bradycardia, or muscle tone loss) is common.

c. Clinical apnea (desaturation, bradycardia, muscle tone loss) is present in as many as 25% of premature infants. It may resolve with stimulation, but the infant may require complete airway support.

E. Cardiovascular system
   1. The neonatal myocardium has fewer contractile elements, making it less compliant and less contractile.
   2. Decreased compliance results in limitation of augmentation of stroke volume if heart rate slows, making cardiac output rate dependent.
   3. Sympathetic innervation is limited, and vagal influences dominate.
   4. Normal heart rate in the neonate is 120 ± 20 bpm, and normal blood pressure is $\pm 70/45$ mm Hg. There is a limited ability to adapt to changes in intravascular volume, and hypovolemia results in decreased cardiac output and hypotension.
   5. Baroreceptor reflexes are absent in anesthetized neonates; thus the systemic blood pressure reflects the intravascular volume.
   6. Pulmonary vessels are very reactive; hypoxemia or acidosis increases pulmonary vascular resistance and decreases pulmonary blood flow, leading to further hypoxemia and increased right ventricular afterload.
   7. Arterial hypoxemia, hypercapnia, or acidosis will reverse transitional circulation to a fetal circulatory pattern.
   8. A patent ductus arteriosus could allow shunting of blood past the lungs. As pressure in the right side of the heart increases, shunting can also occur via the foramen ovale, resulting in a state of persistent fetal circulation.
F. Renal system
   1. Neonates have a lower glomerular filtration rate (GFR) and reduced tubular function. This results in an inability to excrete a fluid or solute overload.
   2. The renal threshold for glucose is low, resulting in hyperglycemia if excess glucose is given.
   3. Hyperglycemia precipitates osmotic diuresis that can lead to hypovolemia, hypotension, electrolyte loss, and decreased cardiac output.
   4. Renal function approximates adult values by the end of the first year.
G. Hepatic system
   1. Metabolic functions of the liver depend on adequate hepatic blood flow.
   2. The capacity to enzymatically break down proteins is depressed at birth.
   3. In the first 4 weeks of life, drug metabolism is less efficient because of the reduced concentration and activity of enzyme systems.

4. Clearance of drugs metabolized in the liver is lower and more variable than in older infants.
5. Protein binding is altered because of decreased plasma levels of albumin and other serum proteins.
6. Hypoglycemia is a significant risk because of decreased glycogen stores.
7. Prothrombin levels can be low, and hemorrhagic disease of the neonate is a risk during surgery. Vitamin K (1 mg) should be administered before surgery.

H. Hematologic system
   1. High fetal hemoglobin (Hgb) levels reduce oxygen-releasing capacity at the tissue level.
   2. Hgb <30% correlates with increased incidence of postoperative apnea in infants <60 weeks' postconceptual age.
   3. A "normal" physiologic anemia occurs as fetal hemoglobin is replaced by adult Hgb.
   4. The neonatal oxyhemoglobin dissociation curve is shifted to the left, and as maturation to adult Hgb occurs, the curve shifts to the right.
   5. Hgb levels stabilize at 2 to 3 years of age.

I. Evaluation of metabolism
   1. Thermoregulation
      a. Hypothermia begins to develop at ambient temperature of 23°C (75°F).
      b. Neonates cannot shiver, and they have underdeveloped sweat glands.
      c. Nonshivering thermogenesis (brown fat metabolism) is a heat-producing, oxygen-consuming mechanism to generate heat.
      d. Cool temperatures and anesthetic agents can convert the thermoregulatory system to poikilothermic.
   2. Glucose
      a. Hypoglycemia is common because of decreased glycogen stores and inadequate gluconeogenesis.
      b. Normal serum glucose is 80 to 120 mg/dl.
      c. Hypoglycemia is defined as a blood glucose level of <35 mg/dl.
      d. Clinical manifestations are tremors, apnea, cyanotic spells, convulsions, limpness, hypothermia, sweating, refusal to feed, and cardiac failure.
      e. Treatment is with 10% dextrose infusion, 5 mg/kg/min, or, if emergent, 50% dextrose (diluted to 10% before injection), 1–2 ml/kg.
      f. Nontreatment can result in neurologic damage in as many as 50% of neonates.

g. Hyperglycemia (blood levels >120 mg/dl) can be due to inadequate insulin release or excess administration of glucose-containing intravenous (IV) fluids.

h. Hyperglycemia can induce an osmotic diuresis resulting in water and electrolyte depletion or osmotic cerebral fluid shifts that could result in cerebral hemorrhage.

3. Calcium
   a. Hypocalcemia is common at birth because of immature parathyroid function and decreased vitamin D stores.
   b. Hypocalcemia is noted when the total serum calcium level is <7 mg/dl or ionized calcium is <4 mg/dl.
   c. Clinical manifestations are jitteriness, twitching, convulsions, and hypotension.
   d. Treatment includes an infusion of 10% calcium gluconate or chloride, 100 to 200 mg/kg, while monitoring the electrocardiogram (ECG).

III. Drug Distribution

A. Differences exist in uptake, distribution, metabolism, and excretion of all drugs.

B. The integrity and maturity of the blood-brain barrier and receptor sensitivity also affect drug performance.

C. Protein binding is decreased because of a decreased amount of total protein, making a larger free fraction of the drug available to penetrate target organs.

D. There is a larger volume of distribution, diluting the plasma concentration of parentally administered drugs and necessitating a larger mg/kg dose to achieve effect.

E. Approximately 30% of the cardiac output is received by the brain, allowing higher concentrations of any lipophilic or inhalational anesthetic to be achieved more quickly than expected.

F. Drugs metabolized by the liver will have a longer half-life because of decreased liver blood flow and immature liver function.

G. Drugs excreted by the kidneys depend on GFR and tubular function, both of which are immature during the first few weeks of life.

IV. Choice of Anesthetic Agents

A. Inhalation agents
   1. A neonate will attain a higher concentration of inhalation agent in the brain and heart, at the same inspired concentration, than an adult.

2. The uptake of inhalants is rapid because of large alveolar ventilation compared to FRC, high cardiac output to vessel-rich organs, and lower blood/gas solubility ratio.

3. Minimal alveolar concentration (MAC) is significantly lower in newborns than in infants. In premature infants, MAC is significantly lower than in full-term infants (see Table 26–2). The result can be severe hypotension and bradycardia because of an unintentional overdose of inhalation agent.

4. Elimination of volatile agents is rapid with adequate cardiorespiratory function.

B. Opioids

1. Neonates and premature infants metabolize opioids more slowly than older infants. Repeated doses for analgesia or anesthesia may lead to accumulation and respiratory depression.

2. When combined with oxygen and a vagolytic agent (atropine or pancuronium), general anesthesia can be achieved with minimal hemodynamic instability. The use of opioids as a primary anesthetic agent will most likely result in postoperative intubation and assisted ventilation (see Table 26–3).

C. Muscle relaxants

1. All nondepolarizing muscle relaxants rapidly and effectively paralyze the neonate.

2. Choice of drug is more often based on the other properties of the relaxant, namely, vagolysis, metabolism, and elimination (see Table 26–4).

3. Neonates are resistant to succinylcholine. Dose requirements are higher, and there is significant risk for many cardiac dysrhythmias, including bradycardia, sinus arrest, nodal rhythms, and ventricular ectopy.

4. Reversal of neuromuscular block can be successful with the same conventional dose requirements for atropine (0.02 mg/kg), glycopyrrolate (0.01 mg/kg), and neostig-

TABLE 26–2. Minimal Alveolar Concentrations of Volatile Anesthetics in Neonates and Infants

Volatile Agent	Preterm Infants	Neonates	Infants
Halothane (%)	0.55	0.87	1.2
Isoflurane (%)	1.3	1.45	1.6
Desflurane (%)	9.16	9.2	9.4
Sevoflurane (%)		3.3	3.2

TABLE 26-3. Intravenous Opioids for General Anesthesia in the Neonate

Drug	Neonate	Advantages	Disadvantages
Fentanyl	5–10 µg/kg: adjuvant 75–150 µg/kg: cardiac surgery	Minimal hemodynamic changes	Bradycardia Chest wall rigidity
Morphine	0.1–0.2 mg/kg	Intraoperative and postoperative analgesia Smoother awakening	Histamine release, vasodilation, hypotension, respiratory depression Crosses blood-brain barrier readily Elimination and clearance prolonged
Meperidine	1–2 mg/kg	Less respiratory depression than morphine	Readily crosses blood-brain barrier
Sufentanil	10–30 µg/kg	5–10 × more potent than fentanyl Long acting Superior to fentanyl in preventing hemodynamic changes intraoperatively	Bradycardia Chest wall rigidity Longer elimination Lower clearance
Alfentanil infusion	20–120 µg/kg/min	Rapid onset Rapid elimination Smaller volume of distribution	Bradycardia Chest wall rigidity
Remifentanil infusion	1–5 µg/kg IV bolus; 0.1–0.8 µg/kg/min	Smaller volume of distribution Rapid onset Rapid elimination	Very short acting Needs supplementation with other opioids for postoperative pain

TABLE 26–4. Muscle Relaxant Doses

Drug	Intubation Dose (mg/kg)*	Maintenance Dose (mg/kg)†
Succinylcholine	2	
Pancuronium	0.1	0.04–0.06
Atracurium	0.3–0.5	0.20
Vecuronium	0.07–0.1	0.02
Mivacurium	0.2	0.1
Cisatracurium	0.2	0.05
Rocuronium	0.6–1.2	0.15

*Two times the effective dose (ED_{95}).
†ED_{95}.

mine (0.05 mg/kg) as in older children. It is advisable to give atropine or glycopyrrolate separately, before neostigmine, to prevent bradycardia.

V. Regional Anesthesia

A. Regional anesthesia can be safely used alone or in combination with general anesthesia.
B. Spinal anesthesia may be useful in preterm or sick neonates with lung disease and an abdominal lesion. The risk of postoperative apnea may be less.
   1. The spinal cord ends at L3, so puncture is performed at L4–5 with a 22-gauge neonatal spinal needle (see Table 26–5 for dose).
   2. The dural space extends to S3–4.
C. Caudal block is safely done for procedures below the umbilicus and for postoperative pain relief.
   1. Landmarks are the tip of the coccyx at midline and the bilateral sacral cornua laterally.
   2. Perform puncture with a 23-gauge or 25-gauge needle directed cephalad at a 45-degree angle to the skin and advanced through the sacrococcygeal ligament (see Table 26–5 for dose).
D. Continuous caudal/epidural analgesia in combination with general anesthesia can be used for major abdominal or thoracic procedures in the neonate, that is, tracheoesophageal fistula repair, abdominal wall defect repair, and minor procedures such as inguinal hernia or pyloromyotomy.
E. Ilioinguinal and iliohypogastric nerve blocks can be done.
   1. These blocks affect innervation to the inguinal and scrotal (L1) area.

TABLE 26–5. Regional Anesthesia/Local Anesthetic Doses for Neonates

Type of Block	Drug	Dose (volume)	Maximum Dose (mg/kg)
Caudal/epidural Below umbilicus Up to T4	Bupivacaine 0.25% with epinephrine 1:200 K	0.5 ml/kg 1 ml/kg	3
Spinal	Tetracaine	1 mg/kg in equal volume $D_{10}W$	1.5
Ilioinguinal/iliohypogastric block	Bupivacaine 0.25%	0.5–1 ml/kg	3
Penile block	Bupivacaine 0.25% *without epinephrine*	1 ml/kg	3
	Lidocaine 1% *without epinephrine*	1–2 ml (total)	7

2. They are done 1 to 1.5 cm superior and medial to the anterior superior iliac crest deep to the external oblique fascia.
F. A penile block can be used to provide complete anesthesia and analgesia for circumcision.
   1. Bilateral injections of lidocaine or bupivacaine (without epinephrine) are given beneath the pubis at the base of the penis at 11 o'clock and 1 o'clock.
   2. A ring block can be done at the base of the penis with lidocaine or bupivacaine without epinephrine.
G. Complications that occur are most often related to local anesthesia toxicity (see Table 26–5).

VI. Premedication

A. Sedative premedication is unnecessary in healthy infants younger than 8 months of age because they have little anxiety and are unable to understand what is going to occur.
B. The exception is the infant who needs major surgery, such as cardiac surgery, and who would benefit from sedation because it will reduce irritability and minimize oxygen consumption.
C. Infants younger than 6 months are more prone to airway obstruction and respiratory depression after sedation.
D. In most neonates the only premedication necessary is

atropine for its vagolytic effect. Atropine, 0.01 to 0.02 mg/kg, or glycopyrrolate, 0.005 to 0.01 mg/kg, is recommended. This is especially important in infants <6 months since their cardiac output is rate dependent.

VII. Fasting

A. Esophageal motility and gastric motility are low, and some degree of reflux occurs continuously. The cardioesophageal sphincter mechanism does not develop until the end of the first year. Up to 40% of any feed may be in the stomach 2 hours later, depending on the type of fluid and the condition of the baby.

B. Prolonged fasting increases the possibility of both hypoglycemia and dehydration.

C. For elective procedures *a milk feed, to include breast milk, may be given up to 4 hours before surgery and clear fluids may be given up to 2 hours preoperatively.*

D. Clear fluids (4-6 oz) can be given up to 2 hours before surgery without increasing the volume of gastric fluid or decreasing its pH.

VIII. Anesthetic Equipment

Anatomic differences in the face and upper airway affect the design of masks, laryngoscopes, and tracheal tubes. Physiologically, the need to minimize resistance and dead space has design implications for breathing systems, connectors, and tubes.

A. Breathing systems

1. The ideal pediatric anesthetic circuit should be lightweight with low resistance and dead space; adaptable to spontaneous, assisted, or controlled ventilation; and readily humidified and scavenged.

2. The Mapleson D or some modification of the Mapleson system is the most common nonrebreathing system. Other common systems are the Jackson-Rees (a modification of the Ayer's T-piece and the coaxial Bain system).

3. Recommendations for necessary fresh gas flow (FGF) to prevent rebreathing vary. Historically, an FGF 2.5 times the patient's minute volume was thought to be necessary to prevent rebreathing during intermittent positive pressure ventilation (IPPV). Other recommendations indicate that lower FGF can be used (see Table 26–6).

4. The standard adult circle system can be modified for use in neonates by incorporating smaller-diameter breathing tubes. It is more economical, but the circuit resistance is higher and the possibility of valve malfunction leads to

TABLE 26–6. Recommended Fresh Gas Flow Formulas to Prevent Rebreathing

Formula (ml/kg/min)	Anticipated ET_{CO_2} (mm Hg)
250	38
500	30

possible risk of increased work of breathing, especially during spontaneous ventilation. The circle system does facilitate end-tidal carbon dioxide monitoring, and there is less mixing of expired and inspired gases than in the T-piece systems.

B. Ventilators
   1. Two methods of mechanical ventilation for the neonate are available:
      a. Conversion of adult to pediatric ventilator: Start with low-set tidal volumes, and progressively increase the delivered tidal volume until chest expansion is appropriate and peak inspiratory pressure (PIP), end-tidal CO_2, and oxygen saturations are adequate.
      b. Volume-controlled ventilation: Start with larger tidal volumes to compensate for the compression volume of the circle system and CO_2 cannister. The risk of volume ventilation is barotrauma. The modern anesthesia ventilators have pressure-limiting valves that can be set to prevent excessive PIP and allow a leak at approximately 30 cm H_2O.

C. Masks
   1. Prevent increasing dead space by obtaining a good fit.
   2. Clear mask to observe for regurgitation.
   3. Do not occlude nostrils with mask (neonates are preferential nasal breathers).
   4. Avoid pressure on the eyes from a mask that is too large.

D. Laryngoscopy/laryngoscopes
   1. If it is anticipated that the intubation will be difficult (e.g., Pierre Robin syndrome), muscle relaxants should be avoided.
   2. If visualization of the glottis is difficult, it can be located by seeing bubbles of saliva as the baby breathes in and out.
   3. It may help to use the bougie, threaded through the endotracheal tube or alone, to locate the glottic opening. If it is used alone, the appropriate endotracheal tube is threaded over the bougie into the trachea.

4. Position is critical. A neutral position (neither flexed nor extended) with a towel under the shoulders (to offset the large occiput) will align the oral and tracheal axes, making the angle less acute and exposure of the glottis easier. Laryngoscopy in the neutral position requires the laryngoscope blade to be at almost a 90-degree angle to the operating room table.

5. The anatomy of the upper airway makes a straight blade preferable. The blade is placed along the right side of the mouth, sweeping the tongue to the left. The epiglottis is picked up with the tip of the blade and the tracheal inlet exposed. The tube is inserted with the convex side to the left. When the tip approaches the glottic opening, rotate the tube 90 degrees counterclockwise. There are several types of straight-bladed laryngoscopes: Anderson-Magill, Seward, Flagg, Robertshaw, and Miller. They should be evaluated based on how well they allow the large tongue of the neonate to be manipulated out of the visual field. There are also modifications of straight blades that allow insufflation of oxygen into the pharynx during intubation.

E. Tracheal tubes
   1. Size
      a. Endotracheal tube size for neonates cannot be calculated by formula because of the rapid growth during the immediate postnatal period. It can be determined from a table based on age (see Table 26–7). It is common for the full-term neonate to accommodate a 3.0 mm oral endotracheal tube and a premature infant (<2 kg) to need a 2.5 mm oral endotracheal tube.
      b. A clinical shortcut is to look at the size of the tip of the fifth (pinkie) finger.
      c. It is wise to select a tube that will result in an air leak at 20 to 30 cm H_2O pressure to avoid postextubation airway edema.
   2. Insertion distance

TABLE 26–7. Recommended Endotracheal Tube Sizes for Neonates and Infants

Patient's Age	Size	Type
Premature neonate	2.0–3.0	No cuff
Full-term neonate	3.0–3.5	No cuff
3 mo to 1 yr	4.0	No cuff

a. The length of the trachea (vocal cords to carina) in neonates and infants up to 1 year varies from 5 to 9 cm. Insertion distance of an oral endotracheal tube should be <10 cm, falling within the 8 to 10 cm range.
3. Cuffed versus uncuffed tubes
   a. Cuffed endotracheal tubes *should not* be used in neonates. Cuffed tubes require that a smaller size be used to accommodate the cuff, and there is an increase in airway resistance and the work of breathing.
   b. The cuff can exert excessive pressure against the walls of the trachea, resulting in tissue damage.

F. Monitors
1. Precordial stethoscope
   a. Listening to the strength of heart tones is an early indicator of changes in cardiac function. A faint heart tone indicates possible decreasing cardiac output and hypovolemia that may manifest itself as hypotension.
   b. When the stethoscope is placed over the left hemithorax, it may indicate displacement of the tip of the endotracheal tube into the right mainstem bronchus.
2. Blood pressure
   a. Accuracy depends on utilization of proper cuff size; the cuff should be 4 cm or one half to three fourths the length of the upper arm.
   b. Inflation and deflation times must be short to avoid venous stasis, petechial hemorrhages, and skin damage.
   c. Automated blood pressure cuffs and manual cuffs with Doppler placed over the brachial or radial artery can be used successfully.
3. Pulse oximetry
   a. Probes placed on the right arm correlate with preductal saturations, whereas lower extremity readings correlate with postductal saturations.
   b. Arterial saturations of 94% to 98% are acceptable, and 92% to 96% saturations are not uncommon in preterm neonates.
4. Capnography
   a. Position of sampling port determines accuracy.
      (1) Side stream: Samples are taken directly from the airway.
      (2) Main stream: Samples are taken at proximal end of breathing system; high gas flows produce dilutional effect, underestimating CO_2.
      (3) Patients with pulmonary shunts (present in congenital heart disease [CHD]) show significant

differences between arterial and expired CO_2, making capnography a trend indicator.

  5. Temperature monitoring
     a. Skin temperature monitors are not accurate; they are only trend indicators.
     b. Esophageal temperatures should be measured in the lower third of the esophagus to avoid false low readings caused by high gas flows into trachea.
     c. Nasopharyngeal probes reflect core temperature; correct insertion distance is measured from nares to auditory meatus.
     d. Tympanic probes are accurate for measuring core temperature; risk is perforation of tympanic membrane.
     e. Rectal probes are reliable; risk is displacement intraoperatively.

IX. Airway Management

  A. Awake intubation, almost universal in the past, is now most often reserved for the sickest neonates. Struggling during intubation risks hypoxia, hypertension, and intraventricular hemorrhage.
  B. Most neonates requiring surgical procedures are intubated under general anesthesia with or without the aid of a short-acting muscle relaxant.
  C. Extubation is performed when the neonate is fully awake (moving all limbs, eyes open, brow furrowed) and when respiratory effort is adequate in rate and depth.
  D. There should be no signs of intercostal retractions or nasal flaring.
  E. The tube is removed with compression of the breathing bag to stimulate the cough reflex and maximally fill the lungs with oxygen.
  F. There may be a period of breath holding, apnea, or even laryngospasm following extubation. This can be managed by a jaw thrust or gentle "fluttering" compression of the reservoir bag. Reintubation may be required.

X. State of Hydration

  A. Determination of hypovolemia through the following clinical signs:
     1. Dry mucous membranes
     2. Depressed anterior fontanelle
     3. Poor skin turgor
     4. Central venous pressure (CVP) <3 cm H_2O

B. Fluid management
   1. Calculate maintenance rate (see Table 26–8) and fluid deficit.
   2. Follow fluid administration plan (see Table 26–9).
   3. Administer glucose at 5 to 7 mg/kg/min (300–420 mg/kg/h) to keep blood glucose concentration <120 mg/dl.
   4. Third-space fluid replacement is 8 to 15 ml/kg/h of lactated Ringer's solution or albumin (determined by amount of tissue trauma).
   5. Normal saline, 0.25%, results in hyponatremia and water overload.
   6. Do not use D_5W and other hypotonic solutions to avoid water overload and seizures.
C. Measuring blood loss
   1. Weigh sponges (4×4 inch *dry* sponge = 10–15 ml; dry lap pack = 100 ml).
   2. Use graduated "mini suction" (total capacity 50–250 ml).
D. Blood replacement
   1. Calculate allowable blood loss (ABL):

$$ABL = \text{Weight (kg)} \times EBV \times \frac{(Hm - He)}{Hm}$$

   where EBV = estimated blood volume, Hm = measured hematocrit, and He = lowest acceptable hematocrit (35%–40%).
   2. Replace whole blood ml for ml with a syringe or pump.
   3. Red blood cells (RBCs) are given as follows: two thirds in RBCs and one third at 3:1 ratio with crystalloid.
   4. Albumin 5% is given at 10 ml/kg.
   5. Include any diluent used in total fluid balance.

TABLE 26–8. Recommended Daily and Hourly Fluid Maintenance Rate

Weight (kg)	Hourly	Daily
<10	4 ml/kg	100 ml/kg
10–20	40 ml + 2 ml/kg for every kg >10	1000 ml + 50 ml/kg for every kg >10
>20	60 ml + 1 ml/kg for every kg >20	1500 ml + 20 ml/kg for every kg >20

TABLE 26–9. Fluid Administration Plan

First Hour	Second Hour	Third Hour	Fourth Hour
One half of fluid deficit + Maintenance*	One fourth of fluid deficit + Maintenance + Third-space loss + Blood loss	One fourth of fluid deficit + Maintenance + Third-space loss + Blood loss	Maintenance + Third-space loss + Blood loss

*The amount of dextrose administered in IV fluids should be limited to 0.5–1 g/kg.

XI. Pain Management

A. Neonates mount an appropriate stress response to pain and surgery

B. Physiologic indicators of pain
   1. Increased heart rate or blood pressure
   2. Increased respiratory rate
   3. Palmar sweating

C. Behavioral indicators of pain
   1. Facial grimacing
   2. Body movements involving active and precise avoidance of pain
   3. Changes in sleep patterns
   4. Changes in cry

D. Pain relief method
   1. Pharmacologic
      a. Opioids (IV)
         (1) Morphine, 50 to 100 µg/kg
         (2) Meperidine, 1 mg/kg
         (3) Fentanyl, 0.5 to 1 µg/kg
         (4) Sufentanil (Sufenta), 0.2 to 0.6 µg/kg
      b. Nonopioids
         (1) Codeine, 1 mg/kg orally
         (2) Acetaminophen, 20 to 40 mg/kg rectally
         (3) Butorphanol (Stadol), 0.01 to 0.04 mg/kg IV
      c. Regional block (see V. Regional Anesthesia)
         (1) Caudal
         (2) Ileoinguinal block
         (3) Penile block
         (4) Local infiltration

2. Nonpharmacologic
   a. Positioning; side or prone
   b. Swaddling or nesting
   c. Nonnutritive sucking (pacifier)
   d. Kinesthetic, vestibular, tactile stimulation (holding, stroking, etc.)

XII. Recovery

A. Neutral thermal environment; incubators or radiant heat warmers
B. Clothing when possible to avoid evaporative heat loss
C. Diligent monitoring of temperature
D. Oxygen via hood (avoid excessive moisture, to prevent overhydration); continuous positive airway pressure
E. Continuous oxygen saturation monitoring
F. Apnea monitoring
G. Ventilation parameters (if indicated)
H. ECG monitoring
I. Noninvasive or invasive blood pressure monitoring

ADDITIONAL READINGS

Bell, C., Hughes, C., & Oh, T. (1991). *The pediatric anesthesia handbook,* St. Louis: Mosby–Year Book.

Cote, C., Ryan, J., Todres, I.D., & Goudsouzian, N. (Eds.). (1993). *A practice of anesthesia for infants and children* (2nd ed.). Philadelphia: W.B. Saunders.

Gregory, G. (1994). *Pediatric anesthesia* (3rd ed.). New York: Churchill Livingstone.

Lake, C.L. (1988). *Pediatric cardiac anesthesia.* Norwalk, CT: Appleton and Lange.

Othersen, H.B. (1991). *The pediatric airway.* Philadelphia: W.B. Saunders.

Steward, D.J. (1990). *Manual of pediatric anesthesia* (4th ed.). New York: Churchill Livingstone.

Anesthesia Care Plans

Kathy Swendner, MSN, CRNA

Premature—Approximate Weight: <3 kg

Endotracheal tube:	2.5 cm
Depth (according to weight):	500 g @ 6 cm
	1000 g @ 7 cm
	2000 g @ 8 cm
	3000 g @ 9 cm
Laryngeal mask airway:	Size 1
Maximum cuff volume:	Up to 4 ml
Atropine (0.01 mg/kg) (0.4 mg/ml):	0.1 mg (0.25 ml)
Succinylcholine (Anectine) (2 mg/kg) (20 mg/ml):	
	According to weight
Epinephrine (0.1 mg/kg) (1:10,000):	According to weight
Blade:	#0 Miller
Bag:	500 ml
System:	Nonrebreathing
Maintenance fluids:	According to weight
Blood pressure (BP) (systolic):	40–60 mm Hg
Heart rate (HR):	120–180/min
Respiratory rate (RR):	50–60/min
Estimated blood volume (EBV):	90 ml/kg
Tidal volume:	6 ml/kg

Newborn—Approximate Weight: 3–4 kg

Endotracheal tube:	3.0–3.5
Depth:	10 cm
Laryngeal mask airway:	Size 1
Maximum cuff volume:	Up to 4 ml
Atropine (0.01 mg/kg) (0.4 mg/ml):	0.1 mg (0.25 ml)
Succinylcholine (Anectine) (2 mg/kg) (20 mg/ml):	8 mg (0.4 ml)
Epinephrine (0.1 mg/kg) (1:10,000):	0.3–0.4 mg (0.3–0.4 ml)
Blade:	#0 Miller
Bag:	500 ml
System:	Nonrebreathing
Maintenance fluids:	16 ml/h + NPO
BP (systolic):	50–70 mm Hg
HR:	100–180/min
RR:	35–40/min
EBV (90 ml/kg):	270–360 ml
Tidal volume (6 ml/kg):	18–24 ml

1 Month—Approximate Weight: 4 kg

Endotracheal tube:	3.5
Depth:	10 cm
Laryngeal mask airway:	Size 1
Maximum cuff volume:	Up to 4 ml
Atropine (0.01 mg/kg) (0.4 mg/ml):	0.1 mg (0.25 ml)
Succinylcholine (Anectine) (2 mg/kg) (20 mg/ml):	8 mg (0.4 ml)
Epinephrine (0.1 mg/kg) (1:10,000):	0.4 mg (0.4 ml)
Blade:	#1 Miller
Bag:	500 ml
System:	Nonrebreathing
Maintenance fluids:	16 ml/h + NPO
BP (systolic):	50–70 mm Hg
HR:	100–180/min
RR:	35–40/min
EBV (80 ml/kg):	320 ml
Tidal volume (6 ml/kg):	24 ml

3 Months—Approximate Weight: 5 kg

Endotracheal tube:	3.5
Depth:	10 cm

Laryngeal mask airway:	Size 1.5
Maximum cuff volume:	Up to 7 ml

Atropine (0.01 mg/kg) (0.4 mg/ml):	0.1 mg (0.25 ml)
Succinylcholine (Anectine) (2 mg/kg) (20 mg/ml):	10 mg (0.5 mg)
Epinephrine (0.1 mg/kg) (1:10,000):	0.5 mg (0.5 ml)

Blade:	#1 Miller
Bag:	500 ml
System:	Nonrebreathing
Maintenance fluids:	20 ml/h + NPO
BP (systolic):	60–110 mm Hg
HR:	100–180/min
RR:	24–30/min
EBV (80 ml/kg):	400 ml
Tidal volume (6 ml/kg):	30 ml

6 Months—Approximate Weight: 7 kg

Endotracheal tube:	3.5–4.0
Depth:	10–11 cm

Laryngeal mask airway:	Size 1.5
Maximum cuff volume:	Up to 7 ml

Atropine (0.01 mg/kg) (0.4 mg/ml):	0.1 mg (0.25 ml)
Succinylcholine (Anectine) (2 mg/kg) (20 mg/ml):	14 mg (0.7 ml)
Epinephrine (0.1 mg/kg) (1:10,000):	0.7 mg (0.7 ml)

Blade:	#1 Miller
Bag:	500 ml
System:	Nonrebreathing
Maintenance fluids:	28 ml/h + NPO
BP (systolic):	60–110 mm Hg
HR:	100–180/min
RR:	25–30/min
EBV (80 ml/kg):	560 ml
Tidal volume (6 ml/kg):	42 ml

12 Months—Approximate Weight: 10 kg

Endotracheal tube:	4.0
Depth:	11 cm
Laryngeal mask airway:	Size 1.5 or 2.0
Maximum cuff volume:	Up to 7–10 ml
Atropine (0.01 mg/kg) (0.4 mg/ml):	0.1 mg (0.25 ml)
Succinylcholine (Anectine) (2 mg/kg)	⌐0 mg (1 ml)
Epinephrine (0.1 mg/kg) (1:10,000'	⌐l)
Blade:	
Bag:	⌐l
System:	ng
Maintenance fluids:	PO
BP (systolic):	Hg
HR:	/min
RR:	/min
EBV (80 ml/kg):	00 ml
Tidal volume (6 ml/kg):	60 ml

2 Years—Approximate Weight: 12 kg

Endotracheal tube:	4.5
Depth:	12.5 cm
Laryngeal mask airway:	Size 2
Maximum cuff volume:	Up to 7 ml
Atropine (0.01 mg/kg) (0.4 mg/ml):	0.1 mg (0.25 ml)
Succinylcholine (Anectine) (1–2 mg/kg) (20 mg/ml):	12–24 mg (0.6–1.2 ml)
Epinephrine (0.1 mg/kg) (1 : 10,000): (0,01mg/kg)	12 mg (1.2 ml)
Blade:	#1 or #2 Miller #1 or #2 Mac
Bag:	1000 ml
System:	Nonrebreathing/circle
Maintenance fluids:	48 ml/h + NPO
BP (systolic):	75–125 mm Hg
HR:	90–150/min
RR:	16–22/min
EBV (70 ml/kg):	840 ml
Tidal volume (7 ml/kg):	84 ml

Ephedrine 1,2 mg (0,1mg/kg)

Epi 0.01mg/kg 0.12mg

Phenylephrine 1-2mcg/kg

Sux 1-2 mg/kg-IV
4-6 mg/kg-IM

Robinul 0,005-0.01mg/kg (0.06-0,12mg)

3 Years—Approximate Weight: 15 kg

Endotracheal tube:	4.5–5.0
Depth:	12 cm
Laryngeal mask airway:	Size 2
Maximum cuff volume:	Up to 7 ml
Atropine (0.01 mg/kg) (0.4 mg/ml):	0.15 mg (0.4 ml)
Succinylcholine (Anectine) (1–2 mg/kg) (20 mg/ml):	
	15–30 mg (0.75–1.5 ml)
Epinephrine (0.1 mg/kg) (1:10,000):	15 mg (1.5 ml)
Blade:	#1 or #2 Miller
	#1 or #2 Mac
Bag:	1000 ml
System:	Nonrebreathing/circle
Maintenance fluids:	50 ml/h + NPO
BP (systolic):	75–125 mm Hg
HR:	90–150/min
RR:	16–22/min
EBV (70 ml/kg):	1005 ml
Tidal volume (7 ml/kg):	105 ml

Ephedrine 0.1mg/kg = 1.5 mg

Epi: 0.01mg/kg = 0.15mg

Phenylephrine 1-2mcg/kg (15-30mcg)

SUX 1-2mg/kg (15-30mg) IV
4-6mg/kg (60-90mg) IM

Glycopyrolate (0.005-0.01mg/kg) = 0.075 - 0.15mg

5 Years—Approximate Weight: 20 kg

Endotracheal tube:	5.0–5.5
Depth:	13–14 cm
Laryngeal mask airway:	Size 2.0 or 2.5
Maximum cuff volume:	Up to 10–14 ml
Atropine (0.01 mg/kg) (0.4 mg/ml):	0.2 mg (0.5 ml)
Succinylcholine (Anectine) (1–2 mg/kg) (20 mg/ml):	
	20–40 mg (1–2 ml)
Epinephrine (0.1 mg/kg) (1:10,000):	2.0 mg (2 ml)
Blade:	#2 Miller
	#2 Mac
Bag:	1000 ml
System:	Ped Circle
Maintenance fluids:	60 ml/h + NPO
BP (systolic):	80–120 mm Hg
HR:	60–140/min
RR:	14–20/min
EBV (70 ml/kg):	1400 ml
Tidal volume (7 ml/kg):	140 ml

Ephedrine 0.1 mg/kg = 2.0 mg

Epi 0.01 mg/kg = 0.2 mg

Phenyleph 1-2 mcg/kg (20-40mg)

SUX 1-2 mg/kg (20-40m)
4-6 mg/kg (80-120mg)

Glycopyrrolate 0.005-0.01 mg/kg (0.1 mg - 0.2mg)

7 Years—Approximate Weight: 30 kg

Endotracheal tube:	5.5
Depth:	15 cm
Laryngeal mask airway:	Size 2.5 or 3.0
Maximum cuff volume:	Up to 14–20 ml
Atropine (0.01 mg/kg) (0.4 mg/ml):	0.3 mg (0.75 ml)
Succinylcholine (Anectine) (1–2 mg/kg) (20 mg/ml):	
	30–60 mg (1.5–2.5 ml)
Epinephrine (0.1 mg/kg) (1:10,000):	30 mg (3 ml)
Blade:	#2 Miller
	#2 Mac
Bag:	1000 ml
System:	Ped Circle
Maintenance fluids:	70 ml/h + NPO
BP (systolic):	90–120 mm Hg
HR:	60–140/min
RR:	14–20/min
EBV (70 ml/kg):	2100 ml
Tidal volume (7 ml/kg):	210 ml

10 Years—Approximate Weight: 40 kg

Endotracheal tube:	6.0 (w/cuff)
Depth:	15–16 cm
Laryngeal mask airway:	Size 3
Maximum cuff volume:	Up to 20 ml
Atropine (0.01 mg/kg) (0.4 mg/ml):	0.4 mg (1 ml)
Succinylcholine (Anectine) (1–2 mg/kg) (20 mg/ml):	
	40–80 mg (2–4 ml)
Epinephrine (0.1 mg/kg) (1:10,000):	40 mg (4 ml)
Blade:	#2 Miller
	#2 Mac
Bag:	3000 ml
System:	Ped Circle
Maintenance fluids:	80 ml/h + NPO
BP (systolic):	90–120 mm Hg
HR:	60–100/min
RR:	12–20/min
EBV (70 ml/kg):	2800 ml
Tidal volume (7 ml/kg):	280 ml

Pharmacologic Agents

John J. Nagelhout, PhD, CRNA, and David Crowninshield MS, CRNA

Acetaminophen

Classification/indications: Analgesic, antipyretic

Dose
1. Oral: 5–10 mg/kg (about 65 mg/kg/d) q4–6 h.
2. Rectal: Up to 25–30 mg/kg
3. Do not exceed five doses in 24 h

Onset: 20–40 min

Duration: 4–6 h

Anesthetic considerations
1. Acetaminophen is the agent of choice for treating fevers in children and adolescents younger than 19 y old
2. Aspirin, but not acetaminophen, carries the risk of the development of Reye syndrome

Albumin

Classification/indications
1. Blood product derivative
2. Plasma volume expansion and maintenance of cardiac output in the treatment of certain types of shock or impending shock

Dose
1. Neonates: 0.5 g/kg per dose
2. Emergency initial dose: 25 g
3. Children, nonemergency: 25%–50% of the adult dose
4. Adult dose: 25 g but no more than 250 g in a 48-h period

Onset: Rapid

Duration: Not applicable

Anesthetic considerations
1. Contraindicated in severe anemia or cardiac failure
2. Rapid infusion may cause vascular overload; observe for signs of hypervolemia

Albuterol Sulfate (Proventil, Ventolin)

Classification/indications
1. A beta$_2$-adrenergic agonist
2. Bronchodilator used in reversible airway obstruction due to asthma or respiratory disease

Dose
1. Oral
   a. 2–6 y: 0.1–0.2 mg/kg, 3 times per day; maximum dose not to exceed 12 mg/d in divided doses
   b. 6–12 y: 2 mg, 3 or 4 times per day; maximum dose not to exceed 24 mg/d
   c. >12 y: 2–4 mg, 3 or 4 times per day; maximum dose not to exceed 32 mg/d in divided doses
2. Inhalation via metered dose inhaler: 90 µg per spray
   a. <12 y: 1 or 2 inhalations 4 times per day as needed
   b. >12 y: 1 or 2 inhalations q4–6h as needed
3. Inhalation via nebulization
   a. >5 y: 1.25–2.5 mg in 2 ml normal saline q6–8h as needed
   b. 5–12 y: 2.5–5 mg q4–6h as needed
   c. >12 y: 2.5 mg 3 or 4 times per day (2.5 mg = 0.5 ml of the 0.5% inhalation solution) in 2.5 ml of normal saline as needed

Onset: Rapid

Duration: 4–6 h

Anesthetic considerations
1. Some adverse reactions may occur more frequently in children 2–5 y of age than in adults or older children
2. Watch for excessive cardiovascular effects when combining inhaled albuterol with long-term oral bronchodilator therapy or halothane anesthesia

Alfentanil HCl (Alfenta)

Classification/indications: Analgesic, anesthesia adjunct

Dose
1. Induction: 8–20 µg/kg
2. Anesthesia maintenance: 3–5 µg/kg

Onset: 1–2 min

Duration: 30 min to 2 h depending on dose

Anesthetic considerations
1. Adverse reaction profile similar to that of adults
2. Children are more prone to respiratory depression, nausea and vomiting, and gastrointestinal (GI) suppressive effects

Alprostadil, PGE$_1$ (Prostin VR)

Classification/indications
1. Prostaglandin
2. Temporary maintenance of patency of ductus arteriosus in neonates until surgery can be performed; defects may include cyanotic (pulmonary atresia, pulmonary stenosis, tricuspid atresia, Fallot tetralogy, transposition of the great vessels) and noncyanotic (interruption of aortic arch, coarctation of aorta, hypoplastic left ventricle) heart disease
3. Investigational use: treatment of pulmonary hypertension in infants and children with left-to-right shunt

Dose
1. Intravenous (IV) continuous infusion into a large vein or through an umbilical artery catheter placed at the ductile opening
2. Give 0.05–0.1 µg/kg/min with therapeutic response; rate is reduced to most effective dose
3. If response is unsatisfactory, rate is increased gradually up to 0.4 µg/kg/min

Onset: Within 30 min

Duration: Several hours

Anesthetic considerations
1. Therapeutic response is indicated by increased pH or Po$_2$ upon therapy

2. Use cautiously in neonates with bleeding tendencies; apnea occurs in 10% to 12% of neonates with congenital heart defects, especially in those weighing less than 2 kg at birth

Aminocaproic Acid (Amicar)

Classification/indications
1. Hemostatic agent
2. Treatment of excessive bleeding from fibrinolysis

Dose
1. Oral/IV: 100 mg/kg or 3 g/m^2 during the first hour followed by continuous infusion at the rate of 33.3 mg/kg/h or 1 g/m^2/h
2. Total dose should not exceed 18 g/m^2 in a 24-h period

Onset: 1–2 h depending on dose

Duration: Not applicable

Anesthetic considerations
1. Contraindicated in disseminated intravascular coagulation (DIC)
2. Use with caution in patients with cardiac, renal, or hepatic disease

Aminophylline

Classification/indications: Bronchodilator

Dose
1. Neonates: Apnea of prematurity
   a. Loading dose: 5 mg/kg for one dose
   b. Maintenance (IV for 0–24 d): Begin at 2 mg/kg/d divided every 12 h, and titrate to desired levels and effects
   c. >24 d: 3 mg/kg/d divided every 12 h; increased dosages may be indicated as liver metabolism matures (usually >30 d of life); monitor serum levels to determine appropriate dosages
2. Treatment of acute bronchospasm
   a. Loading dose (in patients not currently receiving aminophylline or theophylline): 6 mg/kg (based on aminophylline) given IV over 20–30 min; administration rate should not exceed 25 mg/min (aminophylline)
   b. Approximate IV maintenance dosages are based on continuous infusions; bolus dosing (often used in children <6 mo of age) may be determined by multiplying the hourly infusion rate by 24 h and dividing by the desired number of doses per day

   c. 6 wk to 6 mo: 0.5 mg/kg/h
   d. 6 mo to 1 y: 0.6–0.7 mg/kg/h
   e. 1–9 y: 1–1.2 mg/kg/h
   f. 12–16 y: 0.7 mg/kg/h
   g. 9–12 y and young adult smokers: 0.9 mg/kg/h
   h. Dosage should be adjusted according to serum level measurements during the first 12- to 24-h period
   i. Avoid using suppositories because of erratic, unreliable absorption

Onset: 30–60 min

Duration: Up to 8 h

Anesthetic considerations
1. Therapeutic range is 10–20 µg/ml
2. Rapid administration may result in central nervous system (CNS) stimulation, nausea and vomiting, and gastric irritation

Atracurium (Tracrium)

Classification/indications: Neuromuscular blocking agent

Dose
1. Children 1 mo to 2 y: 0.3–0.4 mg/kg; then 0.08–0.1 q20–45min after initial dose to maintain block
2. Children 2 y to adults: 0.4–0.5 mg/kg; then 0.08–0.1 mg/kg q20–45min to maintain neuromuscular block

Onset: Immediate

Duration: 45–90 min depending on dose

Anesthetic considerations: Histamine release especially with rapid administration may result in hypotension and tachycardia

Atropine Sulfate

Classification/indications
1. Anticholinergic agent
2. Preoperative medication to inhibit respiratory secretions, attenuate vagal responses
3. Treatment of sinus bradycardia
4. Antidote for organophosphate poisoning

Dose
1. Children
    a. Preanesthetic (intramuscular) [IM]/IV/subcutaneous [SQ]
    b. <5 kg: 0.02 mg/kg 30–60 min preoperatively, then q4–6h as needed
    c. >5 kg: 0.01–0.2 mg/kg to a maximum 0.4 mg 30–60 min preoperatively; minimum dose: 0.1 mg
2. Bradycardia: IV, intratracheal: 0.02 mg/kg q5min
3. Minimum dose: 0.1 mg (if administered via endotracheal tube, dilute to 1–2 ml with normal saline before endotracheal administration)
4. Maximum single dose: 0.5 mg (adolescents: 1 mg)
5. Total maximum dose: 1 mg (adolescents: 2 mg)
6. When using atropine to treat bradycardia in neonates, reserve use for those unresponsive to improved oxygenation
7. Organophosphate or carbonate poisoning: IV: 0.02–0.05 mg/kg q10–20min until atropine effect (dry flushed skin, tachycardia, mydriasis, fever) is observed, then q1–4h for at least 24 h
8. Ophthalmic, 0.5% solution: Instill 1 or 2 drops twice daily for 1–3 d before the procedure

Onset: Rapid

Duration: 2–3 h

Anesthetic considerations: May cause dry mouth, difficulty swallowing, blurred vision, or rash with high doses

---

Bupivacaine HCl (Marcaine, Sensorcaine)

Classification/indications: Amide type of local anesthetic

Dose
1. Caudal block: 1–3.7 mg/kg
2. Epidural block: 1.25 mg/kg
3. Peripheral nerve block: up to 3 mg/kg maximum

Onset: 20–60 min depending on type of block

Duration: 4–12 h depending on type of block

Anesthetic considerations
1. Not approved for use in children under 12 y of age
2. Solution for spinal anesthesia should not be used in children under 18 y of age

Caffeine

Classification/indications: CNS stimulant/respiratory stimulant

Dose: Apnea of prematurity: oral: 10–20 mg/kg loading dose; 5–10 mg/kg maintenance dose

Onset: 20–60 min

Duration: 4–8 h

Anesthetic considerations
1. Therapeutic range: 3–15 μg/ml
2. Administer with caution in cardiac patients

Calcium Chloride

Classification/indications
1. Electrolyte/cardiac arrest
2. Electrolyte abnormalities, including hypocalcemia, hyperkalemia, hypermagnesemia
3. Calcium channel blocker overdose

Dose
1. Cardiac arrest with hyperkalemia or hypocalcemia, magnesium or calcium channel blocker toxicity: Infants and children: 10–20 mg/kg IV; may repeat in 10 min if necessary
2. Hypocalcemia: Infants and children: 10–20 mg/kg IV; repeat q4–6h prn
3. Tetany: Infants and children: 10 mg/kg over 5–10 min; may repeat after 6 h or follow with an infusion with a maximum dose of 200 mg/kg/d

Onset: Rapid

Duration: 4–6 h depending on use

Anesthetic considerations
1. Calcium chloride is irritating to veins
2. Administer slowly IV to avoid overstimulation of the cardiovascular system
3. Calcium chloride provides 3 times more calcium than an equal amount of calcium gluconate

Calcium Gluconate

Classification/indications
1. Treatment and prevention of hypocalcemia, tetany, cardiac arrest associated with hyperkalemia
2. Calcium channel blocker toxicity

Dose
1. Hypocalcemia
   a. Neonates: 200–400 mg/kg/d as a continuous infusion or in 4 divided doses
   b. Infants and children: 200–1000 mg/kg/d as a continuous infusion or in 4 divided doses
2. Calcium channel blocker toxicity: Infants and children: 100 mg/kg per dose
3. Tetany
   a. Neonates: 100–200 mg/kg; may follow with 500 mg/kg/d in 3 or 4 divided doses or by infusion
   b. Infants and children: 100–200 mg/kg over 5–10 min; may repeat after 6 h or follow with an infusion of 500 mg/kg/d
4. Cardiac arrest: Infants and children: 100 mg/kg q10min as needed

Onset: Rapid

Duration: 4–6 h

Anesthetic considerations: Less irritating than calcium chloride; however, yields 3 times less calcium per treatment

Chloroprocaine HCl (Nesacaine)

Classification/indications: Ester type of local anesthetic

Dose
1. Up to 20 mg/kg maximum depending on type of block
2. Caudal block in children: 0.4–1 ml/kg

Onset: Rapid

Duration: Approximately 1 h

Anesthetic considerations
1. Not used for spinal anesthesia
2. Rapid onset, short duration blockade

Cimetidine (Tagamet)

Classification/indications: Histamine$_2$ antagonist

Dose
1. Neonates: 5–10 mg/kg/d IV in divided doses q8–12h
2. Infants: 10–20 mg/kg/d IV in divided doses q6–12h
3. Children: 20–30 mg/kg/d IV in divided doses q6h

Onset: 15–30 min

Duration: 4–6 h

Anesthetic considerations: May inhibit the metabolism of liver-dependent drugs

Cisatracurium (Nimbex)

Classification/indications: Nondepolarizing neuromuscular blocking agent

Dose: Age 2–12 y; 0.1 mg/kg IV

Onset: 2–3 min

Duration: 45–90 min depending on dose

Anesthetic considerations
1. Similar to atracurium but without histamine release
2. Good for children with hepatic or renal disease

Cocaine HCl

Classification/indications: Ester type of local anesthetic

Dose: Up to 1 mg/kg topical

Onset: 5–10 min

Duration: 30 min to 2 h depending on dose

Anesthetic considerations
1. For topical administration in mucous membranes
2. Watch for signs of CNS stimulation

Codeine

Classification/indications: Narcotic analgesic

Dose
1. Oral/intramuscular (IM)/subcutaneous (SQ): children >2 y: 0.5–1 mg/kg q4–6h as needed
2. Maximum: 60 mg

Onset: 20–40 min depending on dose

Duration: 3–6 h

Anesthetic considerations
1. Children especially prone to respiratory depression
2. The usual considerations for the use of opium agonists are indicated

Cromolyn Sodium (Gastrocrom, Intal, Crolom)

Classification/indications
1. Antiasthmatic, prophylactic prevention of bronchospasm
2. Long-term management of asthma and allergic rhinitis

Dose
1. Inhalation (>2 y): 20 mg 4 times per day
2. Nebulization solution (>5 y): 2 inhalations 4 times per day by metered spray
3. Exercise prophylaxis: 2 inhalations
4. Children >4 y: ophthalmic, 1 or 2 drops 4–6 times per day

Onset: 20 min to 1 h depending on route of administration

Duration: 4–6 h

Anesthetic considerations
1. Not useful for acute bronchospasm
2. Must be taken long term to achieve full benefit

Dantrolene Sodium (Dantrium)

Classification/indications: Antidote, malignant hyperthermia, neuroleptic malignant syndrome

Dose
1. Oral: 4–8 mg/kg/d in 4 divided doses
2. IV: 1 mg/kg; may repeat dose up to a cumulative dose of 10 mg/kg (mean effective dose is 2.5 mg/kg)

Onset
1. Oral: 1–2 h
2. IV: Immediate

Duration
1. Oral: 8–9 h
2. IV: 3 h

Anesthetic considerations
1. Use with caution in patients with impaired cardiac, pulmonary, and hepatic functions
2. Avoid use with calcium channel blockers and monoamine oxidase (MAO) inhibitors

Desflurane (Suprane)

Classification/indications: Inhalation anesthetic/general anesthesia

Dose: Minimum alveolar concentration (MAC) = 6%

Onset: Immediate

Duration: 15–30 min after cessation of anesthetic

Anesthetic considerations
1. Slight respiratory irritation limits usefulness for inhalation induction
2. Rapid induction and emergence may be useful for children and young adults

Desmopressin (DDAVP)

Classification/indications
1. Antihemophilic agent
2. Hemostatic agent
3. Synthetic desmopressin analog

Dose
1. Diabetes insipidus
    a. 3 mo to 12 y: intranasal, 5 µg/d divided once 2 times per day
    b. Range: 5–30 µg/d divided once 2 times per day

2. Hemophilia: >3 mo: IV, 0.3 µg/kg by slow infusion; may repeat prn
3. Nocturnal enuresis
   a. >6 y old: intranasal, initial 20 µg
   b. Range: 10–40 µg

Onset: Rapid

Duration
1. IV: 6–20 h
2. Intranasal: 8–20 h

Anesthetic considerations: Monitor fluid and electrolyte balance since the drug may affect water balance

Dexamethasone (Decadron)

Classification/indications
1. Corticosteroid
2. Antiemetic
3. Antiinflammatory

Dose
1. Antiemetic (before chemotherapy): 10 mg/m^2 for first dose; then 5 mg/m^2 q6h as needed
2. Antiinflammatory immunosuppressant: Oral, IM, IV: 0.03–0.15 mg/kg/d or 0.6–0.75 mg/m^2/d in divided doses q6–12h
3. Extubation or airway edema: Oral, IM, IV: 0.5–2 mg/kg/d in divided doses q6h beginning 24 h before extubation and continuing for 4–6 doses afterward
4. Cerebral edema: loading dose: 1–2 mg/kg as a single dose; maintenance: 1 mg/kg/d (maximum: 16 mg/d) in divided doses q4–6h for 5 d, then taper for 5 d, then discontinue
5. Bacterial meningitis in infants and children >2 mo: IV: 0.6 mg/kg/d in 4 divided doses for the first 4 days of antibiotic treatment; start dexamethasone at the time of the first dose of antibiotic
6. Inhalation
   a. Oral: 2 inhalations 3 or 4 times per day to a maximum of 8 inhalations per day
   b. Intranasal: 6–12 y: 1 or 2 sprays into each nostril twice daily to a maximum of 8 sprays per day

Onset: 5 min to 1 h

Duration: 1–2 d depending on route of administration

Anesthetic considerations: May induce adrenocorticoid insufficiency with rapid withdrawal after long-term administration

Digoxin (Lanoxin)

Classification/indications: Cardiac glycoside/antidysrhythmic

Dose

Age	Total Digitalizing Dose (μg/kg)		Daily Maintenance Dose (μg/kg)	
	PO	IV or IM	PO	IV or IM
Preterm infant	20–30	15–25	5–7.5	4–6
Full-term infant	25–35	20–30	6–10	5–8
1 mo–2 y	35–60	30–50	10–15	7.5–12
2–5 y	30–40	25–35	7.5–10	6–9
5–10 y	20–35	15–30	5–10	4–8
>10 y	10–15	8–12	2.5–5	2–3

Onset: 3–6 h

Duration: 24–48 h

Anesthetic considerations
1. Monitor serum digoxin and potassium levels
2. May produce atrioventricular (AV) block or other cardiac abnormalities with toxic levels

Diphenhydramine (Benadryl)

Classification/indications: Antihistamine (nonselective)

Dose: Oral, IM, IV: 5 mg/kg/d or 150 mg/m²/d in divided doses q6–8h; not to exceed 300 mg/d

Onset: Rapid

Duration: 4–6 h

Anesthetic considerations: May cause sedation and drowsiness

Dobutamine HCl (Dobutrex)

Classification/indications
1. Inotrope
2. Short-term management of cardiac decompensation

Dose
1. Neonates: 2–15 μg/kg/min; titrate to desired response
2. Children: 2.5–15 μg/kg/min; titrate to desired response

Onset: Immediate

Duration: Wears off shortly after cessation of administration

Anesthetic considerations: Hypovolemia should be corrected before use

Dopamine HCl (Intropin)

Classification/indications
1. Catecholamine/treatment of shock
2. Cardiac decompensation

Dose: IV infusion: neonates, children: 1–20 μg/kg/min continuous infusion; titrate to desired response

Onset: Immediate

Duration: Must be given by continuous infusion

Anesthetic considerations: Hypovolemia should be corrected before administration

Doxapram HCl (Dopram)

Classification/indications: CNS stimulant, respiratory stimulant

Dose
1. IV: Neonatal apnea (apnea of prematurity)
   a. Initial: 1–1.5 mg/kg/h
   b. Maintenance: 0.5–2.5 mg/kg/h, titrated to the lowest rate at which apnea is controlled

Onset: Rapid

Duration: 5–15 min after acute administration

Anesthetic considerations
1. Safety in children <12 y not established
2. May cause severe CNS toxicity, seizures
3. Should be used with caution in newborns because the U.S. product contains benzyl alcohol (0.9%); recommended doses for neonates will deliver 5.4–27 mg/kg/d of benzyl alcohol; large amounts of benzyl alcohol (>100 mg/kg/d) have been associated with fatal toxicity (gasping syndrome); use in newborns should be reserved for neonates who are unresponsive to the treatment of apnea with therapeutic serum concentrations of theophylline or caffeine

Droperidol (Inapsine)

Classification/indications
1. Antipsychotic
2. Tranquilizer
3. Antiemetic
4. Preoperative medication

Dose
1. Children 2–12 yrs: Premedication: 0.03 mg/kg IM; smaller doses may be sufficient for control of nausea and vomiting
2. Anesthesia induction: 0.08–0.165 mg/kg
3. Nausea and vomiting: 0.05–0.06 mg/kg IM, IV q4–6h as needed

Onset: 5–10 min

Duration: 4–6 h

Anesthetic considerations: May produce extrapyramidal reactions, respiratory depression, or hypotension

Edrophonium Chloride (Enlon, Reversol, Tensilon)

Classification/indications
1. Anticholinesterase agent
2. Used for diagnosis and treatment of myasthenia gravis

Dose
1. Infants: initially 0.1 mg IV, followed by 0.4 mg; if no response, total dose 0.5 mg
2. Children: For reversal of neuromuscular blockade:
   a. 0.5 mg/kg preceded by atropine or glycopyrrolate
   b. May repeat once for a total dose of 1 mg/kg
   c. Must be given with either atropine, 0.015 mg/kg, or glycopyrrolate, 0.01 mg/kg
3. Children: For diagnosis of muscle disorders:
   a. 1 mg for children <34 kg or 2 mg for children >34 kg followed by 1 mg q30–45s
   b. If no response to a maximum total dose of 5 mg for children <34 kg or 10 mg for children >34 kg
4. Children: For oral anticholinesterase therapy: 0.04 mg/kg once; if strength improves, an increase in dose is indicated

Onset: Rapid

Duration: 30–60 min

Anesthetic considerations: Use caution in administration to avoid cholinergic side effects

Ephedrine Sulfate

Classification/indications
1. Adrenergic agonist
2. Hypotension

Dose
1. 3 mg/kg/d or 100 mg/m²/d IV/SQ in 4–6 divided doses
2. 50–200 µg/kg IV for hypotension

Onset: Immediate

Duration: 2–3 h

Anesthetic considerations
1. May cause hypertension dysrhythmias
2. Can interact with halothane to produce cardiac dysrhythmias

Epinephrine HCl, Racemic (Adrenalin Chloride)

Classification/indications: Bronchodilator treatment for anaphylaxis, cardiac arrest, and shock

Dose
1. Neonates: Cardiac arrest: 0.01–0.03 mg/kg (0.1–0.3 ml/kg 1:10,000 solution) IV or intratracheally q3–5min as needed
2. Children
   a. Bronchodilator: 10 µg/kg SQ (single doses not to exceed 0.5 mg); injection suspension (1:200): 0.005 ml/kg to a maximum of 0.15 ml q8–12h
   b. Cardiac arrest: 0.01 mg/kg (0.1 ml/kg) of 1:10,000 solution (to maximum 5 ml) IV or intratracheally q3–5min as needed; infusion rate, 0.1–4 µg/kg/min
   c. Refractory hypotension (refractory to dopamine and dobutamine): Start infusion of 0.1 µg/kg/min; titrate to desired effect
   d. Hypersensitivity reaction: 0.01 mg/kg SQ q15min for 2 doses; then q4h as needed (single doses not to exceed 0.5 mg)

Onset: Rapid

Duration: 15 min to 3 h depending on route of administration

Anesthetic considerations: Use caution when administered during halothane anesthesia; cardiac dysrhythmias may occur

Esmolol (Brevibloc)

Classification/indications: Beta-receptor blocker/tachycardia

Dose
1. Loading dose: 250 µg/kg IV by slow titration followed by 10–50 µg/kg/min infusion; titrate to effect
2. Average dosage range: 50–200 µg/kg/min

Onset: Rapid

Duration: 10–20 min

Anesthetic considerations: Avoid in children with asthma, diabetes, congestive heart failure (CHF), and severe peripheral vascular disease

Ethacrynic Acid (Edecrin)

Classification/indications
1. Diuretic
2. Treatment of increased intracranial pressure (ICP) and CHF

Dose
1. Orally: 25 mg/d initial dose, adjust in increments of 25 mg to desired effect
2. IV: 0.25–0.5 mg/kg

Onset: 5–30 min

Duration: 2 h IV; 6–10 h orally

Anesthetic considerations: May lead to hypokalemia, hypovolemia, and hypotension with long-term administration

Etidocaine HCl (Duranest)

Classification/indications: Amide type of local anesthetic/regional, epidural anesthesia

Dose: 0.4–0.7 ml/kg of 0.25%–0.5% (for L2–T10 level of anesthesia)

Onset: 20–40 min depending on type of block

Duration: 4–8 h

Anesthetic considerations: Not for spinal use

Etomidate (Amidate)

Classification/indications: General anesthetic/induction of general anesthesia

Dose: 0.2–0.3 mg/kg IV

Onset: 30–60 s

Duration: 15–30 min

Anesthetic considerations
1. Safety in children <4 y not established
2. Use with caution in patients with focal epilepsy

Famotidine (Pepcid)

Classification/indications
1. Histamine (H_2) antagonist
2. Aspiration prophylaxis

Dose
1. 1–2 mg/kg/d orally/IV divided into 1 or 2 doses
2. Maximum dose: 40 mg

Onset: 5–20 min depending on route of administration

Duration: 6–12 h

Anesthetic considerations: Reduce dosage in patients with cardiac and renal disease

Fentanyl (Sublimaze)

Classification/indications: Opioid agonist/analgesia, anesthesia

Dose
1. 1–5 µg/kg for analgesia
2. 10–100 µg/kg for anesthesia (+ N_2O)

Onset: 1–3 min

Duration: 30–60 min

Anesthetic considerations: Monitor for apnea, bradycardia, chest wall rigidity, and hypotension

Flumazenil (Romazicon)

Classification/indications
1. Benzodiazepine-receptor antagonist
2. Benzodiazepine reversal

Dose: 1–3 μg/kg

Onset: 1–2 min

Duration: 45–90 min

Anesthetic considerations
1. Do not use until neuromuscular blockade is reversed
2. Monitor for resedation
3. May cause seizures

Furosemide (Lasix)

Classification/indications: Loop diuretic/diuresis

Dose
1. IV: 0.1–1 mg/kg, given slowly
2. Orally: 1–2 mg/kg, up to 6 mg/kg q6h

Onset: 5 min

Duration: 2 h

Anesthetic considerations: Monitor fluid and electrolyte balance

Glucagon

Classification/indications
1. Hormone
2. Antidiabetic agent (antihypoglycemic)
3. Hypoglycemia

Dose
1. Neonates: 0.3 mg/kg; maximum 1 mg
2. Children: 0.025–0.1 mg/kg per dose, not to exceed 1 mg per dose; repeat q20min as needed

Onset: <5 min

Duration: 10–30 min

Anesthetic considerations
1. Monitor serum glucose levels
2. Rapid IV bolus may cause hypotension

Glucose

Classification/indications: Carbohydrate/hypoglycemia

Dose: 200 mg/kg IV followed by 4 mg/kg/min infusion

Onset: Rapid

Duration: 2–6 h

Anesthetic considerations: Monitor serum glucose levels

Glycopyrrolate (Robinul)

Classification/indications
1. Anticholinergic
2. Antisialagogue
3. Treatment of bradycardia
4. Blockade of muscarinic effects of anticholinesterases

Dose: 0.04–0.01 mg/kg as antisialagogue

Onset
1. IV: <1 min
2. Inhalation: 3–5 min
3. IM/SQ: 15–30 min
4. Orally: 1 h

Duration
1. Antisialagogue: 7–12 h
2. IV vagolysis: 2–3 h
3. Oral vagolysis: 8–12 h

Anesthetic considerations: Tachycardia, dry mouth, blurred vision

Granisetron (Kytril)

Classification/indications
1. Selective serotonin receptor antagonist
2. Nausea and vomiting

Dose: 10 µg/kg IV given over 5 min for ages 2–16 y

Onset: Rapid

Duration: Up to 24 h

Anesthetic considerations: Not studied for use in children less than 2 y of age

Halothane (Fluothane)

Classification/indications: Inhalation anesthetic/general anesthesia

Dose
1. Induction: 1%–4%
2. Maintenance: 0.5%–1.5%

Onset: 5–10 min to achieve surgical anesthesia

Duration: up to 30 min after discontinuation

Anesthetic considerations
1. Rapid, smooth, pleasant induction
2. Myocardial sensitization to catecholamines
3. Avoid in patients with liver disease

Heparin (Liquaemin Sodium, Panheparin)

Classification/indications: Anticoagulant

Dose
1. Initial: 50–100 U/kg IV, then 50–100 U/kg q4h
2. Infusion: Initial 50 U/kg IV, then 15–25 U/kg/h; increase dose by 2–4 U/kg/h q6–8h as required
3. Titrated to partial thromboplastin time (PTT) and specific indication

Onset
1. IV: Immediate
2. SQ: 20–30 min

Duration: 1–2 h

Anesthetic considerations
1. Monitor PTT; check for bleeding
2. Contraindication to using regional anesthesia

Hyaluronidase (Wydase)

Classification/indications
1. Enzyme
2. Adjunct to increase absorption and dispersion; hypodermoclysis; subcutaneous urography

Dose
1. Adjunct: 150 units to injection medium IV
2. Hypodermoclysis: 150 units SQ before clysis or injected into clysis tubing near needle for every 1000 ml clysis solution
3. Subcutaneous urography: 75 units SQ over each scapula

Onset: Immediate

Duration: 30–60 min

Anesthetic considerations: Use with caution in patients with coagulopathies or hepatic or renal disease

Hydralazine (Apresoline)

Classification/indications
1. Direct-acting arterial vasodilator
2. Hypertension

Dose: 0.05–0.1 mg/kg IV

Onset: 15 min

Duration: 2–4 h

Anesthetic considerations: May cause hypotension with excessive dosing and a reduced response to epinephrine

Hydrocortisone Sodium Succinate (A-Hydrocort, Solu-Cortef)

Classification/indications
1. Corticosteroid
2. Steroid replacement therapy

3. Adrenal suppression
4. Asthma

Dose:
1. 1–2 mg/kg bolus IV
2. Oral: 2.5–10 mg/kg/d
3. Shock: 50 mg/kg q4h

Onset: IV/IM 5 min

Duration: 1.25–1.5 d

Anesthetic considerations: Acute adrenal insufficiency may occur with abrupt withdrawal

Insulin Regular (Humulin R, Novolin R, Regular Iletin II)

Classification/indications
1. Hormone
2. Hyperglycemia

Dose: 0.5–1 U/kg/d in divided doses

Onset: 30–60 min

Duration: 5–7 h

Anesthetic considerations: Monitor serum glucose levels frequently

Isoflurane (Forane)

Classification/indications: Inhalation anesthetic/general anesthesia

Dose: MAC 1.15%; titrate to effect

Onset: Rapid

Duration (emergence time): 15 min

Anesthetic considerations
1. May trigger malignant hyperthermia
2. Respiratory irritant, not ideal for inhalation induction

Ketamine HCl (Ketalar)

Classification/indications
1. CNS agent, general anesthetic
2. Sole anesthetic agent for diagnostic and short surgical procedures; induction of anesthesia

Dose
1. 1–2 mg/kg IM sedation
2. 5–10 mg/kg IM anesthesia
3. 6 mg/kg oral sedation

Onset
1. 1–2 min IV
2. 3–8 min IM

Duration
1. 5–10 min IV
2. 12–25 min IM

Anesthetic considerations
1. Emergence delirium
2. Hypertension and tachycardia
3. Excessive secretions

Ketorolac Tromethamine (Toradol)

Classification/indications: Nonsteroidal   antiinflammatory/analgesia

Dose: 0.8–1 mg/kg IV

Onset: 30 min

Duration: 4–6 h

Anesthetic considerations
1. Platelet inhibition
2. GI distress

Labetalol (Normodyne, Trandate)

Classification/indications
1. Beta-adrenergic antagonist
2. Tachycardia, hypertension

Dose: 0.1–0.5 mg/kg IV q5min

Onset: 1–3 min

Duration: 0.25–2 h

Anesthetic considerations: Use with caution in asthmatic, diabetic, and congestive heart failure (CHF) patients

Lidocaine HCl (Xylocaine)

Classification/indications
1. Amide type of local anesthetic
2. Ventricular dysrhythmias
3. Topical and regional anesthesia

Dose
1. Ventricular dysrhythmias: 1–1.5 mg/kg IV; 15–50 µg/kg/min infusion
2. Topical anesthesia: 3–4 mg/kg intratracheal

Onset: 3–5 min IV

Duration: 30 min to 3 h depending on application

Anesthetic considerations: May cause seizures, sedation, burning on injection

Magnesium Sulfate

Classification/indications
1. Electrolyte
2. Anticonvulsant
3. Prevention and control of seizures
4. Treatment of acute hypomagnesemia

Dose: Neonates: 25–50 mg/kg (0.2–0.4 mEq/kg) q8–12h for 2 or 3 doses

Onset
1. Rapid IV
2. Less than 1 h IM

Duration
1. 30 min IV
2. 3–4 h IM

Anesthetic considerations
1. Monitor serum magnesium levels.
2. Potentiates effects of muscle relaxants
3. Monitor urine output and respiratory function.

Mannitol (Osmitrol)

Classification/indications
1. Osmotic diuretic
2. Increased ICP, diuresis

Dose
1. 0.25–1 g/kg IV
2. 2 g/kg IV as 15%–20% solution over 30–60 min to treat cerebral edema, over 2–6 h to treat edema and ascites

Onset
1. Reduction of ICP: 15–30 min
2. Diuresis: 1–3 h

Duration: 3–8 h

Anesthetic considerations
1. Monitor serum osmolarity, electrolytes
2. Discontinue if urine output low

Meperidine HCl (Demerol)

Classification/indications
1. Synthetic opioid agonist/analgesia
2. Preoperative sedation
3. Postoperative pain

Dose
1. 0.2–1 mg/kg IV
2. 1–2 mg/kg IM

Onset: 1–5 min

Duration: 2–4 h

Anesthetic considerations
1. Potent respiratory depressant
2. May cause dysrhythmias when administered with halothane
3. Contraindicated in patients taking MAO inhibitors

4. Prolonged administration may result in accumulation of metabolite normeperidine

Mepivacaine HCl (Carbocaine, Isocaine, Polocaine)

Classification/indications
1. Amide type of local anesthetic
2. Regional anesthesia

Dose
1. Concentration 1%; maximum dose 300–500 mg
2. Varies with procedure

Onset: 3–5 min after infiltration

Duration: 0.75–1.5 h after infiltration

Anesthetic considerations
1. May cause seizures, sedation
2. Burning on injection

Methohexital Sodium (Brevital Sodium)

Classification/indications: Ultra short-acting barbiturate/anesthesia, sedation

Dose
1. 1–2 mg/kg IV for anesthesia
2. 25–30 mg/kg per rectum (PR) (10% solution) for sedation/anesthesia

Onset: Rapid

Duration: 15–30 min

Anesthetic considerations
1. Apnea, hypotension, myoclonia, hiccups
2. Not compatible with lactated Ringer's solution

Methylprednisolone

Classification/indications
1. Steroid
2. Status asthmaticus

Dose: Status asthmaticus: 2 mg/kg IV loading dose, then 0.5–1 mg/kg q6h up to 5 d

Onset: 1–2 h

Duration: 1–1.5 d

Anesthetic considerations: Used primarily as an antiinflammatory or immunosuppressant agent

Metoclopramide (Reglan)

Classification/indications
1. Dopamine-receptor antagonist
2. Antiemetic
3. Stimulant of upper GI mobility/diabetic and postsurgical stasis
4. Prevention of postoperative nausea and vomiting, gastroesphageal reflux

Dose
1. <6 y of age: 0.1 mg/kg IV
2. 6–14 y of age: 0.2–0.5 mg IV

Onset: 1–3 min

Duration: 2–3 h

Anesthetic considerations
1. Extrapyramidal reactions
2. Do not use in patients with history of seizure disorder, pheochromocytoma, or GI hemorrhage, obstruction, or perforation

Midazolam (Versed)

Classification/indications
1. Benzodiazepine
2. Hypnotic; sedative
3. Sedation; induction of anesthesia

Dose
1. 0.05–0.1 mg/kg IV sedation
2. 0.2–0.3 mg/kg IM (10-min onset)
3. 0.5–0.75 mg/kg orally (30-min onset)

Onset
1. 1–5 min IV
2. 5 min IM
3. <10 min orally

Duration: 0.5–2 h

Anesthetic considerations
1. Respiratory depression
2. Bitter taste

Mivacurium (Mivacron)

Classification/indications: Nondepolarizing neuromuscular blocking agent

Dose
1. 0.1–0.2 mg/kg IV over 5–10 s
2. 0.2–0.3 mg/kg IV intubation
3. 10–20 μg/kg/min infusion

Onset: 2 min

Duration: 10–20 min

Anesthetic considerations
1. Histamine release
2. Apnea

Morphine Sulfate (Astramorph, Duramorph)

Classification/indications: Opioid agonist/analgesia

Dose
1. 0.05–0.2 mg/kg IV
2. 0.1–0.2 mg/kg IM/SQ

Onset
1. Rapid IV
2. 10–20 min IM

Duration: 4–5 h

Anesthetic considerations
1. Histamine release
2. Apnea

Nalmefene HCl (Revex)

Classification/indications
1. Opiate antagonist
2. Reversal of respiratory depression, overdose

Dose: 0.25 µg/kg IV q2–5min until desired reversal is reached

Onset: Within 2 min IV

Duration: 8–12 h

Anesthetic considerations: May precipitate acute withdrawal symptoms in opiate-dependent patients

Naloxone HCl (Narcan)

Classification/indications
1. Opioid antagonist
2. Reversal of respiratory depression, overdosage

Dose: 5–10 µg/kg IV/IM/SQ q2–3min until desired reversal is reached

Onset
1. 1–2 min IV
2. 2–5 min IM/SQ

Duration: 1–2 h IV/IM/SQ

Anesthetic considerations
1. May precipitate acute withdrawal symptoms in opiate-dependent patients
2. Monitor for renarcotization

Neostigmine Methylsulfate (Prostigmin)

Classification/indications
1. Anticholinesterase agent
2. Neuromuscular blockade reversal

Dose: 0.05–0.07 mg/kg IV

Onset: <3 min IV

Duration: 45–90 min

Anesthetic considerations
1. May cause bradycardia, increased secretions
2. May increase postoperative nausea and vomiting
3. Administer with atropine (0.015 mg/kg) or glycopyrrolate (0.01 mg/kg)

Nitroglycerin

Classification/indications
1. Peripheral vasodilator
2. Venodilation, myocardial ischemia

Dose: 0.5–2 µg/kg/min IV

Onset: 1–2 min

Duration: 3–5 min

Anesthetic considerations: Hypotension, tachycardia

Nitroprusside Sodium (Nipride)

Classification/indications
1. Peripheral vasodilator
2. Hypertension, controlled hypotension

Dose: Infusion: Start 0.3–0.5 µg/kg/min, titrate to effect; usual dose: 3 µg/kg/min; rarely need >4 µg/kg/min; maximum: 10 µg/kg/min

Onset: Rapid

Duration: 1–3 min

Anesthetic considerations
1. Cyanide toxicity
2. Hypotension, reflex tachycardia

Nitrous Oxide (N_2O)

Classification/indications
1. Inhalation anesthetic
2. Component of balanced anesthesia

Dose
1. Induction: 70% with O_2
2. Maintenance: 70% with O_2
3. Analgesia: 20%–30%

Onset: 1–5 min

Duration: 5–10 min after cessation of continuous inhalation

Anesthetic considerations
1. Rapid diffusion into air-containing cavities
2. Bone marrow suppression

Norepinephrine Bitartrate (Levophed)

Classification/indications
1. Catecholamine
2. Hypotension
3. Inotrope

Dose: 0.05–0.1 µg/kg/min IV

Onset: Rapid

Duration: 2–10 min

Anesthetic considerations
1. Dysrhythmias
2. Excessive vasoconstriction at infusion site

Ondansetron HCl (Zofran)

Classification/indications
1. Gastrointestinal agent
2. Serotonin (5-HT$_3$) receptor antagonist
3. Antiemetic
4. Prevention and treatment of postoperative nausea and vomiting

Dose
1. 0.05–0.1 mg/kg IV
2. Maximum dose 4 mg

Onset: 30 min

Duration: 12–24 h

Anesthetic considerations: Use with caution in children <3 y of age

Pancuronium (Pavulon)

Classification/indications
1. Nondepolarizing neuromuscular blocking agent
2. Neuromuscular blocker

Dose: 0.08–0.15 mg/kg IV

Onset: 1–3 min

Duration: 40–65 min

Anesthetic considerations
1. Tachycardia
2. Apnea
3. Prolonged emergence

Phenylephrine (Neo-Synephrine)

Classification/indications
1. Synthetic noncatecholamine that stimulates $alpha_1$-adrenergic receptors
2. Hypotension

Dose:
1. 10 µg/kg IV bolus q10–15min as needed
2. Infusion: 0.1–0.5 µg/kg/min

Onset: Rapid

Duration: 15–20 min

Anesthetic considerations
1. Hypertension
2. Reflex bradycardia

Phenytoin (Dilantin)

Classification/indications
1. Anticonvulsant
2. Seizures

Dose: 10–15 mg/kg IV loading dose slow infusion

Onset: 3–5 min

Duration: 12–24 h

Anesthetic considerations
1. Mix with normal saline; use 0.22 µm IV filter
2. Potential for nystagmus, hypotension, bradycardia

Procaine HCl (Novocain)

Classification/indications
1. Ester type of local anesthetic
2. Local anesthesia

Dose: Dosage varies with procedure, concentration 1%

Onset
1. Infiltration/spinal: 2–5 min
2. Epidural: 15–25 min

Duration
1. Infiltration: 0.25–0.5 h
2. Spinal/epidural: 0.5–1.5 h

Anesthetic considerations
1. Seizures, sedation
2. Burning on injection
3. Dysrhythmias

Prochlorperazine Maleate (Compazine)

Classification/indications
1. Phenothiazine
2. Antiemetic

Dose
1. 0.2 mg/kg/d IV/IM in divided doses q6h
2. 0.4 mg/kg/d PO or PR in divided doses q6–8h

Onset
1. Rapid IV
2. 10–20 min IM
3. 30–40 min PO
4. 60 min PR

Duration: 3–4 h IV/IM/PO/PR

Anesthetic considerations
1. IV not recommended in children <10 kg or <2 y of age
2. Injection contains sulfites

Promethazine HCl (Phenergan)

Classification/indications
1. Phenothiazine
2. GI agent
3. Antiemetic, antivertigo agent
4. Antihistamine, H_1-receptor antagonist
5. Sedative or adjunct to analgesics
6. Antiemetic, sedation, analgesic adjunct

Dose: 0.25–0.5 mg/kg IV/IM q4–6h

Onset
1. Rapid IV
2. 15–30 min IM

Duration: 2–5 h IV/IM

Anesthetic considerations: Do not use in children <2 y of age

Propofol (Diprivan)

Classification/indications: Anesthetic induction agent/anesthesia

Dose
1. 2–3 mg/kg IV
2. 25–200 µg/kg/min IV infusion

Onset: Rapid

Duration: 5–20 min

Anesthetic considerations
1. Respiratory depression
2. Contraindicated in patients with egg or soybean allergy or history of seizures
3. Pain on injection

Protamine Sulfate

Classification/indications
1. Heparin antagonist
2. Heparin neutralization

Dose: 1 mg IV for every 100 units of heparin to be neutralized

Onset: Within 5 min

Duration: 2 h

Anesthetic considerations
1. Hypotension, bradycardia
2. Monitor PTT or activated clotting time (ACT)
3. Solution preserved with benzyl alcohol may cause toxicity in neonates.

Pyridostigmine Bromide (Mestinon, Regonol)

Classification/indications
1. Anticholinesterase agent
2. Reversal of nondepolarizing muscle relaxants

Dose
1. 0.05–0.15 mg/kg IV
2. Maximum single dose: 10 mg
3. Must be preceded by atropine

Onset: 5–10 min IV

Duration: 90 min IV

Anesthetic considerations: Bradycardia, secretions

Ranitidine (Zantac)

Classification/indications
1. H_2-receptor antagonist
2. Gastric pH control

Dose: Age 2–18 y old: 0.1–0.8 mg/kg IV piggy back infused over 5 min. Give 1 h before induction.

Onset: 30–60 min

Duration: 8–12 h

Anesthetic considerations: Rapid IV infusion may cause bradycardia and hypotension

Remifentanil (Ultiva)

Classification/indications
1. Opiate analgesic
2. Mu-receptor agonist
3. Perioperative analgesia

Dose
1. Infusion only
2. Induction: 0.5–1 µg/kg/min
3. Maintenance: 0.05–0.8 µg/kg/min

Onset: Rapid

Duration: Effects rapidly dissipate 2–5 min after discontinuation of infusion.

Anesthetic considerations
1. May cause apnea, nausea and vomiting, muscle rigidity
2. Administer longer-acting analgesic for postoperative pain management (needed before discontinuing infusion)

Rocuronium (Zemuron)

Classification/indications: Nondepolarizing neuromuscular blocking agent

Dose
1. IV intubation: 0.6–1 mg/kg
2. IV maintenance: 0.08–0.12 mg/kg

Onset: 60–90 sec with intubating dose

Duration: 45–120 min depending on dose

Anesthetic considerations: Agent of choice for nondepolarizing rapid sequence induction

Scopolamine

Classification/indications
1. Anticholinergic
2. Premedication
3. Antisialagogue

Dose
1. 6–10 µg/kg IV/IM
2. Maximum dose: 0.3 mg

Onset
1. Rapid IV
2. 30 min IM

Duration
1. 30–60 min IV
2. 2–3 h IM

Anesthetic considerations
1. May cause tachycardia, blurred vision, dry mouth
2. Use with caution in patients with chronic pulmonary disease

Sevoflurane (Ultane)

Classification/indications: Inhalation anesthetic/general anesthesia

Dose
1. MAC 2%
2. Titrate to effect

Onset: Rapid

Duration: 15 min after discontinuation

Anesthetic considerations: Avoid in patients with renal disease because of fluoride ion release

Sodium Bicarbonate

Classification/indications
1. Electrolyte
2. Metabolic acidosis

Dose: 0.5–1 mEq/kg IV

Onset: Rapid

Duration: 1–2 h

Anesthetic considerations: Rapid administration may lead to hypernatremia, decreased cerebrospinal fluid (CSF) pressure, and intracranial hemorrhage.

Sodium Citrate (Bicitra)

Classification/indications
1. Nonparticulate neutralizing buffer
2. Prophylaxis for aspiration pneumonitis

Dose: 5–15 ml diluted in 5–15 ml water orally or 1 mEq/kg orally

Onset: Rapid

Duration: Maximally effective when given less than 60 min preoperatively

Anesthetic considerations: Contraindicated in patients with severe renal disease or acute dehydration

Succinylcholine (Anectine)

Classification/indications
1. Depolarizing skeletal muscle relaxant
2. Neuromuscular blocker

Dose
1. 1–2 mg/kg IV
2. 2–4 mg/kg IM

Onset: Rapid

Duration: 5–10 min

Anesthetic considerations
1. Pretreat with atropine because of incidence of bradycardia
2. Should not be used routinely in children <12 y of age
3. Malignant hyperthermia trigger; may cause bradycardia, hyperkalemia

Sufentanil Citrate (Sufenta)

Classification/indications
1. Opioid agonist
2. Analgesia, anesthesia

Dose
1. 0.1–0.5 µg/kg IV bolus anesthesia, with N_2O
2. 5–10 µg/kg IV; 0.01–0.05 µg/kg/h infusion anesthesia; no N_2O

Onset: Rapid

Duration: 30–60 min

Anesthetic considerations
1. Respiratory depression, apnea
2. Bradycardia, chest wall rigidity, nausea, vomiting

Terbutaline Sulfate (Brethaire, Brethine, Bricanyl)

Classification/indications
1. Beta$_2$-adrenergic agonist
2. Bronchodilator

Dose
1. 0.005–0.01 mg/kg per dose IV; may repeat in 15–30 min
2. Do not exceed 0.5 mg in 4–6 h

Onset: 15 min

Duration: 1–4 h

Anesthetic considerations: May cause tachycardia, hypertension

Tetracaine HCl (Pontocaine)

Classification/indications
1. Ester type of local anesthetic
2. Local, spinal, and topical anesthesia

Dose: Varies with procedure, 1% concentration

Onset: 5–10 min

Duration: 1–3 h depending on type of block

Anesthetic considerations: Seizures, sedation, burning on injection

Thiopental Sodium (Pentothal)

Classification/indications
1. Ultra–short acting barbiturate
2. Induction of anesthesia

Dose: 3–5 mg/kg IV

Onset: 39–60 s

Duration: 20–30 min

Anesthetic considerations
1. Respiratory depression, apnea
2. Contraindicated in variegate or acute intermittent porphyria
3. Use with caution in asthmatic patients

Vasopressin (Pitressin)

Classification/indications
1. Antidiuretic hormone
2. Treatment of diabetes insipidus
3. Upper GI bleeding

Dose
1. 2.25–5 units IM/SQ q6–8h
2. 1–3 mU/kg/h IV
3. GI bleeding: 0.01 units/kg/min IV

Onset: 1 h

Duration
1. Antidiuretic effects 2–8 h after IM or SQ
2. Pressor effects 30–60 min after IV

Anesthetic considerations
1. Use large vein
2. Monitor epilepsy and asthma patients closely
3. Severe vasoconstriction may be hazardous in cardiac patients

Vecuronium (Norcuron)

Classification/indications: Nondepolarizing neuromuscular blocking agent

Dose
1. 0.07–0.2 mg/kg IV
2. 0.8–1 µg/kg/min infusion

Onset: 1–3 min

Duration: 30–90 min

Anesthetic considerations: Monitor response with peripheral nerve stimulator

Vitamin K, Phytonadione (Aquamephyton)

Classification/indications
1. Vitamin, water soluble
2. Prevention and treatment of hypoprothrombinemia caused by drug or anticoagulant-induced vitamin K deficiency or hemorrhagic diseases of newborn

Dose
1. Newborn hemorrhage: 0.5–1 mg IM/SQ
2. Anticoagulant reversal in infants: 1–2 mg IV/IM/SQ q4–8h

Onset
1. 1–3 h IV/IM/SQ
2. 4–12 h orally

Duration: 6–48 h depending on dose and route of administration

Anesthetic considerations
1. Severe anaphylaxis may occur with IV route
2. Use only in emergency
3. Inject slowly IV
4. Monitor prothrombin time

Warfarin (Coumadin)

Classification/indications
1. Anticoagulant
2. Prophylaxis of thromboembolism

Dose: Adjusted to PT and international normalized ratio (INR)

Onset: 5–7 d

Duration: 5–7 d

Anesthetic considerations
1. Regional anesthesia contraindicated
2. Monitor prothrombin time

Resuscitation Guidelines

Tammy Dukatz, MSN, CRNA

I. Neonatal Resuscitation

A. According to the American Heart Association, neonates are more likely to need resuscitation than any other age-group. Although the following guidelines are specific for care in the delivery room, the considerations are applicable for the newborn in the operating room as well.

   1. Figure C–1 gives an overview of resuscitation in the delivery room.
   2. Ninety compressions and 30 ventilations are done in a 1-minute period. Use two fingers to depress the lower third of the sternum ½ to ¾ inch.

B. Table C–1 gives medications for neonatal resuscitation.

II. Pediatric Resuscitation

A. The American Heart Association and the American Academy of Pediatrics have published specific measures for the treatment of cardiopulmonary arrest in children. These algorithms provide for rapid assessment and intervention by health care professionals.

   1. Anaphylaxis, drowning, sudden infant death syndrome, and a foreign body in the airway are common causes that lead to shock or respiratory failure in children.
   2. Anesthetists are more likely, however, to encounter multiple trauma or one of the following situations related to anesthesia: laryngospasm, bronchospasm, bradycardia, hypotension, hyperkalemia, malignant hyperthermia.
   3. Prevention is the first line of therapy, but should one of these conditions occur, rapid recognition and appropriate management are essential.
   4. If pulseless asystole ensues, the outcome is nearly always poor.
   5. Table C–2 summarizes basic life support (BLS) maneuvers in infants and children.

B. Pediatric advanced life support: algorithms and considerations for the anesthetist.

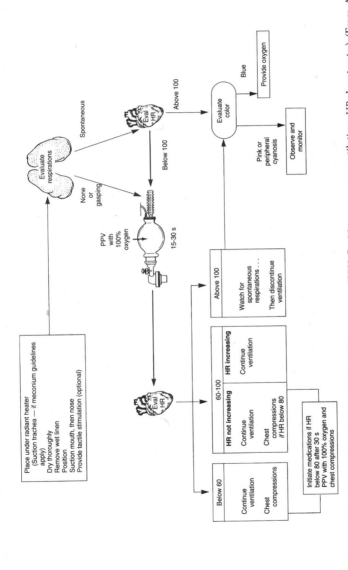

FIGURE C-1. Overview of resuscitation in the delivery room. (*PPV*, Positive pressure ventilation; *HR*, heart rate.) (From American Academy of Pediatrics. *Textbook of neonatal resuscitation.* Elk Grove Village, IL: Author. Used with permission of the American Academy of Pediatrics.)

TABLE C-1. Medications for Neonatal Resuscitation

Medication	Concentration to Administer	Preparation	Dosage/Route*	Total Dose/Infant			Rate/Precautions
Epinephrine	1:10,000	1 ml	0.1–0.3 ml/kg IV or ET	Weight (kg)		Total (ml)	Give rapidly
				1		0.1–0.3	May dilute with normal saline to 1–2 ml if giving ET
				2		0.2–0.6	
				3		0.3–0.9	
				4		0.4–1.2	
Volume expanders	Whole blood 5% Albumin-saline Normal saline Ringer's lactate	40 ml	10 ml/kg IV	Weight (kg)		Total (ml)	Give over 5–10 min
				1		10	
				2		20	
				3		30	
				4		40	
Sodium bicarbonate	0.5 mEq/ml (4.2% solution)	20 ml or two 10 ml pre-filled syringes	2 mEq/kg IV	Weight (kg)	Total Dose (mEq)	Total (ml)	Give *slowly*, over at least 2 min
				1	2	4	Give only if infant is being effectively ventilated
				2	4	8	
				3	6	12	
				4	8	16	

			Weight (kg)	Total Dose (mg)	Total (ml)	
Naloxone hydrochloride	0.4 mg/ml	1 ml	0.1 mg/kg (0.25 ml/kg) IV, ET IM, SQ			Give rapidly IV, ET preferred IM, SQ acceptable
			1	0.1	0.25	
			2	0.2	0.50	
			3	0.3	0.75	
			4	0.4	1	
	1 mg/ml	1 ml	0.1 ml/kg (0.1 ml/kg) IV, ET IM, SQ		0.1	
			1	0.1	0.1	
			2	0.2	0.2	
			3	0.3	0.3	
			4	0.4	0.4	

			Weight (kg)		Total (µg/min)	
Dopamine			Begin at 5 µg/kg/min (may increase to 20 µg/kg/min if necessary) IV			Give as a continuous infusion using an infusion pump Monitor heart rate and blood pressure closely Seek consultation
			1		5–20	
			2		10–40	
			3		15–60	
			4		20–80	

$$6 \times \frac{\text{Weight (kg)} \times \text{Desired dose (µg/kg/min)}}{\text{Desired fluid (ml/h)}} = \frac{\text{mg of dopamine}}{\text{per 100 ml of solution}}$$

From American Academy of Pediatrics. (1994). *Textbook of neonatal resuscitation.* Elk Grove Village, Il.: Author. Used with permission of the American Academy of Pediatrics.
*IM, Intramuscular; *ET,* endotracheal; *IV,* intravenous; *SQ,* subcutaneous.

TABLE C-2. Summary of Basic Life Support (BLS) Maneuvers in Infants and Children

Maneuver	Infant (<1 y)	Child (1–8 y)
Airway	Head tilt–chin lift (if trauma is present, use jaw thrust)	Head tilt–chin lift (if trauma is present, use jaw thrust)
Breathing		
Initial	Two breaths at 1–1½ s per breath	Two breaths at 1–1½ s per breath
Subsequent	20 breaths per minute (approximate)	20 breaths per minute (approximate)
Circulation		
Pulse check	Brachial/femoral	Carotid
Compression area	Lower half of sternum	Lower half of sternum
Compression width	2 or 3 fingers	Heel of one hand
Depth	Approximately one third to one half the depth of the chest	Approximately one third to one half the depth of the chest
Rate	At least 100/min	100/min
Compression/ ventilation ratio	5:1 (pause for ventilation)	5:1 (pause for ventilation)
Foreign body airway obstruction	Back blows/chest thrusts	Heimlich maneuver

Reproduced with permission. *Pediatric advanced life support*, 1997. Copyright American Heart Association.

1. A decision tree for tachycardia with poor perfusion is given in Figure C–2.
2. Clinical considerations for tachycardia and poor perfusion.
   a. A heart rate that is above the normal range for a child's age is tachycardia.
   b. In a child under 2 years, the upper normal sleeping heart rate is 160 bpm, whereas 90 bpm is the upper normal sleeping rate for a child older than 2 years.
   c. Normal upper awake rates range from 205 bpm in the newborn to 140 bpm in the 10-year-old child.
   d. The most frequent explanations for increases in heart rate in children under anesthesia include a response to a surgical stimulus or administration of a beta-adrenergic or parasympatholytic medication. Deepening the anesthesia will blunt the response to pain and subsequently lower the heart rate.
      (1) The appropriate dose of atropine or glycopyrrolate

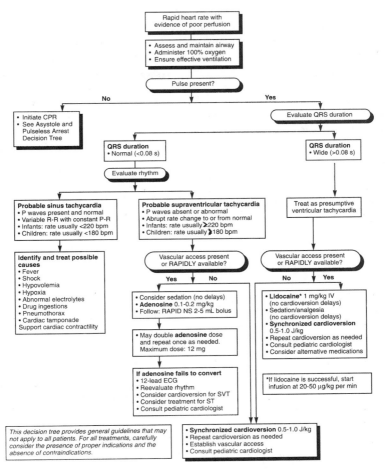

FIGURE C–2. Decision tree for tachycardia with poor perfusion. (Reproduced with permission. *Pediatric advanced life support,* 1997. Copyright American Heart Association.)

rarely increases the heart rate above the high normal awake rate.

(2) Epinephrine or cocaine given locally by the surgeon may lead to tachycardia and ventricular ectopy when used with the inhalation agents, especially halothane.

e. If tachycardia is not accounted for by these means, then the other causes listed in the algorithm should be carefully considered.

   f. Supraventricular tachycardia (SVT) is caused by a reentry mechanism via an aberrant pathway.
   g. Ventricular tachycardia (VT) occurs mainly in children with underlying cardiac anomalies or QT syndrome; but it may be caused by hypoxemia, acidosis, electrolyte imbalance, drug toxicity, and poisons. If cardiovascular instability is present, the most rapid and effective treatment is synchronized cardioversion.
   h. Hyperkalemia caused by malignant hyperthermia or succinylcholine administration should be considered in ventricular dysrhythmias.
3. A bradycardia decision tree is given in Figure C–3.
4. Clinical considerations for bradycardia.
   a. Bradycardia can occur during anesthetic induction.
   b. Hypoxia caused by airway obstruction, laryngospasm, or prolonged apnea with intubation can rapidly lead to cardiovascular compromise as evidenced by a decreased heart rate.
   c. Effective ventilation and oxygenation must be immediately established. Greater depths of anesthesia with halothane or sevoflurane during inhalation induction can result in a disturbance in atrioventricular (A-V) node conduction.
   d. Vagal stimulation during intubation has also been associated with bradycardia.
   e. Parasympatholytic medication such as atropine is often given both preemptively and responsively to maintain cardiac output, which is predominantly heart rate dependent.
   f. If the patient is unresponsive to atropine or severe bradycardia has ensued, the inhalation agent should be discontinued and epinephrine given as outlined in Figure C–3.
   g. Cardiac compressions may be needed.
5. An asystole and pulseless arrest decision tree is given in Figure C–4.
6. Considerations for identifying causes of asystole and pulseless arrest are given in the box on p. 473.
7. Drugs used in pediatric advanced life support are given in Table C–3.

III. Technical Procedures in Pediatric Advanced Life Support

   A. Venous access in pediatric resuscitation
      1. Children are frequently anesthetized before the establishment of venous access.

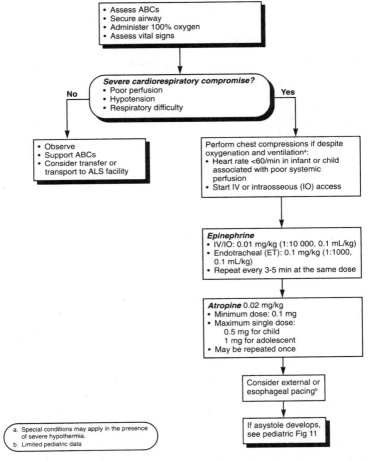

FIGURE C–3. Bradycardia decision tree. (Reproduced with permission. *Pediatric advanced life support,* 1997. Copyright American Heart Association.)

2. Rarely an IV line infiltrates or becomes disconnected without immediate detection.
3. If access must be rapidly obtained for resuscitation, the American Heart Association recommends a maximum of three attempts at a peripheral IV line or a lapse of no more than 90 seconds of time (whichever comes first).
4. The anesthetist should then consider alternative means of

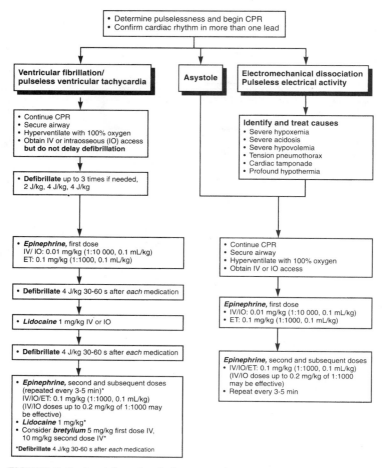

FIGURE C–4. Asystole and pulseless arrest decision tree. (Reproduced with permission. *Pediatric advanced life support,* 1997. Copyright American Heart Association.)

venous access and medication administration as outlined in Figure C–5.
B. Central line placement
1. Before any central line placement, the anesthetist should
   a. Scrub hands.
   b. Position the patient appropriately.
   c. For cannulation of the neck and chest the child should be placed in 30-degrees head-down position.

Considerations in Identifying Causes of Asystole and Pulseless Arrest

Severe Hypoxemia
Airway obstruction
Bronchospasm
Laryngospasm
Aspiration
Atelectasis
Bronchopulmonary
  dysplasia
Cyanotic heart disease
Sickle cell crisis
Inadequate reversal of
  muscle relaxant on
  emergence

Severe Acidosis
Secondary to hypoxemia
Hyperglycemia in diabetes
Sepsis
Pyloric stenosis (with
  hypochloremia)
Massive transfusions
  (trauma, liver transplant)
Anaphylaxis
Unclamping of a major
  vessel/release of a
  tourniquet
Malignant hyperthermia

Severe Hypovolemia
Major blood loss
Major insensible loss
Sepsis
Anaphylaxis

Tension Pneumothorax
Chest trauma (rib fractures)
Placement of a central venous
  access catheter
Barotrauma (history of lung
  disease such as bronchopulmonary dysplasia)
Jet ventilation (catheter or
  stylet displacement)

Cardiac Tamponade
Chest trauma (especially
  penetrating injury)
Cardiac surgery

Profound Hypothermia
Environmental exposure
Trauma
Rapid administration of cold
  fluids or blood
Neonatal surgery

Hyperkalemia*
Malignant hyperthermia
Succinylcholine induced
  (history of muscular
  dystrophy, trauma,
  burns)

*Hyperkalemia is not listed as a cause for arrest in the *Pediatric advanced life support (PALS)* algorithm. However, there have been several documented incidences of dysrhythmias and arrests associated with extrajunctional potassium release. Hyperventilation with the administration of calcium salts, sodium bicarbonate, glucose plus insulin, and epinephrine promotes the intracellular transfer of potassium and reverses cardiotoxicity by decreasing membrane excitability.

TABLE C–3. Drugs Used in Pediatric Advanced Life Support

Dosage (Pediatric)	Remarks
ADENOSINE 0.1–0.2 mg/kg Maximum single dose: 12 mg	Rapid IV bolus
ATROPINE SULFATE* 0.02 mg/kg	Minimum dose: 0.1 mg Maximum single dose: 0.5 mg in child, 1 mg in adolescent
BRETYLIUM 5 mg/kg; may be increased to 10 mg/kg	Rapid IV
CALCIUM CHLORIDE 10% 20 mg/kg	Give slowly.
DOPAMINE HYDROCHLORIDE 2–20 µg/kg/min	Alpha-adrenergic action dominates at ≥15–20 µg/kg/min
DOBUTAMINE HYDROCHLORIDE 2–20 µg/kg/min	Titrate to desired effect
EPINEPHRINE FOR BRADYCARDIA* IV/IO: 0.01 mg/kg (1:10,000, 0.1 ml/kg) ET: 0.1 mg/kg (1:1000, 0.1 ml/kg)	
EPINEPHRINE FOR ASYSTOLIC OR PULSELESS ARREST* **First Dose** IV/IO: 0.01 mg/kg (1:10,000, 0.1 ml/kg) ET: 0.1 mg/kg (1:1000, 0.1 ml/kg) IV/IO doses as high as 0.2 mg/kg of 1:1000 may be effective **Subsequent Doses** IV/IO/ET: 0.1 mg/kg (1:1000, 0.1 ml/kg); repeat every 3–5 min IV/IO doses as high as 0.2 mg/kg of 1:1000 may be effective	
EPINEPHRINE INFUSION Initial at 0.1 µg/kg/min Higher infusion dose used if asystole present	Titrate to desired effect (0.1–1.0 µg/kg/min)

TABLE C-3. Drugs Used in Pediatric Advanced Life Support
   Continued

Dosage (Pediatric)	Remarks
LIDOCAINE* 1 mg/kg	
LIDOCAINE INFUSION 20–50 µg/kg/min	
NALOXONE* If ≤5 yr old or ≤20 kg: 0.1 mg/kg If >5 yr old or >20 kg: 2.0 mg	Titrate to desired effect
PROSTAGLANDIN E$_1$ 0.05–0.1 µg/kg/min	Titrate to desired effect
SODIUM BICARBONATE 1 mEq/kg per dose or 0.3 × kg × base deficit	Infuse slowly and only if ventilation is adequate

*For ET administration dilute medication with normal saline to a volume of 3–5 ml and follow with several positive pressure ventilations.

Reproduced with permission. *Pediatric advanced life support,* 1997. Copyright American Heart Association.

    d. If there is no cervical spine injury, hyperextend the neck by placing a roll under the shoulders.
    e. Cover the area with a sterile drape.
    f. Anesthetize the skin with 1% lidocaine if the child is responsive to pain.
    g. Flush the needle, syringe, and catheter with sterile saline.
 2. Pediatric sizes in catheters over the wire or through introducing sheaths
    a. <10 kg: 4.0F–4.5F; 6 cm long (0.53 mm wire diameter) with 20-gauge needle
    b. 10–40 kg: 5.0F–6.5F; 13 cm long (0.64 mm wire diameter) with 19-gauge needle
    c. >40 kg: 7.0F–8.0F; 13 cm long (0.89 mm wire diameter) with 18-gauge needle
 3. Procedure
    a. Using sterile technique, attach the appropriate-size needle to a 3 ml syringe and slowly advance the needle into the vein by the chosen route (internal jugular, subclavian, or femoral vein).
    b. When a free flow of blood is obtained, disconnect the

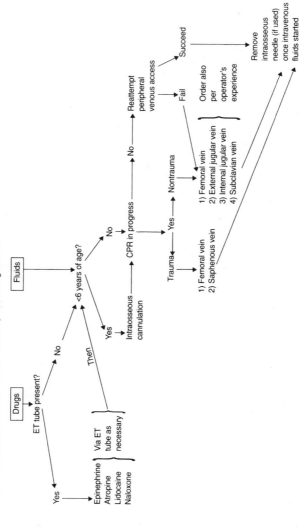

FIGURE C-5. Priorities for vascular access. (Reproduced with permission. *Pediatric advanced life support,* 1997. Copyright American Heart Association.)

syringe and place a finger over the needle hub to prevent entrainment of air.

    c. Insert the appropriate-size guide wire through the needle during a spontaneous exhalation or a positive pressure breath.

    d. Pass a catheter or catheter-introducing sheath over the wire. The guide wire or introducer can then be removed and an infusion set attached. Secure in place with a suture.

    e. Auscultate for bilateral breath sounds. Obtain a chest radiograph to verify that the catheter tip is in the correct place.

4. Internal jugular vein

    a. The right side of the neck is preferable since it is the more direct route to the right atrium. Also there is minimal risk of injury to the thoracic duct and the dome of the right lung is lower than the left lung. Bilateral breath sounds should be checked before the procedure.

    b. Anterior route: Palpate the carotid artery medially at the anterior border of the sternocleidomastoid muscle. Introduce the needle at the midpoint of the anterior border at a 30-degree angle with the coronal plane. Direct the needle caudad in the sagittal plane toward the ipsilateral nipple.

    c. Central route: Identify the triangle formed by the two portions of the sternocleidomastoid muscle with the clavicle at its base. Introduce the needle at the apex of this triangle at a 30-degree angle to the coronal plane. Direct the needle caudad to the ipsilateral nipple. If the vein is not entered, withdraw and redirect the needle more toward the ipsilateral shoulder.

    d. Posterior route: Introduce the needle deep into the sternal head of the sternocleidomastoid muscle at the junction of the middle and lower thirds of the posterior margin (above where the external jugular vein crosses this muscle). Direct the needle toward the suprasternal notch.

    e. Figure C–6 shows the internal jugular vein and its relationship to the surrounding anatomy.

5. Subclavian vein

    a. Identify the junction of the middle and medial thirds of the clavicle.

    b. Introduce the needle toward a fingertip that is placed in the suprasternal notch.

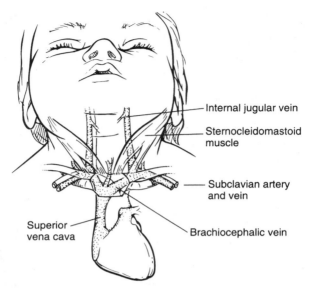

Internal jugular vein

Sternocleidomastoid muscle

Subclavian artery and vein

Superior vena cava

Brachiocephalic vein

FIGURE C-6. The internal jugular vein and its relationship to the surrounding anatomy. (Reproduced with permission. *Pediatric advanced life support,* 1997. Copyright American Heart Association.)

    c. The needle should be parallel to the frontal plane, directed medially and slightly cephalad, beneath the clavicle toward the posterior aspect of the sternal end of the clavicle.

  6. Femoral vein

    a. Identify the femoral artery by palpation.

    b. If there is no pulse, locate the midpoint between the anterior superior iliac spine and the symphysis pubis.

    c. Insert the needle one finger's breadth below the inguinal ligament, just medial to the femoral artery.

    d. Direct the needle toward the umbilicus at a 45-degree angle.

    e. Figure C-7 shows the femoral vein anatomy and cannulation technique.

C. Intraosseous cannulation

  1. If venous access cannot be achieved in 90 seconds or after three peripheral attempts during cardiopulmonary resuscitation, then intraosseous cannulation should be performed in the child 6 years of age or younger.

  2. Any medication that can be given intravenously may be

administered intraosseously (into the intramedullary sinus).

3. Equipment

    a. A specifically designed intraosseous needle, or a large-bore (Jamshidi-type) bone marrow needle

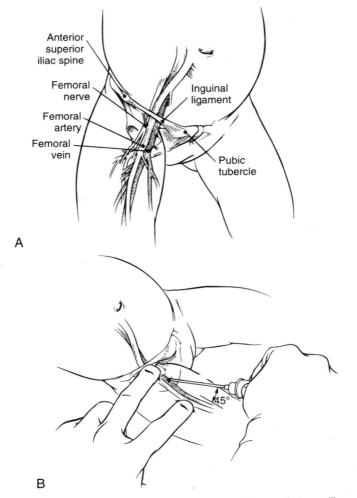

A

B

FIGURE C–7. **A,** Femoral vein anatomy. **B,** Cannulation technique. (Reproduced with permission. *Pediatric advanced life support,* 1997. Copyright American Heart Association.)

      b. An 18-gauge spinal needle may be used if the above are not available, but it may be too flexible

      c. Antiseptic solution

      d. Local anesthetic if the child is responsive to pain

      e. Sterile saline (30 ml vial)

      f. 10 ml syringe

  4. Landmarks

      a. Palpate the tibial tuberosity.

      b. The intraosseous cannulation site is about 1 to 3 cm below this tuberosity on the anteromedial surface.

  5. Procedure

      a. Restrain the leg.

      b. Cleanse the skin with antiseptic solution.

      c. Inject local anesthetic if child is responsive.

      d. Locate the above landmarks, and direct the needle perpendicular to the long axis of the bone or slightly caudad to avoid the epiphyseal plate.

      e. Use a boring or screwing motion until penetration into the bone marrow is achieved.

      f. A decreased resistance or a "give" is felt after the needle passes through the bony cortex.

      g. The needle should stand upright without support at this point.

      h. The stylet should be removed, and bone marrow can be aspirated into the 10 ml syringe filled with normal saline.

      i. A test injection of normal saline should be administered, and then the needle can be attached to standard IV tubing.

      j. Observe the site when the IV fluid is flowing freely; there should be no evidence of infiltration if the needle is correctly placed.

      k. Secure the needle and tubing with tape.

      l. Add a bulky dressing for support.

  6. Figure C–8 shows the intraosseous cannulation technique.

D. Percutaneous cricothyrotomy

  1. Cricothyrotomy is indicated for complete upper airway obstruction when standard methods of ventilation have failed.

  2. Standard methods of securing an airway include ventilation with a bag-valve mask system, laryngeal mask airway, or tracheal intubation.

  3. Cricothyrotomy can be a life-saving procedure in patients with foreign body aspiration, epiglottitis, airway tumors, laryngeal fracture, or severe orofacial injuries.

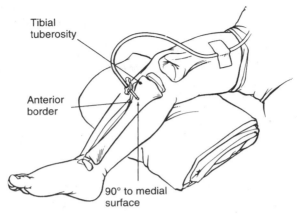

Tibial
tuberosity

Anterior
border

90° to medial
surface

FIGURE C–8. Intraosseous cannulation technique. (Reproduced with permission. *Pediatric advanced life support,* 1997. Copyright American Heart Association.)

4. Procedure.
  a. Place a rolled towel under the child's shoulder allowing extension of the child's neck.
  b. Stand to the left of the child and stabilize the trachea with the right hand.
  c. Palpate the cricothyroid membrane with the index finger of the anesthetist's left hand.
  d. The cricothyroid membrane lies under the indentation between the thyroid cartilage and the cricoid cartilage.
  e. Initially a small-bore (20- or 22-gauge) needle that is attached to a 3 ml syringe can be inserted through the cricothyroid membrane. If air is easily aspirated, the small needle is removed.
  f. A 12- to 14-gauge IV catheter needle should then be inserted at a 45-degree angle caudally. The needle is removed, and air is aspirated to confirm placement in the trachea.
  g. The catheter can then be attached to a 3 ml syringe with the plunger removed. A no. 7.0 mm endotracheal tube adapter will fit into the barrel of the syringe and may be attached to the breathing circuit or other ventilating device. Alternatively a no. 3.0 mm endotracheal tube adapter will attach directly to the ventilating device.

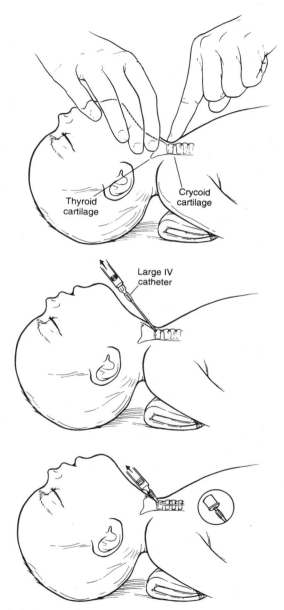

FIGURE C–9. Percutaneous cricothyrotomy. (Adapted from Coté et al. (1988). *Critical Care Medicine, 16,* 615–619. Lippincott Williams and Wilkins.)

5. Figure C–9 shows how to perform a percutaneous cricothyrotomy.
6. Ventilation via a cricothyrotomy.
   a. The small diameter of the IV catheter (when compared to an appropriate-size endotracheal tube) creates high resistance to air flow.
   b. The pop-off valve of the Ambu bag must be disabled to provide the high inflation pressures necessary.
   c. Fresh gas flows of 100% oxygen should be approximately 100 ml/kg or 1 to 5 L when the Ambu bag or anesthesia breathing circuit is used.
   d. Moderate hypercarbia can develop with either the Ambu bag or breathing circuit.
   e. High flow jet ventilators can ventilate effectively to maintain normocarbia.
   f. However, if the catheter migrates from the tracheal lumen, a pneumothorax is a likely complication.
   g. Observation of the chest rising and falling is essential in preventing barotrauma.
   h. It may be necessary to pause between insufflations to allow for passive exhalation.
7. The cricothyrotomy is a temporary emergency airway.

ADDITIONAL READINGS

Bloom, R.S., & Cropley, C. (Eds.). (1995). *Textbook of neonatal resuscitation.* Elk Grove Village, IL: American Academy of Pediatrics.

Chameides, L.C., & Hazinski, M.F. (Eds.). (1997). *Textbook of pediatric advanced life support.* Dallas: American Heart Association.

Crosby, J. (1988). Guidelines for intraosseous infusions. *Journal of Emergency Medicine,* (6), 143–146.

Larach, M.G., Rosenberg, H., Gronert, G.A., & Allen, G.C. (1997). Hyperkalemic cardiac arrest during anesthesia in infants and children with occult myopathies. *Clinical Pediatrics,* 36(1), 9–16.

Zaritsky, A. (1993). Pediatric resuscitation pharmacology. *Annals of Emergency Medicine,* 22(2), 445–455.

Index

Note: Page numbers in *italics* refer to illustrations; page numbers followed by t refer to tables.

486 *Index*

V

Vasopressin, 462
VATER association, 130
Vecuronium, 25, 462–463
   in neonatal anesthesia, 401, 403, 403t
Venous access, 97
   in advanced life support, 472, 475, 477–478, *478, 479*
Venous air embolism, during neurosurgery, 174–175, *175*
Ventilation, in postoperative care, 384, 385t
   monitoring guidelines for, 65, 66–67
Ventilators, 58
   for neonatal anesthesia, 406
Ventricular hypertrophy, in bronchopulmonary dysplasia, 256
Ventricular septal defect, 191–192, 229–231
Ventriculoperitoneal shunt, 185–186

Visual evoked potentials, monitoring guidelines for, 68
Vital capacity, 11t, 245
Vitamin K, 463
Volume expansion, in neonatal resuscitation, 466t
Volvulus, 135
Vomiting, in ear, nose, and throat surgery, 111, 115
   postoperative, 385t, 388t

W

Wakefulness, recovery of, 384, 385t
Wake-up test, in spinal surgery, 156–157
Warfarin, 463
Warming blanket, 60
Warming devices, 59–60
Water. See also *Fluid therapy.*
   body distribution of, 84–85, 85t
   requirement for, 84
Waterston shunt, 193
Wilms' tumor, 143